U. F. Gruber

# Blood Replacement

Translated by
L. Oxtoby and Dr. R. F. Armstrong, F.F.A.R.C.S. (Eng.)

With 20 Figures

Springer-Verlag Berlin Heidelberg GmbH 1969

*PD Dr. med. Ulrich F. Gruber*
*Oberarzt*
*Department of Surgery, University of Basel*
*(Chairman: Prof. Dr. M. Allgöwer)*
*Bürgerspital Basel*
*Switzerland*

ISBN 978-3-642-49504-5 ISBN 978-3-642-49790-2 (eBook)
DOI 10.1007/978-3-642-49790-2



Originally published by Springer-Verlag Berlin Heidelberg in 1969
Softcover reprint of the hardcover 1st edition 1969

Library of Congress Catalog Card Number 69-16845



Title-No. 1551

*Dedicated to my wife Lisa*

Es wurde fertig in Deiner Hut.
Bleib Du mir auf dieser Erden,
so soll alles fertig werden.

THOMAS MANN

# Foreword

The manifold problems of shock are still of great importance, diagnostic and therapeutic experience of the "severely ill" being supplied with new information almost every month. In the 5 periodicals which have found their way to my desk during the past few days there are no less than 10 interesting articles on questions concerning shock research [see Bibliography *41 b, 53 a, 60 a, 192 a, 242 a, 350 b, 810 a, 941 a, 1069 a, 1082 a*]. The most urgent point still is to maintain as complete as possible the objective catalog of the various shock manifestations found in man and in animals — yet at the same time to view interpretations of these phenomena in their relative and temporal "truth".

Problems of shock research are not only interesting for their scientific value but also for their clinical implication. In particular, almost every practicing physician is facing problems of blood replacement very frequently. The effective or circulating blood volume remains an important theoretical and therapeutic problem in the shock field. For years, U. F. GRUBER has pursued this question clinically and experimentally. This volume deals with the world literature in an exceptionally thorough manner. This book is made more than a compilation by including a long list of original work done with F. D. MOORE in Boston, in the Surgical Department in Chur, with L. E. GELIN and S. E. BERGENTZ in Göteborg and in the Laboratory for Experimental Surgery in Davos; judgements are made on the basis of original studies, and essential points are separated from unimportant ones.

This volume will be welcomed by the medical profession because it carefully treats vital questions concerning this complicated, much-discussed, and in part contested field, considering that today, along with various forms of blood and several plasma preparations, there are more than 40 different plasma replacement substances available with various physico-chemical, biological and pharmacological properties. Older preparations have been abandoned, others modified, and new ones appear.

A comparative evaluation of the chemical characteristics, the range of indication and the therapeutic effectiveness of these solutions suggests itself particularly at this time because in recent years the use of large amounts of balanced electrolyte solutions tended to reverse the principles of blood replacement in the U.S.A.

It is agreed today that this procedure can sometimes lead to amazingly good results. As several recent papers [*1591, 1783, 1785, 1792, 1805, 1813,*

*1844*; cf. *1611 a, 1703, 1796*] have shown, the previous attempts to explain these methods of treatment are based partly upon misinterpretation of isotope dilution studies. It has been shown in various laboratories working independently of each other that no unproportional reduction of the interstitial space occurs in hemorrhagic shock. The main source of error was non-consideration of the prolonged equilibration time for the radioactive substances used (e. g. $^{35}SO_4$) for measuring the extracellular space.

These methods are difficult to use and easily misinterpreted. Although the results drawn from the above-mentioned studies were definitely overrated, "blood volume therapy including the interstitial space" is appropriate so long as the blood volume and the interstitium for the most part become proportionally larger or smaller. A combined therapy with water, electrolyte *and* colloids, however, still seems to be the more physiologically sound and clinically simpler method, provided that adequate non-toxic colloids are available.

With tireless effort, U. F. GRUBER has been able to present a survey which is remarkably easy to understand and for which the reader will be grateful.

Basel, November 1967

M. ALLGÖWER
Professor of Surgery
University of Basel

## Contents

# Abbreviations

| | |
|---|---|
| ACD solution | Acid citric dextrose solution, citrate solution in preser' blood |
| BP | blood pressure |
| BV | blood volume |
| bw | body weight |
| CO | cardiac output |
| dextran 40 | dextran with an average molecular weight $\overline{M}_w$ of appr 40,000 |
| dextran 70 | dextran with an average molecular weight $\overline{M}_w$ of appr 70,000 |
| ECS | extracellular space |
| EV | erythrocyte volume |
| Hb | hemoglobin |
| Hct | hematocrit |
| HDP | human dried plasma |
| HO-ethyl starch | hydroxyethyl starch |
| IS | interstitial space |
| m | molar |
| MFG | modified fluid gelatin |
| MW | molecular weight: method of determination unspecifi |
| $\overline{M}_n$ | number average molecular weight |
| $\overline{M}_w$ | weight average molecular weight |
| $n$ | number of experiments |
| $\eta$ | viscosity; various symbols, see p. 55 |
| OPG | oxypolygelatin |
| PPS | pasteurized plasma protein solution |
| PV | plasma volume |
| PVP | polyvinyl pyrrolidone |
| REAC | relative erythrocyte aggregating capacity |
| RES | reticuloendothelial system |
| $R^{131}IHSA$ | radioactive marked $^{131}$ iodine human serum albumin |
| SR | sedimentation rate |
| SRC | Swiss Red Cross |
| T-1824 | Evans blue, blue dye for plasma volume determinatio |

# Introduction

Blood replacement presents problems in most fields of medicine. While the human organism can compensate for small blood losses by means of spontaneous refilling of the vascular system, larger blood losses must be replaced by means of infusions of blood, plasma, artificial colloids or electrolyte solutions. If the lost volume has reached a certain degree and cannot be replaced immediately, a syndrome arises which is termed shock.

Few concepts in medical terminology are so controversial and so often criticised as that of *shock* [*182, 1042, 1278, 1311*]. Even specialists in this field have contributed to the confusion, for more than one hundred different forms of shock have been described in the literature [*642*]. Several symposia on shock [*182, 371, 400, 1021, 1311*] have been held, with the intention of bringing about clarity in terminology, and to create a generally comprehensible and binding definition of shock, even to go so far as to bury the word. To this date, however, none of these attempts has achieved the expected result.

Clinicians generally understand very well what is meant when a patient is said to be in shock. The clinical picture of a cold, hypotensive patient with a tachycardia, which is implied by this term has remained unchanged despite all later changes in shock theory. *Hemorrhagic shock,* i. e. shock caused by loss of blood, presents no difficulty in *definition* [*1833*]. Today this term denotes the complex of symptoms of an acute hemodynamic disturbance, caused by a reduction in the circulating blood volume as a result of blood loss. The extent of this disturbance is such that the metabolic processes in vital organs are affected, resulting in functional and later morphological disturbances.

The importance of immediate and complete replacement of lost fluid is now generally recognized and documented in the treatment of all forms of hypovolemic shock [*1742, 1750, 1756*]. In practice, however, the implementation of this principle often presents difficulties; i. e.

1. Early replacement may not be possible, e. g. in rescue operations in remote areas, where much time is needed for transport and when specialists or the necessary materials are absent from the scene of accident.

2. The assessment as to whether complete replacement has actually been achieved is not so easy as is often assumed in spite of the fact that we now have relatively simple diagnostic aids at our disposal. In addition to the traditional measurements of blood pressure, pulse, skin colour and hourly urine output we may also measure central venous pressure and determine

the blood volume with electronic semi automatic devices. The use of th aids for diagnosis and control of therapy, however, has not yet beco generally accepted because the value and the interpretation of the resu thereby obtained are contested in part [1]. Protracted conditions of und transfusion and, less often, overtransfusion therefore still occur [*349*].

The *time factor* plays an important part in shock pathogenesis. T longer a massive hypovolemia lasts, the poorer the prognosis, since secon ary changes occur which are very difficult or even impossible to treat.

*Thus states of shock still present the clinician all too often with co siderable problems* [*1125*]. *Recently there has been increasing doubt co cerning the opinion that administration of blood exclusively in all stages hemorrhagic shock and in all circumstances represents the best therapy.*

Apart from the question of indication, there are many situations which little or *no blood* is *available*. In this context one can think not on of war conditions [*663, 725*], but also of the increasing number of traf and sport accidents and of mass catastrophes in civilian life. There are al the situations in small hospitals without a large blood bank of their ow and of large heart, vascular and cancer centers whose surgical programr places a great strain on the best organized blood banks.

*Thus there is a real need for so-called blood substitutes.* Research h provided important knowledge in this field. On the one hand *human plasn preparations* have been improved. On the other, *artificial colloids* sho therapeutically interesting *pharmacological effects* along with their physic chemical characteristics as volume substitutes. In some circumstances the effects provide certain advantages over blood and its derivatives. Since tl ideal plasma substitute has not yet been found, new preparations are beir developed and old ones modified according to the latest information avai able. For a long time there have been advocates of the theory that bloc may be replaced to a large extent by simple *electrolyte solutions*. More now being heard about this subject following the assumption that in tl treatment of shock it is not so much a matter of replacing lost blood volun but of replenishing the interstitial space.

*What, how much and when? These are the questions raised in tl therapy of blood loss and in the treatment of the various stages of hemo rhagic shock.* What objective proof is there for the superiority of certai forms of therapy in particular clinical situations? What are the decisi mechanisms at work? This book attempts to answer these questions on tl basis of related literature and original investigations.

---

[1] Important arguments concerning the value of the determination of *bloc volume or of central venous pressure* in shock are to be found in the followir references: [*134, 190, 241, 289 b, 367, 369, 437, 439, 443, 474, 602, 625, 724, 74 812, 939, 940, 989, 990, 1040, 1101, 1202, 1358, 1409, 1500, 1534, 1621, 169 1701, 1703*].

*In Part I* hemodynamic and metabolic changes which occur in hemorrhagic shock are briefly summarized and criteria to be taken into account during therapy are mentioned.

*In Part II* blood and plasma preparations and the artificial colloidal and crystalloid solutions available today are discussed. In describing those preparations for which no references are given, the manufacturer's data has been used (package information sheets and brochures). Detailed information is given about the volume effect of all solutions listed. This is followed by a summary of animal experiments and clinical results obtained in the management of shock.

*In Part III* these results are discussed. An attempt is made to draw conclusions and to present a survey of the trend and goals of modern shock research.

*Part IV* is a summary of the whole material covered. In addition to the bibliography some of the literature is listed under different subject headings. *Note that references with numbers higher than [1584] are contained in the list of additional literature (p. 256 f.).*

PART ONE

# Pathophysiology of Blood Loss

## A. Pathophysiology of Hemorrhagic Shock

In 1920 J. C. AUB [*89*] and later A. BLALOCK [*164*] emphasized decisive importance of *volume loss* (cf. also [*297*]). Before that, *nerv factors and toxins* were held responsible for the occurrence of shock (surv in [*40*] and WIGGERS [*1513*]). Extensive blood loss of more than 20% the blood volume leads to *regional vasoconstriction* [*305*], *decrease central venous pressure* [*296*] *and in venous return* [*541*], *as well as reduction of the cardiac output* [*626*]. The heart rate rises, the temperat in the periphery drops, and the skin is pale and moist. Obvious sympto of increased sympathetic activity are present, but because of the volu deficit no hypertension occurs [*1257*].

Compared with other circulatory beds *vasoconstriction* in humans probably directed to a disproportionately high degree to skin, kidneys a the splanchnic bed [*1144*]; because of this, a redistribution of the card output occurs favoring heart [*946*] and brain. If vasoconstriction persi long enough, lack of oxygen in the tissues increases and metabolism th continues anerobically [*1810*]. Accumulation of acid metabolites such pyruvic and lactic acid occurs [*1809*], leading to a *metabolic acido* This in turn increases the sympathetic activity [*948*]. The contract arterioles react more weakly to endogenous *catecholamines* and practica not at all to exogenous ones [*247*]; finally the sphincters relax, causing reduction in tonus first on the precapillary side [*884, 1000*]. Because of t the capillaries dilate and *prestasis* occurs. If the *filtration pressure* in t capillaries increases, intravascular fluid may be lost [*1241*]. Thus the pe pheral resistance will depend, vice versa, on the capillary permeabil [*1205, 1412*]. This process does not occur everywhere in the same phase a with the same intensity [*1781*]; for this reason even a single organ may irregularly perfused with blood [*1459*, cf. *1597*].

Many of these findings are confirmed in animal experiments only a species differences can be important (cf. [*144*]). Whereas in dogs necrosis the *intestinal mucosa* occurs first, it cannot be said with any certainty what extent the *intestinal tract* [*618*] *and liver* [*1693*] play a decisive p in humans.

The condition of "*irreversibility*" begins when adequate transfusion alone can no longer save an animal [*438, 1513*]. This definition is derived from shock research in animals — for in clinical medicine the term can be used only retrospectively at most [*340*]. The *causes* which lead to this condition are not yet clear [*539 a*]; in the long run *lack of oxygen* probably plays an essential part. *Cardiac factors* [*1264, 1492, 1640*] and *neurogenic stimuli* [*211*] are also of importance, and in turn adequate oxygen supply to the myocardium and central nervous system is decisive. Furthermore the sudden rise in *blood sugar* [*415, 1652*] is unexplained, and even today a consistent explanation is lacking for the decrease of *serum iron, serum transferrin and iron binding capacity* which follows extreme blood loss [*1323*].

During the first hours after blood loss a tendency toward *hypercoagulation* with simultaneous *activation of fibrinolysis* can be noted [*126, 193*], whereas the return to normal or reduced coagulability begins with decreased fibrinolysis. The decrease of fibrinogen in lymph is due to an increased catabolism of fibrinogen [*1724*]. The number of thrombocytes decreases. The first phase is indicative of the origin of microthrombi [*643, 644, 645, 646, 647, 648, 649, 717, 1179, 1784*]; their importance in the impairment of pulmonary function likewise needs explanation [*649 a, 1641*].

With low perfusion rates, prestasis in the capillaries and the hypercoagulability will favor the reversible aggregation of formed blood elements [*248, 498, 504, 507, 641, 832, 1005, 1404, 1405, 1737, 1746, 1747*], whereby primarily old cells are sequestrated [*140*], as a result the viscosity of the blood increases [*515, 516, 1507*].

The *kidney* produces less urine or none at all; *sodium* excretion decreases due to increased resorption in the proximal tubules [*492*], whereas excretion of *potassium* increases [*495, 1389*]. Electrolyte changes are determined by increased *secretion of aldosterone* [*1816*]. Two mechanisms are probably responsible for this: The *volume receptors*, even today not clearly identified and perhaps under neurogenic control [*295, 496*], and the *renin-angiotensin system* [*1540*]. In addition *vasopressin (ADH), ACTH*, adrenalin and noradrenalin, and perhaps also erythropoëtin, participate in volume regulation [*330, 905, 1043, 1044*]. The combination of sodium and water retention after severe trauma, with simultaneous decrease of the serum-sodium causes one to consider a migration of water and especially sodium, into the ground substance and eventually into the intracellular space [*431*]. The latter phenomenon, however, has not been shown in pure blood loss [*219, 352*].

Nor are various research groups in agreement about the role of *bacterial factors* in the pathogenesis of shock. On the basis of the investigations of Fine [*438, 442*], it was long believed that irreversible shock was due to the action of an endotoxin [*1667*], not only in septic but also in hemorrhagic shock. Today, however, justifiable doubts about this theory can be raised since the irreversible phase occurs just as soon, if not sooner, in germfree animals than in normal animals. It is even assumed that certain bacteria sometimes provide a protective effect (survey in [*618*]). The contribution of FINE to shock research is that he recognized the importance of the intestinal tract and the reticulo-endothelial system, and at an early date indicated the importance of other than hemodynamic factors in shock.

This short survey shows that in serious hemorrhagic shock practically all organs are affected in order to maintain homeostasis. Further data about the individual aspects are found in the books and articles compiled at the end of the bibliography.

With regard to the vast area which is still to be investigated by research workers in shock it seems sensible for an individual to stake out a limited area and investigate this as thoroughly and carefully as possible. Therefore we have concentrated our efforts in this volume primarily on the problems of therapy and circulatory homeostasis — with the thought that this represents the most important aspect for the successful management of hemorrhagic shock. Additional measures are touched upon insofar as they have a connection with volume replacement. Selected problems of shock pathogenesis are taken up when they are specifically influenced by the volume replacement solutions discussed here.

## B. Spontaneous Regulation Processes of the Organism Following Blood Loss

The proper understanding of the therapeutic principles of volume replacement in hemorrhagic shock requires that the *spontaneous regulation mechanisms of the organism after blood losses of varying degree are known.* The most essential of these data are summarized in the following.

Normally a balance exists in the capillaries between the influx and eflux of fluids. The lymph circulation participates considerably in the return of interstitial fluid to the intravascular space. Considerable regional differences exist for the permeability of colloids [*983*]; it is high in the intestine, liver, lungs, and perhaps also in the heart [*1111, 1179*]. The capillary arteriovenous pressure gradient is approximately 4 mm Hg; according to STARLING [*1379*] the hydrostatic pressure in the capillaries is greater than the colloid osmotic pressure; from recently published results concerning indirect measurements in the mesenteric vessels of the frog and rat [*768*] it has become known that under normal conditions approximately 70—80% of the capillaries lose fluid, and therefore, their blood hydraulic pressure was higher than colloidal osmotic pressure.

## I. Losses of 500—1000 ml of Blood

In a healthy young person a volume loss of 500—1000 ml in general causes no essential hemodynamic changes [*1706*]. In blood donors [*1795*] a slight and transient increase in pulse rate can occur [*1427*]. Skillman has shown that venous hemorrhage causes a greater and more prolonged drop in blood pressure than does arterial hemorrhage of 15% of b. w. [*1815*]. As a result of this blood loss, an inflow of fluid containing protein begins, with an initial volume of the order of 100 ml/hr (= 0.5—2.0 ml/min) [*1814*]. This amount then decreases exponentially; within 18—48 hours the blood volume has been spontaneously replenished to its normal level [*376, 1043, 1044*]. This filling takes place through the capillaries as well as through the lymphatic system [*298*], and depends upon the state of hydration of the individual [*333, 767, 1508*]. The erythrocytes are regenerated at a rate of 15—50 ml (i. e. approx. 5—16 g Hb) per day, provided that sufficient iron is available. If in addition tissue trauma is present, then the process of normalization of the blood volume lasts longer, taking up to 6 days [*957*]. Other authors [*359*] assume that the spontaneous intravascular refilling occurs in two phases: According to them the first phase has already finished at the end of the period of hemorrhage and is characterized by the entry of protein-free interstitial fluid, which however is quickly lost through the kidneys. They maintain that the entry of protein-rich fluid begins between 2 and 24 hours following the occurrence of hypovolemia.

It is interesting that the transcapillary filling occurs without particular hypoalbuminemia [*886*] and that both noradrenalin [*904*] and angiotensin [*329, 330*] impair the normal entry process of interstitial fluid [*291, 1268*]. One research group [*520*] is of the opinion that administration of catecholamines does not influence the transcapillary refilling; but no information concerning blood volume determinations is available.

## II. Larger Blood Losses

For obvious reasons there is little data available concerning spontaneous regulation mechanisms in humans after larger blood losses: here we are dependent upon data gained in animal experiments [*1817*].

In the *dog* for example, after a *30% reduction in blood volume* there is still no replenishment of the erythrocyte volume up to 48 hours after blood loss although the plasma volume returns to normal after 24 hours, and the entire BV after 48 hours. The intravascular albumin pool is restored to 88% after 24 hours and to 92% after 48 hours. As the fine work of Birke *et al.* [*160, 1787*] shows the albumin pool is replenished by albumin flooding from the interstitium and not by increased synthesis (cf. also [*1195 a*]).

In *rats, cats* and *rabbits* spontaneous volume replacement occurs much more quickly [*314, 1200, 1318*]. In the case of rats for example, replenishment of the plasma volume was observed within 4 hours independent of the extent of bleeding and the state of hydration [*1113*].

In *dogs* it has been shown [*993, 994*] that *no mobilization of intracellular water* is effected by measures such as bleeding of 50% of the BV (occurring once), repeated bleeding of small amounts until profound shock occurs, blood loss in fractures, or infusion of unphysiologically high doses of adrenal cortical steroids. In these situations as well, all fluid displacement refers to the extracellular space. In the adrenalectomized animal without steroid substitution, spontaneous refilling brings about a plasma volume above normal while the blood pressure remains low. Six hours after administration of hydrocortisone *and* aldosterone the extracellular space becomes enlarged due to mobilization of cellular water. Simple administration of hydrocortisone enlarges the plasma volume while this effect is not seen after aldosterone alone. The effect of hydrocortisone is possibly determined by its activity on the peripheral vessels [*995*] (cf. also [*275, 276*]. The presence of angiotensin is a prerequisite for the spontaneous replenishment of the vascular system [*905*].

In blood loss averaging 66% (62—74%) of the BV, the survival rate of dogs is 50%, the compensatory hemodilution being 10% [*31*] (cf. also [*91, 277, 849, 1163, 1401, 1473, 1474*]).

The mortality rate of rats from which 3.9—4.0% of the body weight in blood has been withdrawn varies between 20—70% [*1393*].

For *humans* an acute loss of approx. 50% of the BV and more is of the greatest danger.

## C. Problems of Oxygen Transport

Hemorrhagic shock means loss of oxygen-carrying erythrocytes *and* plasma. The therapy must take both of these components into account, as the main task is to provide tissues with an adequate supply of oxygen. This depends not only upon the number of circulating erythrocytes but also on many other factors, whose importance is discussed in the following paragraphs.

### I. Rest Conditions

Under conditions of rest the following values are found in a normal adult [*821*]:

$O_2$: Consumption 250 ml/min
$CO_2$: Production and release, each, 200 ml/min
Heat: Production and loss, each, 40 cal/m$^2$/hr *

In the human body the total oxygen store amounts to about 1.5 litres [*1769*]. Since the normal tissue requirements are about 250 ml $O_2$/min the

* Body surface of an adult of 160 cm and 70 kg = 1.73 m$^2$.

*safety factor* for the oxygen supply is only about 3 (as not all the oxygen is available for use). This is quite low in comparison to all other vital substances. If ventilation, arterial oxygen content and blood flow are sufficient to cover the $O_2$ requirement, the organism is generally also provided with adequate amounts of all other substances so long as no irreversible changes are present.

## II. Jeopardy of Adequate Oxygen Supply

In hemorrhagic shock adequate oxygen supply of the organism is threatened for various reasons:

1. As a result of the reduction in the total amount of circulating hemoglobin the *arterial oxygen content* falls [*1722*, *1769*]. Every gram of hemoglobin can carry 1.34 ml $O_2$. Normally 100 ml of arterial blood thus contains about 20 ml $O_2$. After a blood loss of 20—30% of the blood volume there is a replenishment of the volume deficit with erythrocyte-free fluid resulting in a fall of the hematocrit to approx. 30 and the Hb to approx. 11 g-%. Thus the oxygen content of the blood is reduced from 20 to 14 ml $O_2$/100 ml blood. Such a reduction can be compensated for by a redistribution of blood flow favoring the heart and brain to the detriment of other tissues such as skin and muscles; it can also be compensated for by a rise in cardiac output and by improved oxygen release to the tissues [*816 a*] (shift to the left of the $O_2$ dissociation curve with pH decrease) [*677*].

2. The *cardiac output* in humans is normally about 5 l/min, the normal heart index 3.2 l/m²/min. The cardiac output is reduced in profound hemorrhagic shock, while in slight blood losses it shows an initial increase.

3. In extensive injuries there may be a reduction in *alveolar ventilation.* Usually this is the result of an increase in dead space with normal or even increased total ventilation and less often with a decrease in total ventilation [*821*].

4. A decrease in *arterial* $pO_2$ may therefore occur because of inadequate ventilation of alveoli well perfused with blood or because of the development of shunts when adequately ventilated alveoli become inadequately perfused.

In this connection the work of LAVER and BENDIXEN [*870*] is worthy of attention. These authors have shown that more or less extensive *atelectasis* occurs in practically all surgical patients and often is the cause of postoperative hypoxia. A contributory factor in the development of atelectasis may be the absence of the intermittent deep sigh seen in normal respiration but eliminated by anaesthesia, artificial ventilation and during the early postoperative period.

5. In spite of normal pressure and cardiac output after blood transfusion for volume replacement, *regional oxygen transport* in certain areas may be inadequate, if the *microcirculation* is already severely damaged (intravascular coagulation phenomena — aggregation of cells — anoxia — death of cells), or if any redistribution of blood flow remains.

## III. Necessity of Erythrocyte Replacement

Here again several factors are involved:

1. Extent of erythrocyte loss: *total amount of hemoglobin.*
2. *Rate* at which erythrocytes are lost.
3. *Oxygen requirement* of the organism (muscular activity).
4. Compensatory increase in *ventilation,* which in turn is dependent upon:
   $O_2$ concentration of inspired air,
   $O_2$ content of the alveoli,
   Perfusion of ventilated alveoli.
   (Hypoxia of slight degree increases ventilation.)
5. Adaptability of the circulation: *cardiac output.*
   (Slight hypoxia increases cardiac output, severe hypoxia lowers it.)
6. Perfusion of *microcirculation.*

With the exception of item 6 one is able today to measure all values quantitatively more or less accurately.

The *rate* at which erythrocytes are lost is very important. Patients with severe anaemia which has developed over a long period of time (e. g. leukaemia, pernicious anaemia etc.) show no signs of reduced tissue oxygenation, and in these cases the entire blood volume is normal, sometimes raised.

Bedridden patients have a reduced oxygen requirement. A hemoglobin content of 8—10 g-% is adequate for them under conditions of rest [*318, 435, 1544*].

In the management of patients with reduced oxygen carriage in the blood, one can make maximum use of the compensatory capability of ventilation by tracheotomy and artificial ventilation with 100% oxygen.

## IV. Evaluation of the Oxygen Supply of the Body

The *normal arterio-venous (a-v) oxygen difference* for the entire organism is about *5 vol.-%,* i. e. the average oxygen content of the mixed venous blood in the right atrium — or better, in the Pulmonary Artery — is approx. *15 vol.-%.* Decreased capillary blood flow is followed by an increase in oxygen extraction by the tissues. The overall extraction by the entire organism, as represented by *the a-v oxygen differences, is not however an indication of the oxygen reserve in the individual vital organs.*

According to the definition of Bendixen *et al.* [*119*], the *oxygen reserve* of any given organ is the difference between the normal oxygen content of the venous blood leaving that organ, and the oxygen content at the critical range of $pO_2$ below which oxygen can no longer be transferred from blood to tissue.

The vulnerability of a given tissue to hypoxemia depends in part upon the amount of oxygen it is able to extract from blood. At rest the heart has the highest a-v $O_2$ difference of any tissue. The selective increase in coronary blood flow in shock prevents the heart from being the first organ to suffer during hypoxemia.

The *clinical symptoms of oxygen deficiency* are
tachycardia,
extrasystoles,
hyperpnea,
fatigue, and altered mental status,
possibly cyanosis.

*However, all of these are nonspecific, and thus they give no reliable basis for the diagnosis of hypoxia.* It is often assumed that the presence of cyanosis is a reliable indication of hypoxia; the occurrence of blue lips, nail beds and mucosa, however, is dependent upon the absolute amount of reduced hemoglobin. *Before cyanosis can be diagnosed clinically, at least 5 g-%/o of reduced hemoglobin must be present.* Thus someone with polycythemia may have more than 5 g-% of reduced hemoglobin and become noticeably blue without the oxygen supply of his tissues being jeopardized. On the other hand a *patient in deep shock* may not have enough circulating hemoglobin to demonstrate cyanosis. *The presence or absence of cyanosis consequently permits no conclusions concerning the supply of oxygen to vital tissue.*

For the evaluation of the oxygen supply of the organism the following parameters are available today:

1. *$CO_2$-exchange in the alveoli: Measurement of $pCO_2$* in the arterial blood,

Normal value: 36—40—44 mm Hg.

With poor alveolar ventilation the values are high and vice versa.

2. *Oxygen uptake in the lung capillaries: Measurement of $pO_2$* in the arterial blood,

Normal values:

| Age | $pO_2$ in mm Hg |
|---|---|
| under 30 | 90—100 |
| 30—40 | 85—95 |
| 40—60 | 75—90 |
| over 60 | 65—80 |
| ($O_2$ saturation 95%) | |

With inhalation of pure $O_2$ the $pO_2$ rises to 610—670 mm Hg.

3. *Arterial oxygen content: direct measurement* [*119*, *1722*] or *computed:* 1.34 ml $O_2$/gram of hemoglobin, multiplied by the Hb concentration times the $O_2$ *saturation of hemoglobin.*

Normal value: 18—21 ml/100 ml.

(With 100% $O_2$: 19.5—22.5 ml.) Example: 1.34×15 g-%×95% = 19 ml $O_2$/100 ml.

4. *Flow: Measurement of cardiac output* with the dye dilution method (indocyanine green, cardiac green).

*In marginal situations* (i. e. low normal values) the *determination* of
blood lactate concentration,
pH and total bicarbonate, as well as
*oxygen content in mixed venous blood* (normal value: 14—15 vol.-%)
provide further clues. If these values are normal, i. e. if no metabolic acidosis is present, then tissue perfusion is in all probability adequate.

5. *Total oxygen delivery: calculation:* cardiac output × arterial oxygen content.

Normal value: 500—600 ml $O_2/m^2$/min.

6. *Perfusion pressure for oxygenation of selected capillary beds.* To check the functional condition of various organs only indirect methods are available clinically:

*ECG:* conclusions about ischemic changes of the *myocardium.*

*EEG:* certain conclusions about ischemic changes of the *brain* can be obtained from changes in mental status and from the EEG.

*Kidney:* normal quantities of urine are a good sign that the pressure and flow in the aorta are adequate for continuing glomerular filtration. Unfortunately, however, the reversed situation does not apply, as flow and pressure reduction in the aorta cannot necessarily be diagnosed on the basis of reduced urine output.

*In the evaluation of experimental and clinical results obtained by using erythrocyte-free blood replacement solutions, it is most important to know to what extent the cardiac output and flow in the microcirculation (also in the lungs!) can be influenced.* One starts with the assumption that experimentally the respiratory factors can be standardized for the most part and can be kept under control under clinical conditions. This applies to all minor blood losses and to most of those cases which are not accompanied by lung diseases or lung injuries.

## V. Flow Properties of Blood

As has already been mentioned above, along with an improvement of cardiac output in management of hemorrhagic shock, the restoration of normal conditions in the terminal part of the vascular system is also of decisive importance, since the essential metabolic processes take place here. The factors which influence flow in any given vascular bed are the pressure gradient $dP$ ($P_{\text{arterial}} - P_{\text{venous}}$) and the peripheral resistance ($R$). The latter is, among other things, dependent upon the vascular wall, the viscosity ($\eta$) [*511*], the radius ($r$) and the length ($l$) of the vessel.

The following equation is valid (POISEUILLE):

$$\text{flow} = \frac{dP}{R} = \frac{dP \cdot r^4 \cdot \pi}{l} \times \frac{1}{\eta} \times \text{constant} \left(= \frac{1}{8}\right).$$

Since blood is a pseudoplastic fluid (survey in [*1180 a*]), the relationship between flow and $\eta$ is not linear [*504, 1505*]. If the flow rate drops below a certain level, then the internal friction of blood rises sharply. Rheologically speaking, blood is a tixotropic system, i. e. the viscosity rises with decreasing shear rates, and vice versa [*353*].

Thus, for example, the viscosity of normal blood with a shear rate (see p. 55) of 0.01 $\text{sec}^{-1}$ is 800 centipoise, but with a shear rate of 1 $\text{sec}^{-1}$, $\eta$ is 20 centipoise [*1180 a, 1849*].

For given shear rates the *viscosity* of blood is in turn influenced by several factors:

1. By the hematocrit, which in turn is influenced by point 3 [*610, 1150, 1180*].

2. By the plasma viscosity, which is mainly determined by the presence of high molecular proteins (esp. fibrinogen [*1632*]) or pathological proteins and nucleic acids. GELIN [*515*] speaks of the so-called viscosity plus-factor.

3. By the internal viscosity of the erythrocytes, which is dependent upon shear force (cf. [*202*]).

4. By the reversible aggregation of erythrocytes which quantitatively is an important factor for the viscous and tixotropic properties of the blood [*512*].

In shock the circulation of the erythrocytes in the capillaries may be retarded [*95, 133, 1325, 1334, 1335, 1399*]. Hence aggregation of erythrocytes increases [*498, 499*], and this is most noticeable in extensive tissue trauma [*513, 1737, 1746*]. Platelet aggregation probably occurs first [*139, 1747*]; the pH fall caused by the deteriorating circulation leads in turn to a further increase in viscosity [*354*]. Immediately following normalization of a deranged capillary circulation, experimentally produced by injection of very high molecular weight dextran, an increase in acidosis can be observed [*913*], i. e. locally the pH drop can probably assume considerable proportions [cf. *1820*]. All of these phenomena are closely connected with the simultaneously occurring changes in the *coagulation mechanism*. These changes are in turn reinforced by thromboplastic material which is released from damaged cells, as well as by *hemolysis* of stagnating erythrocytes [*583, 584*].

The difficulties in methodology in this field are extremely great, and there is little quantitative data available. To determine platelet aggregation, which is clinically important [*1665*], one may measure thrombocyte adhesiveness on a glass surface, according to HELLEM [*698*], or photometrically after addition of ADP as described by BORN [*409*]. In addition there is measurement of the screen filtration pressure according to SWANK [*1406*]. Viscosity measurements of the blood permit further insight into these processes.

Today it is not yet known to what extent the individual components such as hypovolemia, platelet or erythrocyte aggregation affect the extremely complex flow relationships. It is certain that an increased tendency toward thrombus formation exists after trauma and blood loss [*251*] with aggregation of formed blood elements [*1746*]; this is reinforced by the hypoxic acidosis [*914, 1821*] and a retardation of wound healing occurs [*1567*].

The phenomena enumerated above are particularly important in the postcapillary venules where the blood flows very slowly [*127*]. Vascular areas with low pressure gradients, such as organ systems with double capillary systems, like kidney, liver, and pituitary gland, are said to be affected most by these relationships [*507, 1767*]. Actually kidney, intestine and liver (survey in [*38, 618*]) play an important part in the occurrence of shock. It can be assumed that in the future one must use better diagnostic methods in order to gain better knowledge of the state of the microcirculation [*159*], and it seems appropriate to employ therapeutic means to counteract such disturbances [*1820*] as are caused by aggregation of platelets and erythrocytes, increased coagulation, acidosis, hemolysis, and increased viscosity [*875, 1710, 1747, 1785*].

## VI. To what Extent May the Blood Volume be Replaced with Erythrocyte-free Solutions?

It has long been known that the organism can do without a certain number of erythrocytes and remain undamaged so long as the total blood volume remains normal. As early as 1883, OTT [*1107*] wrote: "The danger of blood losses of up to $^2/_3$ of the total blood volume lies in the disproportion of vascular size and vascular content caused by the loss, and the volume of fluid infused counteracts this danger, no matter whether the fluid contains erythrocytes or not, so long as it is not directly injurious, but rather is indifferent."

This theory was later confirmed by further experiments. AMBERSON [*46*], in his plasmaphoresis experiments, repeatedly took small amounts of blood from dogs and cats, washed the erythrocytes and reinfused part of these mixed with saline or artificial colloid solutions. The animals survived if the erythrocyte volume was not less than 30% of normal.

It has been shown that dogs can stand an acute hemodilution with dextran 75 * down to an Hb of 3 g-% (oxygen content 4 vol.-%) so long as they are ventilated adequately with air. A still greater hemodilution to 2 g-% and less (Hct 2—4%) is possible if pure oxygen is provided [*656, 788 a, 1236*]. In other experiments the observations were continued over a longer period. Seven out of 10 dogs survived without symptoms. The cardiac index rose to 170% [*459, 460*]. The acid-base relationships were fully normalized after 24 hours. In one week the Hct had returned to approx. 50% of the original value [*494, 1414, 1415, 1416, 1417*].

Wise and co-workers [*1545*] found that both dextran and plasma were equally suitable for the transport of dissolved oxygen in cases of extreme hemodilution (identical mortality in exchange transfusions). They observed adequate compensation mechanisms until the Hb had dropped to half of the original value (cf. [*1577*]). Hunt et al. [*1700*] have recently shown, that $pO_2$ in subcutaneous tissue is more a function of blood volume than of hematocrit (cf. [*1715, 1716*]).

Murray et al. [*1068*] assume, however, that the hemodynamic adaptation mechanisms, in normovolemic anemia in the dog, are not sufficient to provide a normal oxygen supply to the tissues. On the other hand they have shown that polycythemia in normovolemia does not cause improvement but rather deterioration of the oxygen supply, since the peripheral resistance increases due to a rise in viscosity; and coronary flow decreases [*1169, 1702*].

Crowell [*320*] brought 67 dogs with initial Hct levels of 12—56 into severe hemorrhagic shock and determined the time required for occurrence of irreversibility. The results were as follows: With Hct levels of up to *35*, the resistance of the animals rises to 5 times that of an Hct of 12%. *A higher Hct, however, lowers the resistance against occurrence of irreversibility.* Animals with Hct values between 20 and 25% surprisingly demonstrate better shock resistance than do those with an Hct between 45 and 50%. In a later article [*321*] the oxygen consumption and transport were measured under similar conditions. Both rise up to an Hct of 42. Higher values, however, lower the $O_2$ consumption, which is explained by the occurrence of increased viscosity. However, the experiments are not convincing because the Hct variations were caused by addition of erythrocytes washed in saline solution and administration of phenylhydrazine hydrochloride. Data concerning blood volume are lacking, and it must be assumed that the anemic animals were hypovolemic (see [*363*]). Of great importance is the knowledge that an oxygen deficiency of 120 ml/kg bw in the dog represents an $LD_{50}$, while an oxygen deficiency of 140 ml/kg bw and more is always fatal [*322*]. Thus a significant correlation exists between the time necessary to develop irreversible shock and the time required to produce an oxygen deficit of 120 ml/kg bw (Jones [*1705*]).

* Dextran with an average molecular weight $\overline{M}_w$ of approx. 75,000.

Important observations on *humans* come from the Korean War [*78*. Wounded soldiers who had lost 50% of their erythrocyte volume wer often treated only with dextran without signs of oxygen deficiency occurrir (Hct between 20 and 30%). In this respect 150 patients were examine carefully, and on the basis of these observations the following guidelines fc the best volume replacement were proposed:

| Amount required for volume replacement, in ml | Proportion |
|---|---|
| 1000—1500 | dextran only |
| 1500—4000 | dextran 1 : blood 1 |
| 4000—7000 | dextran 1 : blood 2 |
| over 7000 | maximum 2500 ml dextran, rest blood |

Up to 1500 ml of dextran could be administered in 15 minutes.

Precise data concerning oxygen metabolism in man are rare, and up now no definite proof is available with regard to how much the Hct ca be lowered in humans in hemorrhagic shock without danger. In spite of th ample clinical experience confirms that losses of the erythrocyte volume up to 25—30% of normal can be sustained as long as the plasma volume soon completely replenished and respiration is adequate. That losses 20—30% of the BV (this amount is approx. 1—1½ litres in a normal ma with a BV of 5 litres) can be replaced without danger with erythrocyte-fr fluids is therefore a view shared by many authors: [*78, 199 a, 318, 363, 47 550, 658, 681, 824, 935, 943, 1013, 1094, 1100, 1141, 1236, 1247, 127 1272, 1274, 1275, 1277, 1278, 1299, 1304, 1319, 1396, 1502, 1532, 155 1556, 1557, 1559, 1617*].

This view is also based upon numerous data from *open heart surge* where the patients today are usually perfused according to the "hem dilution method" [*917, 1081, 1207, 1208, 1339, 1410 a, 1774*].

Gollub [*535*] performed open heart surgery without any sort of blo transfusion on 5 Jehovah's Witnesses. Immediately postoperatively the H lay between 16.5 and 32.5%; the patients went through prolonged co valescence, but all recovered.

Murphy [*1066*] reports on the *kidney function of dogs* in massive hem dilution with starch, dextran and saline solutions (see section on star p. 142, and [*1763*]).

*All of these data indicate that Hct levels of approx. 30% are genera tolerated without danger of reduced oxygen supply so long as the circul ing blood volume remains normal.*

No proof has been found for the theory that anemia leads to poor *wound healing*. The reduction of wound healing under conditions of anemia reported by SANDBLOM (quoted in [*1567*] can be explained by hypovolemia, according to ZEDERFELDT [*1567*]. ZEDERFELDT has shown experimentally that completely normal healing of wounds occurs when the circulating blood volume is kept normal with dextran 70 — this too, when the Hb content is only 30% (see also [*535, 777*]).

In this connection it is also important to know that *erythrocyte-regeneration* is increased after acute blood losses (increase of reticulocytes), and that well-nourished individuals with sufficient protein and iron supply produce erythrocytes for much more than 1 litre of blood in about a month (cf. [*1510*]).

Because of the risk involved in blood transfusion (see below), the principle is generally valid that blood should not be administered without definite reason. *Blood is not required in the following situations* [*550, 943, 1051*]:

1. In blood losses of up to 10% of the BV (= approx. 500 ml in a normal healthy person),

2. in anemias which can be managed with medication (iron, vitamin $B_{12}$),

3. for symptomatic treatment in incurable diseases.

With this procedure valuable blood can be saved for those patients who really need it [*318, 319, 1476*].

It has been shown that a quick correction of chronic anemias preoperatively impairs pulmonary function [*10, 1374*]. If one is forced to take such steps, erythrocyte concentrates should be used.

## D. Summary and Conclusions: Pathophysiology of Blood Loss

1. Irreversibility in hemorrhagic shock occurs when the oxygen deficit has reached a certain level (in dogs 140 ml/kg bw).

2. It has not yet been definitely established whether certain organ systems of the human suffer more in shock than others. It is also unknown to what extent secondary factors which occur as a result of reduced circulation contribute toward irreversibility by increasing the oxygen deficit, or whether certain organs lose their normally present protective function with lack of oxygen.

3. Blood losses of 500—1000 ml (10—20% of the BV) in humans lead to a sudden influx of water, salt, and albumin into the circulatory system. This process lasts 18—48 hours, according to the state of hydration. Refilling takes place very quickly at first and diminishes considerably with time. The plasma volume replaced equals the sum of plasma plus erythrocytes

lost. Corresponding data in larger blood losses have been available up to now only from animal experiments.

4. The main task in the therapy of hemorrhagic shock lies in supplying the tissues with adequate amounts of oxygen.

5. Evaluation of results with erythrocyte-free replacement solutions depends primarily upon knowing to what extent these solutions are capable of raising cardiac output and improving capillary perfusion and thus of releasing oxygen into the surrounding tissues.

6. To what extent the BV in hemorrhagic shock in man can be replaced with erythrocyte-free solutions without danger is not yet proved with any certainty using metabolic data. Considerable clinical experience, however, shows that blood losses of up to 1000 or 1500 ml (reduction of the Hct after replenishment of the BV to approx. 30) in previously healthy individuals can be replaced with erythrocyte-free solutions without any particular risk to the oxygen supply.

PART TWO

# Various Methods of Volume Replacement

## A. Volume Replacement Using Blood

With the discovery of blood groups and subgroups, together with the introduction of reliable preservation processes, blood transfusions have become routine therapy in all hospitals (review in [*1797*, *1798*]). On the principle that lost fluid should be replaced with similar fluid, blood is administered in many places, even after small blood losses. The replacement of blood losses with stored citrated blood is a very effective method of treatment [*747*]. Without doubt it represents the greatest and most important progress in the management of hemorrhagic shock in this century [*1342*].

In recent years, however, there have been more and more warnings of the hazards involved in unnecessary blood transfusion [*694*, *981*, *1525*, *1704*]. In minor blood loss particularly no blood should be transfused [*552*, *1396*]. The disadvantages and dangers have become increasingly recognized [*1845*], and in many places have led to a very strict stand being taken with regard to the indications for blood transfusion [*163*]. On the basis of retrospective investigations it is assumed that 35—50% of all blood transfusions are unnecessary [*522*, *743*] and that only 1% are given on vital indication [*335*].

Therefore the disadvantages and dangers are to be discussed first in this chapter. Heparinized, decalcified (resin-collected) and, more recently, deep-frozen blood is sometimes transfused. Here, however, only the administration of ACD-blood [*748*] is to be discussed, since the overwhelming majority of all blood transfusions is in the form of citrated blood.

Various new preservatives are in the trial stage [*215*] and have already produced promising results, but they are not yet in routine use. In his foreword to Hurn's "Storage of blood" (London: Academic Press Inc. Ltd. 1968) Greaves recently stated: "It is surprising that twenty years after the war no further improvements in blood storage have been introduced.... A further week of storage could probably be achieved now, but it would not be easy to prove its clinical efficiency was as good as the present stored blood about which there is overwhelming evidence as to its safety and clinical efficiency. In a way the present situation is highly satisfactory, but looked at from another point of view it is very inhibitory to further progress. The ultimate aim should be indefinite storage. So far, all attempts to freeze-dry whole blood have failed, but considerable success has followed *freezing and storage at very low temperatures.* Two basic methods are used. One involves the use of an intracellular additive such as glycerol or dimethylsulphoxide with relatively slow freezing; the other involves the use of an extracellular additive such as polyvinylpyrrolidone (PVP) or sugars, followed by relatively rapid freezing. The introduction of liquid nitrogen storage containers enables storage of the frozen blood at very low temperatures of —170° to —196° C at which temperatures storage should be indefinite. — Both methods have been used successfully for storing red cells of rare groups for blood typing, and both methods have been used for preserving blood for transfusion. The disadvantages of the glycerol process are mainly due to the difficulty of removing the glycerol after thawing. These difficulties seem largely to have been overcome by HUGGIN's method of agglomeration [*748*], and it is of interest that this method is being used by the U.S. forces for transfusions in Vietnam. The PVP frozen blood must be thawed very rapidly, but is immediately available for transfusion without further processing and would thus be ideal in an emergency were it not for the fact that about 4% of cells are haemolysed by the process and that there are doubts as to the safety of injection of the PVP. The relative merits and disadvantages of the two processes must be further elucidated. The glycerol frozen blood would seem to be ideal for the premeditated transfusion; the PVP frozen blood for sudden emergencies. But although a permanently preserved blood by avoiding wastage would improve the economics of transfusion, this advantage would be greatly outweighed by the increased cost of processing and storage. Even now this increase would probably be justified for the storage of rare bloods and stockpiling against emergencies, particularly if these low temperature storage facilities were also used for storage of certain tissues for transplantation surgery." Moss [*1758*] has recently reported the clinical experience with using frozen blood in combat casualties in Vietnam.

## I. Disadvantages and Dangers of Blood Transfusion

### 1. Mortality

Mortality as a result of blood transfusion is about 0.1—1‰ [*335, 358, 550, 672, 1282*]. The chief legal adviser of the American Medical Association asserts that these figures are comparable to the mortality resulting from appendicitis or anesthesia alone [*716*]. In 1960 he assumed that about

3000 persons die annually in the USA as a consequence of blood transfusions.

In this respect one must consider that probably many cases remain unreported, and that deaths as a direct result of the infusion of plasma expanders commonly used today are probably most rare [*53*]. Of course these two situations are not strictly comparable, since blood often *must* be administered upon vital indication.

*However, one must never forget that blood transfusions involve a certain percentage of mortality.*

## 2. The Transmission of Disease

The transmission of disease represents the greatest risk of blood transfusions today (cf. [*669*; with 155 references]).

The most important of the transmitted diseases are generally considered to be

viral hepatitis,
syphilis,
malaria,
trypanosomiasis.

The transmission of brucellosis is less important today [*630*]. It is quite possible that still other diseases specifically caused by viruses are transmitted without knowledge, because these organisms cannot be traced, and the causal connection is not clear.

With the exception of hepatitis most of these diseases can be shown by laboratory tests and can be treated chemotherapeutically. But in order to stop transmission really successfully, the respective tests would have to be carried out in *all* units, which unfortunately is very far from reality. The frightening increase of veneral diseases in recent years (cf. [*606*]) as well as the intensification of international travel make contamination of preserved blood with spirochetes and organisms of tropical diseases more likely than ever, even in non tropical areas; this represents a danger when using *fresh blood* (stored less than 72 hours) [*887*].

Even at an early date the *transmission of viral hepatitis* was considered to be *one of the greatest problems in transfusion practice.* For many years, however, the danger received insufficient attention. The risk of transmission of hepatitis is the major concern of many authors who advise a strict standpoint with regard to indication of blood transfusions [*294, 1655, 1689*].

In order to evaluate this problem, precise data concerning the frequency of transfusion hepatitis are necessary. Until recently the importance of *non-icteric hepatitis* was not recognized properly; for this reason data concerning the frequency of the *icteric* form are to be discussed first. The following is a list of articles which refer to this problem.

| Author | Year | Reference |
|---|---|---|
| J. G. ALLEN et al. | 1959 | [*26*] |
| J. G. ALLEN and W. A. SAYMAN | 1962 | [*27*] |
| J. G. ALLEN | 1966, 1966 | [*28, 29*] |
| W. BEHRENDS and N. STEINHARDT | 1961 | [*117*] |
| S. N. COHEN and W. J. DOUGHERTY | 1963 | [*286*] |
| S. CRONBERG et al. | 1963 | [*315*] |
| E. A. FRIEDMAN and G. E. THOMSON | 1966 | [*475*] |
| G. F. GRADY et al. | 1964 | [*548*] |
| A. HÄSSIG et al. | 1953, 1955, 1963, 1966 | [*662, 664, 669, 675*] |
| H. HEISTÖ | 1958 | [*696*] |
| G. C. HILL | 1965 | [*709*] |
| P. I. HOXWORTH et al. | 1959 | [*743*] |
| R. KATZ et al. | 1957 | [*811*] |
| J. J. KREBS and P. SCHARENBERG | 1959 | [*839*] |
| C. M. KUNIN | 1959 | [*843*] |
| S. MADSEN | 1954 | [*942*] |
| G. MAURER | 1965 | [*970*] |
| G. S. MIRICK et al. | 1965 | [*1024*] |
| L. NORGREN | 1966 | [*1093*] |
| M. ODIN | 1954 | [*1098*] |
| J. PROCHAZKA | 1957 | [*1145*] |
| O. RAMGREN and J. E. TENGBERG | 1960 | [*1157*] |
| H. REISSIGL | 1956 | [*1174*] |
| K. W. SCHNEIDER | 1965 | [*1278*] |
| A. W. SCHWENZER | 1954 | [*1302*] |
| J. R. SENIOR | 1965 | [*1315*] |
| N. SHIMADA et al. | 1965 | [*1327*] |

### *a) The Frequency of Transfusion Hepatitis*

**Icteric Form.** The information in various articles and statistics varies greatly; the frequency lies between *0—25%*.

The reasons for this great variation are as follows:

1. The criteria applied in follow-up checks range from written questionnaires to personal examination of each case, including tests of liver function. This should also explain those results which show no cases of transfusion hepatitis whatsoever [*1174*].

2. Many follow-up studies are admittedly incomplete [*548*]. Because of the incubation time which sometimes lasts up to 6 months the patients are often no longer traceable. Either they have in the meantime changed their

place of residence or they see no connection with the transfusion when hepatitis occurs and consult a different physician. A large number of transfusions are prescribed by surgeons. Because of the hepatitis symptoms the patients usually consult a general practitioner or a physician who is not always able to recognize the connection with a blood transfusion, as the patients themselves do not even know that they have received blood. Even today it is not possible to make a differential diagnosis between infectious and serum hepatitis.

3. Various methods of computing hepatitis frequency are used, but the examination series are often too small, and only few statistics include control groups.

4. Transfusion centers which pay their donors show a higher hepatitis frequency since unreliable individuals do not report previous hepatitis because of the money which they can earn relatively easily [*26*, *29*, *843*].

5. The general standard of the transfusion service and the criteria for selecting donors vary considerably from one country to another. In Japan, where there is a majority of paid donors the incidence of hepatitis is 25% [*1445*].

6. Although blood donors are paid in Sweden, that country has a relatively low frequency of post-transfusion hepatitis [*1093*]. Apparently there are also great differences in the geographical distribution of the hepatitis virus.

7. The ratio of icteric to non-icteric hepatitis is also dependent on regional and seasonal fluctuations [*1818*].

8. The incubation period of transfusion hepatitis does not always differ from that of infectious hepatitis. Transfusion hepatitis can occur after 14 days [*7*, *678*, *720*, *1093*, *1315*, *1484*].

9. Its frequency varies according to age, sex, race, and underlying disease.

10. The absolute risk of transfusion hepatitis increases with increasing number of transfusions [*29*, *312*, *1024*].

In taking these points into consideration one must assume that transfusion hepatitis occurs more frequently than many of the statistics listed would tend to indicate. More recent articles generally show higher figures.

**Overall Incidence of Transfusion Hepatitis.** New extremely careful and complete follow-up studies with repeated transaminase determination and liver biopsies show the following figures for the frequency of post-transfusion hepatitis (icteric plus non-icteric cases):

| | | |
|---|---|---|
| CREUTZFELDT et al. | [*312*] | 14.0% |
| HOLLAND et al. | [*720*] | 14.9% |
| REDECKER | [*1164*] | 17.5% |
| RUBINSON et al. | [*1226*] | 12.0% |

In the investigation by CREUTZFELDT the incidence of hepatitis was 10.6% after a single blood transfusion whereas in patients with more than 10 transfusions the incidence reached 28.6%.

It is not easy to make the *diagnosis of non-icteric hepatitis;* it is possible only with repeated transaminase determinations and liver biopsies [*1818*]. Thus it is understandable why this disease was not observed more often previously. In addition it generally occurs during the convalescence after serious disease or large operations and is often hard to distinguish from the basic ailment because of its nonspecific symptoms. However, during convalescence the occurrence of additional complications is particularly undesirable. Such patients should not be subjected to additional burdens, especially iatrogenic and avoidable ones.

According to the information available at this time there is no reason to believe that non-icteric hepatitis is less dangerous than the icteric type. On the contrary, CREUTZFELDT was able to prove by means of liver biopsies that non-icteric transfusion hepatitis can result in cirrhosis. A non-icteric hepatitis is thus by no means harmless; in addition its course is often very prolonged [*294*].

### *b) Mortality of Transfusion Hepatitis*

In *icteric transfusion hepatitis* the mortality is about 1—12% according to various sources [*312, 1378 a, 1689*].

*Table 1* gives a survey of some results published recently. Here too one must give consideration to the points mentioned above with regard to variations amongst the results.

Table 1. *The mortality after transfusion hepatitis*

| Author | Mortality of patients with transfusion hepatitis | Year of publication |
|---|---|---|
| P. I. HOXWORTH et al. [*743*] | 9% | 1959 |
| J. G. ALLEN and W. A. SAYMAN [*27*] | 25% | 1962 |
| G. F. GRADY et al. [*548*] | 12% | 1964 |
| T. C. CHALMERS et al. [*271*] | 6—28% | 1965 |
| J. R. SENIOR [*1315*] | 10—12% | 1965 |
| W. CREUTZFELDT et al. [*312*] | 12% | 1966 |

### *c) Measures for Preventing Transfusion Hepatitis*

The problem of preventing transfusion hepatitis remains unsolved [*669*]. At present, in spite of precise inquiry and examination of all blood donors, one cannot exclude all virus carriers. Many cases of hepatitis, especially non-icteric ones, run their course undiagnosed, and thus remain unknown to the patient and his physician alike. It has been shown that not even all virus carriers of icteric hepatitis can be determined by the usual questioning as to whether they have had jaundice, and donors who have had the non-icteric type of hepatitis, which occurs four times as frequently, cannot be determined at all. A greater number of virus carriers could be excluded by checking the liver function of all donors before they donate blood. There are, however, no specific tests which would make it possible to recognize previous hepatitis with certainty. From results available today no binding conclusions can be drawn concerning the value of transaminase determination [*675*]. Besides, the organizational problems connected with such plans are practically insurmountable in view of the present situation in most blood donor centers.

Therefore it is understandable that continuous research is being carried out to find new methods for reducing the alarmingly high frequency of hepatitis and its consequences. It is still not clear how useful the prophylactic *administration of gamma globulin* may be. CREUTZFELDT [*313*] believes that a protective effect can be obtained with intravenous administration, but according to his own statements, the number of patients who have been examined is still too small for valid conclusions. HOLLAND [*720*], on the other hand, is of the opinion that gamma globulin is completely useless in this respect; MIRICK [*1024*] assumes that prophylactic administration of gamma globulin merely changes icteric cases to non-icteric ones, depending upon dosage and when it is administered.

If larger series should show that prophylactic i. v. administration of gamma globulin actually succeeds in creating significant protection for certain cases (probably only in small transfusions), then new problems would arise. How should the world's supply of gamma globulin be sufficient to cover the tremendous demand? Gamma globulin is also derived from preserved blood; thus production depends on donors. In addition these preparations are exceedingly expensive. For these reasons it is hard to imagine that important progress can be made in this direction.

The excellent investigations by HUGGINS [*748*] concerning *deep-frozen blood* (—85° C) show another possibility. Until now no cases of icteric hepatitis have occurred in 2229 cases after transfusion of such deep-frozen blood but the figures are not yet conclusive. If it should be shown that a certain protection is afforded by washing the erythrocytes, as is necessary during thawing, then formidable technical problems would have to be solved here as well, for the expensive apparatus for deep-freezing blood will be reserved only for certain centers for many years to come (see p. 20). It is possible that immunoglobulin assay may provide a useful screening procedure for potential blood donors [*1608*].

Thus today, the only practical possibilities for reducing the risk of hepatitis are by the following well established methods:

1. Extremely strict selection of blood donors (NORGREN et al. [*1093*] exclude all donors whose blood was used in a patient who later developed hepatitis). This means that it will become more and more difficult to procure whole blood in the near future if no effective measures can be found for destroying the hepatitis virus [*1140*].

2. Absolute restriction to blood transfusions deemed urgent [*1140*].

Excellent surveys concerning the questions of transfusion hepatitis are by MOSLEY and BULL [*1052*], GRINDON et al. [*1689*] and by HAUSSMANN [*677 a*].

## 3. Reactions due to Bacterial Contamination

Serious, sometimes lethal reactions due to bacterial contamination of preserved blood have often been described [*187, 204, 205, 206, 380, 381, 385, 987, 1030, 1097, 1388*]. It is generally assumed that *approximately 2% of preserved blood is bacterially contaminated* even with strict control [*156, 204, 721, 778, 1031, 1134*] and that the number of serious reactions resulting from infusion of bacterially contaminated blood is greater than the complications caused by incompatibility [*335, 987*].

LITWIN et al. [*912*] have pointed out the synergistic toxic effect of gram-negative bacteria and free hemoglobin. They recommend the use of *fresh* compatible blood for the treatment of shocked patients, especially those who suffer from a serious infection caused by gram-negative bacteria. With the slightest suspicion of hemolysis, one should not use preserved blood in such cases.

## 4. Incompatibility

A compatible blood transfusion is a successful *homotransplantation*, wherein the survival time of transfused compatible erythrocytes corresponds to that of the host erythrocytes.

Today incompatibility is understood to be any reduction in survival time of red blood cells, of donor erythrocytes as well as host ones [*676*]. The half-life for transfused erythrocytes is considered to be 34 days [*245, 621*]. In approx. 30% of all blood transfusions, especially in patients who are transfused several times, the erythrocytes survive only 14—16 days and then disappear from the vascular system [*145*]. This means that in about $^1/_3$ of all cases the tests for blood group incompatibility in use today are inadequate. Thus patients may be sensitised several times which can have serious results in later transfusions.

Incompatibility is not identical to the occurrence of hemolytic transfusion reactions. The latter occur much less frequently. With serological compatibility tests one protects the patient from infusion of incompatible blood. Anesthesia often suppresses the symptoms of incompatibility [*1458*].

The reported frequency of incompatibility reactions is 0.2‰—0.7% [*634, 676*]. In 3900 blood transfusions Huestis [*758*] observed immunohematological problems in 3.5% of the cases and requires new crossmatching before *every* blood transfusion.

The frequency of *heat-active irregular antibodies* is about 0.5—1.0‰ in individuals *without* previous transfusions and pregnancies. In persons *with* previous transfusions and after pregnancies the frequency is approximately 10 times greater [*672*], whereby the number of persons thus isoimmunised continually increases. The risk of isoimmunization is additive and is approx. 1% per blood transfusion. 2/3 of these new erythro-antibodies are blood group specific [*921*].

Immunization processes against thrombocyte and leucocyte agglutinins play a part to an increasing degree [*819, 1122*].

Regarding problems occurring after transfusions of universal donor blood see [*1599*].

## 5. Hemolytic Reactions

Hemolytic complications are caused by *ABO incompatibility* and can usually be traced back to poor organization (mistakes!) [*787, 1031, 1567*].

Under ideal conditions they occur in 0.2—0.3‰ of the cases or even less frequently [*467, 481, 676, 1387*]. But most often they are more frequent, for example as determined according to new data, in 1‰ of all transfusions [*1282*].

Doberneck [*358*] reports on 17 cases of his own involving acute renal failure after hemolytic complications; 2 patients died. According to Spielmann [*1372*] 1 patient in 10,000—30,000 transfusions dies from this cause.

With regard to the synergistic effect of free hemoglobin and gram-negative bacteria see p. 26, "reactions due to bacterial contamination" [*912*].

## 6. Allergic Reactions

The various articles on this subject are difficult to evaluate since varying criteria are used.

The most frequently observed urticarial and asthmatic reactions usually occur in only a few percent of cases and are rarely of clinical importance [*552*]. More serious asthmatic reactions or laryngeal edemas are said to occur in 0.1—0.2% [*1157, 1458*]. Horatz and Langer [*725*] report a total side-effect figure of 6.92% after blood transfusions. According to a more recent compilation [*1282*], a total of 430 transfusion reactions (including hemolytic complications) occured in 28,273 whole blood transfusions, i. e. 1.52%.

## 7. Citrate Toxicity

Preserved blood contains *100—120 ml ACD solution* (solutio anticoagulans). This is made up of the following:

6.7 mval citric acid,
13.4 mval sodium citrate,
13.9 mMol glucose (Ph. H. V.).

The addition of larger amounts of sodium citrate at first causes a metabolic acidosis, especially if the citrate cannot be broken down immediately in the liver, as for example in severe shock, serious liver disease, and in infants. A rise in the plasma potassium concentration accompanies the decrease in pH. In the situations mentioned above, larger amounts of citrated blood administered rapidly can lead to tetaniform cramps and cardiac arrhythmias [*236*].

With intact liver function, sodium citrate is changed to sodium bicarbonate in the liver, leading to "post-transfusion alkalosis" which as a rule is clinically unimportant [*911*]. This alkalosis can occur even after a few hours but normally in 1—3 days according to the condition of the liver function as well as the amount and rate of blood administered. Bicarbonate is further broken down into $CO_2$ and water — sometimes a rather considerable surplus of sodium remains, which can lead to a rise in sodium in the extracellular fluid. One must think of these large amounts of sodium when determining the daily electrolyte requirement after large transfusions.

It is generally assumed today that one can administer *2 litres of citrated blood in approx. 20 min* in an adult without danger of citrate intoxication [*1031*]. If a larger amount must be infused even more rapidly, or if reduced citrate breakdown is to be taken into consideration (serious liver damage, hypothermia, shock, neonates), 1 g of calcium gluconate is usually given per litre of citrated blood [*1550*].

Howland [*735, 736, 737, 738, 740*] is against giving *calcium* routinely. In a large investigation series, the mortality resulting from ventricular fibrillation following addition of calcium was higher than in the group of patients without calcium therapy, even when 5 litres and more were transfused. Although these investigations do not stand up against all criticism — the series were not carried out simultaneously — Howland and his coworkers have shown that large amounts of citrate without additional calcium can be infused in a short period, without the likelihood of citrate intoxication or disturbance of the calcium metabolism. Several facts in these articles emphasize that addition of calcium is not necessary and can sometimes even be dangerous. It is pointed out that the calcium reserves of the body are extremely large and that serum calcium only makes up about 1% of them.

The effect of citrate on bacterial resistance is discussed in the respective chapter (see p. 31).

## 8. Acidity of Preserved Blood

BAUE and co-workers [*108*] and BOYAN [*197*] see a further danger in this point, especially when the preserved blood is not warmed before use.

ACD blood has a pH of less than 6.8 after being stored for 3 days; after 3 weeks the pH is at 6.7 and continues to drop [*215, 1571*]. HOWLAND and SCHWEIZER [*739*] assume that preserved blood contains an average of about 5 mval of acid; they found maximal levels of 8 mval/unit. With the use of warmed blood metabolic acidosis never occurred, even after massive transfusions [*1301*]. They were able to reduce the mortality further by routinely giving bicarbonate in the warmed preserved blood to patients who required 20 or more transfusions [*741*].

*In practice the following procedure has proved useful:* If more than 3 units of blood are to be transfused rapidly, the blood is warmed from the fourth unit on. 44.6 mval of *sodium bicarbonate* are given i. v. for every 5 units of blood, i. e. approx. 3.75 g (1 g sodium bicarbonate = 11.9 mval sodium) [*742*].

## 9. Temperature Drop after Addition of Larger Amounts of Cold Blood

The specific heat of blood is 0.87 cal [*1002*]. Therefore 0.5 litres of blood stored at 4° C requires $0.5 \times 33 \times 0.87 = 14.4$ kcal to be warmed to body temperature.

If anesthetized patients with a reduced thermoregulatory capability are infused rapidly with large amounts of cold blood, the heart and body temperatures [*195, 735, 881, 938, 1228, 1229*] fall; at the same time the oxygen consumption rises sharply [*1209*], which is absolutely undesirable during and after surgery. *Children* especially cannot produce the required amount of heat in a short time; ventricular fibrillation and cardiac arrest are observed as complications. BOYAN [*195*] determined a decrease in body temperature after the rapid infusion of more than 3—4 units of blood.

With consideration of these facts, BOYAN and HOWLAND [*196, 197, 198*] more recently use *warm blood* exclusively for massive transfusions and in this way are able to sharply reduce the incidence of cardiac arrhythmia and cardiac arrest. With transfusions of 20 units of blood and more, the mortality rate with cold blood is 50%, with warmed blood 20%.

The general condition of patients who have received warmed blood is also much better; they have warm, dry skin of normal color; but with patients who have received cold blood it is often difficult to measure pulse and blood pressure, the patients are cold, often cyanotic and have poor peripheral circulation.

The same conclusions have been reached by other authors as well [*152, 374, 470, 831, 1108*] who have developed simple devices for warming the blood during transfusion.

Of more theoretical interest is the fact that a massive reduction in body temperature is also undesirable for rheological reasons, in that the viscosity rises threefold with a temperature drop from 38° C to 8° C with a constant hematocrit [*397*].

## 10. Blood Coagulation Disturbances after Massive Blood Transfusions

The most common disturbances in the coagulation mechanism of patients who require massive transfusions during surgery are a marked *reduction in the number of thrombocytes as well as a decrease of factors V and VIII.* Fibrinolysis can occur as a serious complication [*742*].

R. F. Wilson [*1539*] observed disturbances in the coagulation system in 34 out of 209 patients who all received 5 litres of blood within 24 hours (cf. also [*1561*]).

## 11. Potassium Intoxication

Potassium intoxication can occur after transfusion of very large amounts of blood which has been stored for several days when given to patients with reduced renal function, e. g. to shocked patients (see also point 7, p. 28).

This conclusion was also confirmed experimentally [*882*]. When blood is stored for 10 days, the plasma potassium concentration of 4—5 mval/l rises to about 15 mval/l. After 21 days levels of 25 mval/l can be reached [*283, 374, 436*].

## 12. Ammonia Intoxication

The *ammonia concentration* of fresh preserved blood is normally approx. 100—150 µg-%. After storage for 20 days this amount rises to 700—800 µg-% [*1369*]. On the other hand, cerebrospinal fluid contains practically no ammonia [*986*]. Even with a liquor concentration of 150 µg-% coma can occur. Since a diffusion coefficient of 0.85 exists between plasma and cerebrospinal fluid, the infusion of a few units of stored blood or "outdated plasma" are sufficient to produce coma in patients with high ammonia concentrations in their plasma as are sometimes found in liver diseases, gastrointestinal bleeding and nephritis. For this reason such patients should receive only fresh blood and plasma. This view, however, is not uncontested [*1096 a*].

## 13. Post-transfusion Hyperbilirubinemia

Post-transfusion hyperbilirubinemia is actually not very dangerous [*1390*] yet undesirable; to avoid it Bergmann [*142*] recommends limitation of the use of preserved blood to 10 days (cf. also [*1131*]).

## 14. Various other Factors

The rise in *inorganic phosphates* is without practical importance. *Free hemoglobin* is not harmful if renal function is adequate and there are no septic complications, provided that large amounts of old blood are not infused quickly.

The longer erythrocytes are preserved, the more pronounced is the shift to the left in the *oxygen dissociation curve* of hemoglobin [*869*].

## 15. Reduction of Bacterial Resistance

ALLGÖWER [*32, 33, 34*] has shown in vitro that transfusion of citrated blood clearly reduces the phagocytic capability of neutrophile leucocytes for bacteria.

OLLODART [*1102*] assumes on the basis of his investigations that the treatment of blood losses with stored homologous citrated blood does not restore the RES function already reduced by shock, and instead makes it worse. These findings perhaps explain in part the many serious infections which are seen after management of severe blood losses.

## 16. Impairment of the Flow Properties of Blood

In hemorrhagic and traumatic shock, platelet aggregation can occur early. At a later stage erythrocyte aggregation may be seen [*1737*] in the areas of stasis in the microcirculation (see p. 5 and 12).

In view of the fact that such *platelet aggregation* often occurs in preserved blood as well, M. SCHNEIDER [*1281*] doubts that whole blood is always the best means for volume replacement. However, these phenomena are important only if volume replacement is made too late. When therapy is begun in time, apparently the restoration of a normal flow is sufficient to relieve this disturbance.

Recently after whole blood transfusion abnormalities in the EEG have been shown [*243*], which could be related to an impairment of microcirculation.

Since the hematocrit of preserved blood is about 36 due to the addition of ACD, generally no great importance is attributed to the *viscosity* so long as a rise in Hct is not produced by massive over-transfusion, or if it is not desireable to reduce a high viscosity following trauma [*127, 130, 132*]. Whole blood is surely not suitable in such cases. This might explain the unfavourable results regarding oxygen extraction in treatment of traumatic shock with blood in man [*1710*] and dogs [*1785*].

The swelling of erythrocytes, as can be observed in preserved blood stored for a longer period, is regarded by ALBERT [*18*] as particularly disadvantageous from the rheological standpoint (see also [*202*]).

## 17. Survival of Transfused Erythrocytes

Dern et al. [*346*] determined the survival time of erythrocytes whic were kept for 21 days in plastic bags and which contained the customary ACD solution as an anticoagulant. 24 hours after autotransfusion in 10 healthy males the survival rate was 78.3±9.2% thus showing a striking variation. The 24 hour survival rate of red cells frozen and thawed in liqui nitrogen averages about 73.5% [*1757*].

In general a *half-life of approx. 34 days* is assumed for transfuse erythrocytes [*245, 621*] (see also point 4, p. 26).

Table 2. *Changes in citrated blood during storage at 4±1° C* (acc. Strumia [*1396*])

| Days | 0 | 7 | 14 | 21 | 28 |
|---|---|---|---|---|---|
| Hemoglobin mg-% | 0—10 | 25 | 50 | 100 | 15 |
| pH | 7,00 | 6,85 | 6,77 | 6,68 | 6,6 |
| Glucose mg-% | 350 | 300 | 245 | 210 | 19 |
| Lactic acid mg-% | 20 | 70 | 120 | 140 | 15 |
| Inorganic phosphate mg-% | 1,8 | 4,5 | 6,6 | 9,0 | 9, |
| Sodium mval/l | 150 | 148 | 145 | 142 | 14 |
| Potassium mval/l | 3—4 | 12 | 24 | 32 | 4 |
| Ammonia µg-% | 50 | 260 | 470 | 680 | – |

A similar table is found in Albert [*18*].

## II. The Volume Effect of Blood Transfusions — Therapeutic Result

The first blood volume measurements of patients in shock were made b Keith [*813*] in 1915. Since then especially the classic investigations of th English (Grant and Reeve [*553*]) and of the American shock teams c World War II (Beecher et al. [*114, 115*]; Emerson [*411*]) and of th Korean War (Artz et al. [*78*]; Howard [*730*]) have shown that the mai cause of hemorrhagic and traumatic shock [*1090*] is to be found in th reduction of the circulating BV [*423*], and that restoration of the BV b means of sufficient blood transfusion can relieve shock if the hypovolemi phase does not remain untreated for too long (survey in Reeve [*1167*]).

Worldwide experience in surgery and general medicine over many yea confirms this fact for the most part. In countless experimental models (se Part Two, Chap. B, C and D) with few exceptions, there was proof of th superiority or equivalence of blood transfusion alone as compared with man other tested infusion solutions in profound hemorrhagic shock. Most of the experiments, of course, have the disadvantage that the experimental situatic does not correspond to clinical conditions. In such experiments the anim is retransfused with its own heparinized blood — an ideal situation which unfortunately does not occur in the hospital, but which perhaps may be used in the future in elective surgery. Corresponding studies are in progress (personal information from M. LAVER, Boston, 1968).

Surprisingly few authors have measured the *volume effect of blood in humans.* COURNAND and co-workers [*306*] have performed detailed circulatory studies after blood transfusion in 10 patients. They point out that although the erythrocytes were retained in all patients, in 2 patients the plasma volume did not increase according to the amount added.

Since 1952 WOLLHEIM and SCHNEIDER have reported several times [*1552, 1554, 1556*] that the blood volume after transfusion increases only in about half of the cases. Their data show however that methodological errors are involved, for the rise of the erythrocyte volume was often not at all measurable, on the other hand there were increases which were far above the amount infused. These authors assume that the volume effect of blood is very much dependent upon the initial volume. More recent results from other authors show that infusions of erythrocyte concentrates into normovolemic individuals regularly give rise to an increase in the erythrocyte volume [*54, 369, 1274*].

AHNEFELD and co-workers [*14*] have demonstrated the volume effect of 400 ml of autologous citrated blood after removal of the same amount in healthy volunteers (see Fig. 16 a).

In the articles of a large number of authors [*578, 761, 927, 1106, 1143, 1178, 1487*] one finds data to show that in a certain percentage of cases the administration of fresh blood or fresh plasma does not lead to the desired volume effect. Others have determined in both clinical work and in carefully controlled experiments that often more blood or plasma must be transfused than was lost in order to maintain a normal plasma volume [*448, 1778*] (see also p. 38). Recent studies by KHO [*1710*] also show a decrease in $O_2$ extraction after blood transfusion in traumatic shock.

At the same time as COURNAND, WILLENEGGER [*1519, 1520*] published an extensive study of his observations on the volume effect of fresh citrated plasma. He writes that "in 6 of 27 cases the thinning effect after plasma transfusion was absent". The citrated plasma used was whole blood after removal of the erythrocytes.

Obviously here is one of the first accurate descriptions of the *"homologous blood syndrome"* which has been studied intensively since the introduction of extracorporeal circulation. The term is attributed to DOW [*361*]. After perfusion with large amounts of homologous blood, massive plasma losses and corresponding hemodynamic changes can occur in certain cases [*61, 484, 485, 486, 487, 488, 489, 529, 908, 909, 910, 1606*].

BLISS [*165, 166, 167, 168*], FREEDMAN [*465*], and HUTCHISON et al. [*759, 760*] showed that deep-frozen homologous plasma leaves the vascular system within 1 hour following infusion in normovolemic dogs and humans. Urticarial phenomena occur in half of the cases. We decided in 1964 to investigate this problem in hypovolemic humans [*609, 612, 615*]. For these experiments 1—2 weeks old citrated plasma was used, as is customary in Sweden for plasma transfusions and as it exactly corresponds to the portion of plasma in preserved blood. In the clinical management of shock it seemed important to know if, after a short time, the portion of plasma in preserved blood leaves the vascular system.

*Fig. 1* shows the experimental setup. The results of our measurements can be seen in *Figs. 2, 3, 4 and 5.* 3 persons out of 9 who received homologous plasma showed allergic reactions: one with chills, two with temporary urticarial symptoms, a serious urticaria occurring in one of the volunteers who at the same time showed a massive plasma loss. Significant changes in pulse, blood pressure and temperature could not be determined (for detailed results see GRUBER [*615*]).

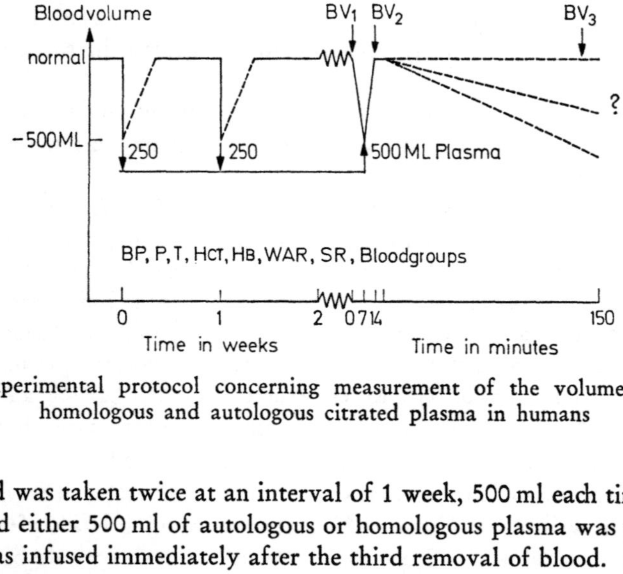


Fig. 1. Experimental protocol concerning measurement of the volume effect of homologous and autologous citrated plasma in humans

Blood was taken twice at an interval of 1 week, 500 ml each time. From this blood either 500 ml of autologous or homologous plasma was produced which was infused immediately after the third removal of blood.

28 healthy men ranging in age from 20—55 volunteered in the investigation; none had ever received blood or plasma transfusions before. During the first two removals the blood was collected in a bottle containing 120 ml of citrate solution and was kept in a refrigerator at 4° C. On the evening before the experiment the plasma was pipetted off and removed from the refrigerator 2 hours before the beginning of the experiment. With each blood removal Hct, Hb, AB0 and rhesus (incl. genotype) blood groups, as well as the Kell, Duffy and Lewis factors were determined. In addition the sedimentation rate, Wassermann, Meinicke and Kline reactions were

checked. The volunteers took no more food or fluid after midnight before the day of the experiment; during the entire experiment they were kept in bed.

Immediately before the third removal of blood, the blood volume was determined by means of the Volemetron-R$^{131}$IHSA-hematocrit technique ($BV_1$). 5 min ($BV_2$) as well as 2$^1/_2$ hours ($BV_3$) after the end of the infusion, new BV measurements were made, and an additional Hct measurement was made 1 hour following termination of the infusion.

The volunteers were checked for allergic reactions several times after the plasma infusion; blood pressure, pulse, and temperature were also measured every half hour. No tourniquet was used in the blood removal for BV and Hct determinations; the 10 min-albumin space was measured. All microhematocrit determinations were made in triplicate, the necessary blood always being taken from the "post-mix" tube of the BV determination.

A control group received an infusion of 500 ml of 6% dextran 70 in 0.9% saline solution in place of plasma.

(GRUBER [*612, 615*]).

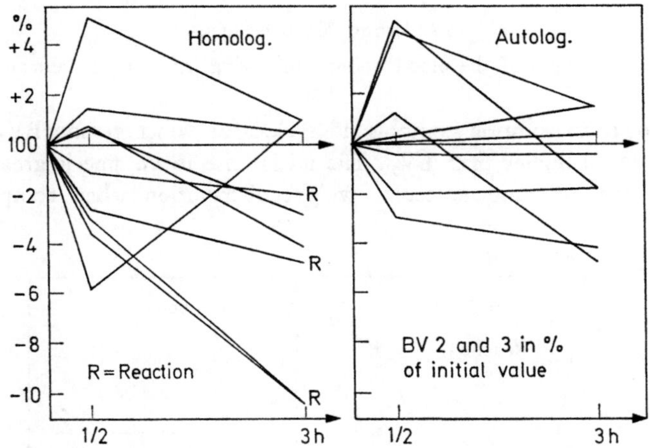


Fig. 2. Results of BV determinations after infusion of homologous or autologous plasma

The initial blood volume ($BV_1$) was assumed as 100% for each individual, and $BV_2$ and $BV_3$ were recorded as a percentage of this value. 2 people who received homologous plasma show a reduction of $BV_3$ of more than 10% of the original value. With an initial BV of 5.74 and 5.64 litres this is a loss which corresponds approximately to the 500 ml of plasma infused. Since the plasma preparation used also contained citrate solution, an average slight reduction of $BV_3$ compared to $BV_2$ is explained

(—62 ml in the autologous group, —79 ml in the homologous group with the exception of 2 persons with massive drop of $BV_3$).

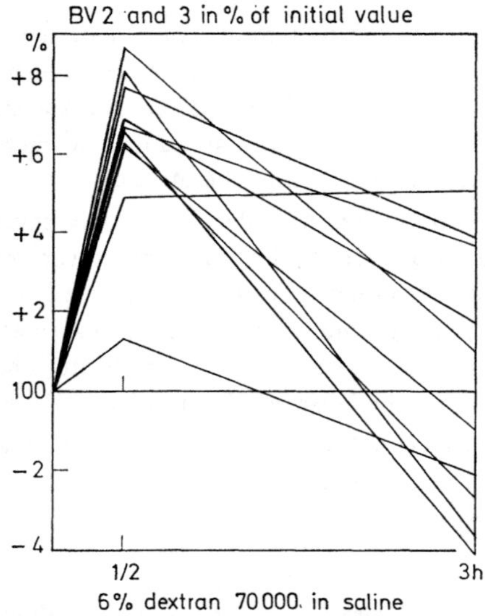


Fig. 3. Changes of the blood volume following infusion of dextran 70

The dextran solution contains no ACD, for which reason $BV_3$ in this group is 11 ml higher than $BV_1$. The initial rise in volume is greater as a result of the different molecular weight distribution when compared to plasma.

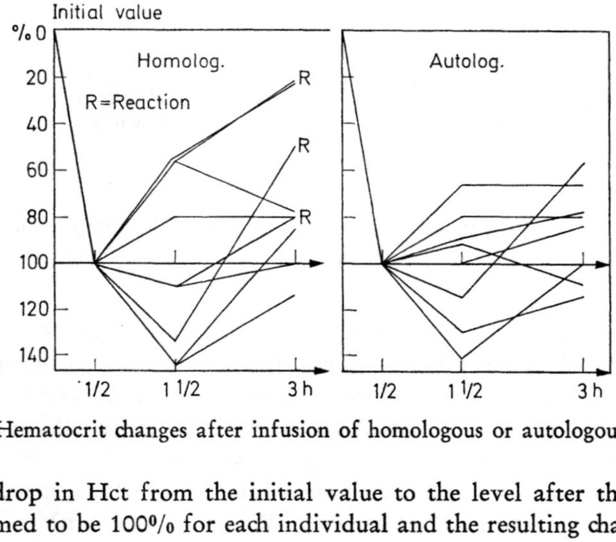


Fig. 4. Hematocrit changes after infusion of homologous or autologous plasma

The drop in Hct from the initial value to the level after the infusion was assumed to be 100% for each individual and the resulting changes were entered in percentages. This figure confirms that the BV reduction in 2 individuals who received homologous plasma is based on a plasma loss, since in these cases a simultaneous massive Hct rise is to be observed. The Hct values in the autologous and in the dextran group (Fig. 5) turned out as expected.

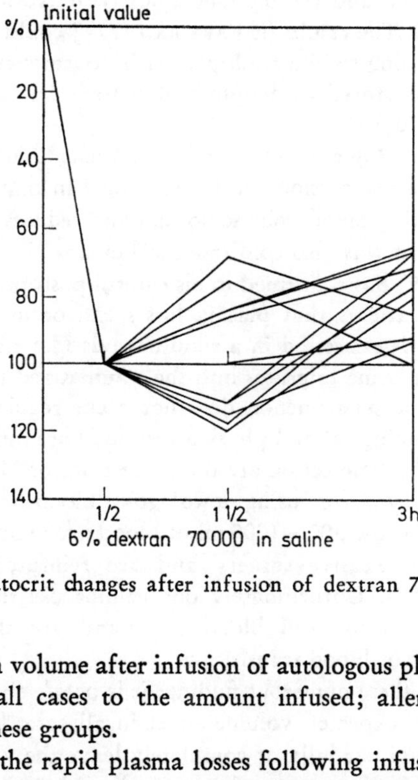


Fig. 5. Hematocrit changes after infusion of dextran 70 (in percent)

The increase in volume after infusion of autologous plasma or dextran 70 corresponded in all cases to the amount infused; allergic reactions were not observed in these groups.

The causes of the rapid plasma losses following infusion of homologous blood or fresh plasma remain unexplained. According to Hässig [*670*] it could be a matter of self-restraining gamma globulins, which because of their affinity to the cell surface may themselves cause anaphylactic reactions at that point. E. L. Smith [*1350*] assumes that this phenomenon arises through the release of a substance during the treatment of the blood *in vitro*.

Melrose [*1001*] and Sykes [*1410*] were able to show that the use of homologous blood in the heart-lung machine leads to the formation of pulmonary shunts. They are inclined to consider that the plasma cells are responsible for this. Similar phenomena of plasma loss after addition of homologous blood were recently reported several times [*343, 538, 686 a, 749, 985, 1126, 1843*], in some cases [*188, 246, 1180, 1206*] without the authors having interpreted their data in this sense.

In severe hemorrhagic shock in dogs, ELIAS et al. [*406*] always found a volume expansion which corresponded to the amount of homologous plasma infused. They assumed that the massive catecholamine output in shock prevents the functional effects of the anaphylactic reaction observed by other authors. Yet in these experiments the blood was heavily centrifuged to obtain the plasma, and the immunologically active leucocytes may thus have been removed. The results of PAREIRA [*1114*] could also be interpreted in this sense. According to him fresh plasma in tourniquet shock in the rat is ineffective, whereas stored or lyophilized plasma has a strong protective effect (see also [*1320*]).

The short-lived volume rise observed by SEAVERS [*1309*] in normovolemic animals after blood transfusion can be explained in that the organism tries to keep the circulating blood volume normal and reduces the plasma volume for that reason. This was also confirmed in humans [*711*]; see also [*1355*].

WILLIAMS [*1529*] has confirmed in his careful postoperative BV measurements on several patients that plasma losses can occur after blood transfusions, which also is expressed in a simultaneous Hct rise (see also [*744*]). It is assumed that plasma migrates into the traumatized tissue, but this does not explain why the phenomenon does not occur regularly. Possibly both mechanisms (immunological and physico-chemical) are mutually involved.

Interesting in this connection are the suggestions of MILLES [*1018, 1019*] and LANGSTON [*861*], for using *autologous* blood more frequently in surgery. For this purpose 500—1000 ml of blood are taken from the patients 1—2 weeks before elective surgery and are reinfused during or after surgery [*1595, 1853*]. Unfortunately one cannot use this procedure with emergency patients who need blood most and are thus most strongly exposed to the risks of blood transfusion.

On the basis of these numerous findings it is possible that blood does not always produce the expected volume effect in all cases because the plasma component can either partially or completely leave the vascular system in a very short time. This phenomenon is not predictable and has nothing to do with the blood groups known up to this time.

## III. Summary and Conclusions: Volume Replacement with Blood

1. The mortality as a result of blood transfusion is about 0.1—1.0‰, perhaps higher (see point 5).

2. The greatest danger of a blood transfusion lies in the risk of transmitting viral hepatitis.

3. The frequency of post-transfusion hepatitis *(non-icteric + icteric cases)* is on an average about *14.5%* on the basis of recent careful and complete follow-up studies. In single transfusions the frequency is about 10%, *and in recipients of more than 10 transfusions* it is up to 30%.

4. Until now there has been *no basis for believing that the non-icteric form is harmless.* It occurs about 4 times more frequently than icteric hepatitis.

5. The *mortality after transfusion hepatitis* is approx. 1—12%.

6. At this time the only certain methods for reducing the hepatitis risk are:

a) extremely strict selection of blood donors.

b) absolute restriction of blood transfusion to cases deemed urgent.

7. Approx. 2% of preserved blood is *bacterially* contaminated. Serious, sometimes lethal reactions occur.

8. The *half-life for transfused erythrocytes* is approx. *34 days.*

9. As a result of immunological processes which cannot be determined with routine methods, the survival time is *often much shorter.* Immunological problems are becoming more important because an increasing number of patients have already been transfused before.

10. *Hemolytic reactions* occur in less than 1‰ of all cases; they are usually due to confusions in distribution (in the AB0 or Rh systems).

11. The *citrate content* is important only in rapid infusion of large amounts in patients in shock, with liver damage, with hypothermia, and in infants. In such cases cardiac arrhythmia can occur.

12. The routine *addition of calcium* is not absolutely necessary and is sometimes even dangerous.

13. In rapid massive transfusions *the acidity* of preserved blood can have a deleterious effect. The addition of 3.75 g of sodium bicarbonate is recommended for 5 units of blood.

14. Where large amounts of blood must be transfused rapidly, it is advisable to *warm* the preserved blood from the fourth unit on, since a temperature drop is undesired. Ventricular fibrillation and cardiac arrest can otherwise occur.

15. After large transfusions the decrease in thrombocytes and in factor V and VIII can lead to *coagulation* disturbances. As a further complication fibrinolysis can occur.

16. The danger of *potassium* intoxication exists only with the infusion of large amounts of old blood in patients with restricted renal function.

17. Patients with liver diseases should receive only fresh blood because of the danger of *ammonia* intoxication.

18. Post-transfusion *hyperbilirubinemia* generally presents no clinical problem.

19. Septic patients should be given fresh blood only because of the sometimes synergistically damaging effect of *free hemoglobin and bacterial products* on the kidney.

20. There is reason to believe that homologous citrated blood impairs the function of the *RES.*

21. Sometimes the cell aggregates and denatured proteins occasionally occurring in preserved blood hamper flow in the *microcirculation,* under low-flow conditions due to increased viscosity.

22. In severe hemorrhagic shock blood transfusion is the most effective therapy. One must take into account the risks coupled with it. Erythrocytes produce a *volume effect* which corresponds to the amount transfused.

23. There are, however, good reasons to believe that the *plasma component leaves the vascular system within about 1 hour in certain cases* (the percentage is not accurately known — it is presumed to be about 20%).

24. The phenomenon known in cardiac surgery as "*homologous blood syndrome*" is probably due to immunologic causes and has nothing to do with the known blood groups.

## B. Volume Replacement with Plasma

As citrated blood can be stored for only 3 weeks, methods for preservation of blood fractions were sought at an early date. Disregarding the excess of citrate, fresh plasma, i. e. citrated blood without erythrocytes, would theoretically be an ideal plasma replacement substance. However this form of plasma likewise can not be stored much longer than whole blood and has the same important disadvantage of transmitting hepatitis. Therefore various processes for producing *stable* plasma preparations with low side-effect rate have been developed in many countries.

In the following section on the plasma preparations in use today, the results of these developments are briefly described.

### I. The Various Plasma Preparations

#### 1. Fresh Plasma

Fresh citrated plasma is usually obtained from refrigerated preserved blood by means of simply drawing off the plasma layer after the erythrocytes have settled. In many countries such plasma is used — exclusively in Sweden — because it can be produced inexpensively without complicated apparatus.

*However as the hepatitis risk with fresh plasma is about as high as that of whole blood, this form of plasma should not be used in the management of shock.*

In American terminology one distinguishes the following kinds of fresh plasma preparations:

*Blood bank plasma:* Plasma separated from the cellular elements by drawing off the supernatant layer within 3 hours of blood donation.

*Fresh plasma:* Plasma separated from the cellular elements by cold centrifugation, within 3 hours of blood donation.

*Fresh deep-frozen plasma:* Fresh plasma frozen at —20 to —30° C.

*Group-specific plasma:* Plasma titrated for anti-A and anti-B antibodies.

The hepatitis risk mentioned above is valid for all these plasma types.

We find extensive experimental and clinical evidence that *allergic reactions* can occur after fresh plasma infusion [*165, 166, 167, 168, 465*].

Hutchison [*759*] observed urticarial reactions in 6 out of 15 normovolemic volunteers after infusion of homologous deep-frozen citrated plasma. In 3 out of 9 persons receiving citrated plasma we ourselves have observed similar symptoms which occurred immediately after the infusion was concluded and lasted for about 30 minutes [*615*]. As with Hutchison, these symptoms were absent after administration of autologous plasma or dextran 70.

These reactions also occur in the transfusion of group-specific plasma, and the cause of such reactions is still unexplained. Along with AB0 and Rhesus factors (including genotype), we have also determined Duffy, Kell and Lewis factors and could find no definite explanation for these phenomena (see also discussion of homologous blood in the chapter "Blood", p. 33). In another investigation symptoms of incompatibility were observed in 3.4% of the cases [*1270*].

## 2. Pooled Plasma (Aged Plasma, Normal, Whole) Stored at 32° C

This economical form of plasma has been used rather frequently in the USA for about 6 years. It was believed that this plasma was relatively free from any hepatitis risk compared with preserved fluids stored at room temperature [*25, 711, 1246*]. The plasma is obtained from any number of donors and is stored in the *liquid state for at least 6 months* at 31—32 °C. This procedure has practically never been used in Europe, since the method of production has the disadvantages of a long storage period, a room necessary for storage, and the risk of bacterial toxin formation [*1476*].

*Allergic side-effects* were observed in 1% or fewer of the cases [*711, 1017*].

Contrary to earlier assumptions, aged plasma is also *by no means free from any hepatitis risk.* This became evident in a very thoroughly executed, comprehensive double blind study (with albumin as control) by Redeker [*1164, 1638*]. He found a *total hepatitis frequency of 10%.* In 50% of these cases it was the icteric type (maximum total serum bilirubin greater than 2.0 mg-%) although only 25% had clinically icteric hepatitis. All patients were followed up with transaminase determinations and liver biopsies. If one compares these figures with the hepatitis frequency after blood transfusion, then it seems justified to assume that a certain prophylactic effect results from the storage period. *However the incidence of hepatitis is still so high that this form of plasma likewise should not be used.*

## 3. Human Dried Plasma = HDP

It was shown at an early date that lyophilized pooled plasma leads to a rather high number of hepatitis cases (up to 25% icteric!), because one single infected bottle can contaminate the entire pool [*662, 876, 1067, 1248, 1327*].

All measures for destroying the hepatitis virus such as by irradiation with ultraviolet [*664*] and x-rays were unsuccessful [*1524*]. In addition the presence of strong antibodies in the pooled plasma proved to be a further disadvantage (see also [*1240*]). For these reasons the Swiss Red Cross went over to the production of *lyophilized plasma from individual donors* [*697*].

The *main advantages* of this plasma preparation are good storage capability which is practically independent of temperature, and the exclusion of all bacterial growth.

*Human dried plasma* SRC* = HDP = lyophilized (freeze-dried) individual donor plasma in bottles of 125 and 250 ml.

| Conc. | Na mval/l | K | Ca | Cl |
|---|---|---|---|---|
| 5.5% | 181 | 4 ** | 5 * | 100 |

* Complex bound by citrate excess.
** Personal information from the SRC, not stated in the pamphlet.

In contrast to this there is the *extremely important disadvantage* that the *hepatitis risk is no less than it is with whole blood* [*729*]. In addition there is a rate of 1% febrile and allergic reactions [*69*] (cf. also [*1282*]). A purely practical disadvantage is that dried plasma must be dissolved before use. The sodium content of 181 mval/l is unphysiologically high. The manufacturer states that cardiac insufficiency, hypertonia and esophageal varices are contraindications to use, but fails to give any reason for these restrictions.

## 4. Pasteurized Plasma Protein Solution = PPS

*Pasteurized plasma protein solution SRC = PPS II* in bottles of 250 ml.

| Conc. | Na mval/l | K | Cl |
|---|---|---|---|
| 4% | 140 | 3.8 | 110 |

Additions: 1% 0.004 molar sodium caprylate as stabilizer.
0.24 ascorbic acid.
$\eta = 1.3$.

* Swiss Red Cross.

The hepatitis virus is inactivated by means of 10-hour pasteurization at 60° C [*665, 667, 1085, 1086*].

*Contraindications:* Same as for HDP.

Febrile transfusion reactions occur in 1—2% of all cases [*670*].

The manufacturer terms PPS II a "complete replacement for human plasma", although the preparation contains no gamma globulins and only traces of $\alpha$ and $\beta$ globulins.

The corresponding preparation in the USA is called *Plasmanate* (Cutter, Berkeley): 5% solution containing 88% albumin, 7% $\alpha$-globulin, 5% $\beta$-globulin in a buffered electrolyte solution (Na 110, K 2.0, Cl 50 mval/l). *In 50, 250 and 500 ml flasks.*

The manufacturer states the following with regard to *hepatitis risk:* "Since there is no known method of proving presence or absence of hepatitis-producing viral agents, no absolute statement can be made concerning their presence or absence from blood plasma preparations."

*Another similar preparation is called Plasma Protein Lösung human,* Immuno GmbH, Heidelberg/Vienna (see also [*1429*]).

Sensitization to this plasma type could not be proved [*151*]. The frequency of transfusion reactions is stated as 1—2% [*151, 1282*].

Infusion of 500—1000 ml of Plasmanate effects no change in bleeding time, coagulation time and prothrombin time. Prothrombin consumption, number of thrombocytes and fibrinogen concentration remain unchanged [*151, 265*].

## 5. Albumin

*Albumin SRC = Albumin solution* in bottles of 70 ml, corresponding to approximately 250 ml of plasma in their oncotic activity.

| Conc. | Na | Glucose |
|---|---|---|
| 15% | 132 mval/l | 3% |

Purity: over 95%.

Additions: Sodium mandelate + sodium caprylate, 0.017 molar each as stabilizers.

Pasteurization process as in PPS [*667, 1086*], therefore free of hepatitis [*873*].

*Contraindications:* the same as for HDP and PPS II.

The manufacturer claims that the solution is low in saline content, but the sodium content approximates to that of normal serum.

*Similar preparations:*

1. *Albumin human* 5% and 20%, Immuno GmbH, Heidelberg/Vienna,
2. *Humanalbumin* "Behringwerke" 5% and 20%,

3. *Humanalbumin* "Biotest" 5% and 20%,
4. *Albumin* (normal serum albumin, human) 25%, 50 ml.

Long [*919*] has shown that the administration of 5 g albumin/kg b.w. or of another colloid (dextran 40) in dogs strongly increases the bleeding time. This is a non-specific effect due to circulatory overloading.

## II. The Volume Effect of Plasma

### 1. Fresh Plasma

Fresh plasma, in all its properties, corresponds to the plasma portion of ordinary citrated blood (compare [*1787*]). For this reason we can refer primarily to the chapter, "Volume effect of blood transfusions", and the viewpoints discussed there. In summarizing here, one should again emphasize that good reasons exist for assuming that fresh plasma leaves the vascular system in a certain unpredictable percentage of the cases within one hour after infusion. The causes of this phenomenon are not clear, and they have no connection with the blood groups known today. The plasma loss is sometimes accompanied by urticarial symptoms, but it can also occur without symptoms. Possibly the phenomenon is connected with the presence of cells or of cellular elements.

### 2. Stored Pooled Plasma

A volume effect corresponding to the amount infused in all cases was proved in a very careful study [*711*].

### 3. Dried Plasma

In 1962 we also tested HDP in the frame of our investigations for judging the volume effect of various plasma replacement substances [*37, 596, 999*]. After removing 400 ml blood (plus 50 ml for BV determinations) we infused 500 ml HDP in 8 healthy volunteers.

Compared with the initial volume, i. e. before removal of the blood, as *Fig. 6* shows, the BV increased 1.3% immediately after the infusion, and was 7.9% higher $2^1/_2$ hours after the infusion was completed. The excessive volume increase is ascribed to the fact that the volunteers were fully hydrated before the beginning of the experiment.

### 4. Pasteurized Plasma Protein Solution

It has been known since 1959 that the volume effect of the American PPS solution, Plasmanate, corresponds to the amount infused for many hours [*151*].

We have also tested the volume effect of Swiss PPS II in the same experimental series as HDP (*Fig. 6*). In all cases we were able to prove a reliable volume effect corresponding to the amount infused.

These data have since been confirmed for other PPS solutions [*14, 1276*].

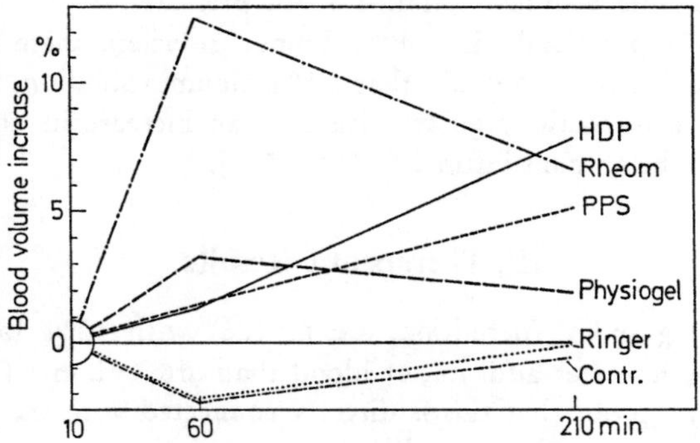


Fig. 6. Volume increase after bleeding (400 ml) and infusion of 500 ml HDP, PPS II, dextran 40, Physiogel or Ringer solution in healthy volunteers. Control group without therapy

The initial BV (before removal of 400 ml blood) for each person is designated as 0%. The average BV increase or decrease for each group ($n=7$ for HDP, 8 for PPS II, 8 for dextran 40, 9 for Physiogel and 7 for Ringer solution) after bleeding and infusion of the test solution is given as a percentage of the initial value. Since more volume was infused than removed, the BV must be 2—3% higher after infusion, if the blood replacement substance remains in the vascular system (Gruber [*601, 604*]).

## 5. Albumin

The first experiments with human albumin were made by Stead and Ebert [*1380*]. They showed that albumin can effectively raise the blood volume (see also [*1587*]). Cournand and co-workers [*306*] made additional measurements of oxygen transport.

In an excellent treatise, Heyl et al. [*705*] have measured the volume effect of a 25% albumin solution in 11 volunteers after removal of up to 1085 ml blood. An average water retention capability of 17.4 ml per g albumin was determined. This figure was confirmed shortly afterwards by Warren and his co-workers [*1485*]. Mild variations in the state of hydration did not affect these findings (dehydration 15 hours before to 20 hours after addition of the albumin compared with additional oral water and salt administration during the experiment). The remark of the authors is interesting, that there are no reasons to believe that there will be any disadvantageous consequences of an infusion of concentrated albumin solution in slightly dehydrated individuals.

K. W. SCHNEIDER and L. PIPPIG [*1271*] have determined the volume effect of 5% albumin in 24 patients. On the basis of their results, they assume that the plasma volume can be increased by means of albumin infusions in patients with low colloid-osmotic pressure.

Since PPS II practically is a 4% albumin solution, these findings are also valid here. There is no doubt that a 5% albumin solution, i. e. approximately blood iso-oncotic, regularly leads to an increase in volume which corresponds to the amount infused [*1713, 1787*].

## III. Therapeutic Results

The bleeding index (definition, see p. 126) with 40% loss of BV is significantly better after addition of blood than after plasma [*703*]. However, there is no proof that this is directly connected with the effectiveness of a preparation under shock conditions.

The results with regard to *fresh plasma* are discussed in the chapter, "Blood". Because of the volume effect which is not reliable in all situations, some therapeutic failures with fresh plasma are also understandable.

The good therapeutic effect in the treatment of hypovolemic shock conditions with pooled plasma, dried plasma, PPS II and albumin have been documented experimentally [*42, 244, 405, 578, 703, 769, 1048, 1115, 1155, 1245, 1470, 1472;* see also *1214*] and clinically [*78, 114, 260, 306, 705, 710, 1509*].

WARREN et al. [*1485*] have shown the effectivity of the albumin therapy by means of careful circulatory analysis. Blood pressure and cardiac output rise, and the arterio-venous oxygen difference decreases.

## IV. Summary and Conclusions: Volume Replacement with Plasma

1. The total hepatitis rate after transfusions of fresh plasma, stored pooled plasma and lyophilized dry plasma is almost the same as that after blood transfusions. Since this is the case, these plasma preparations should not be used for management of shock. The total hepatitis rate for stored plasma is 10%, i. e. compared with blood (14.5%) the frequency is somewhat reduced by the process of storage. Careful follow-ups which detect all cases of hepatitis do not exist for fresh plasma and dried plasma but the existing evidence leads one to assume that the hepatitis frequency after infusion of these plasma preparations corresponds to that of blood transfusions.

2. There is no basis for assuming that hepatitis is transmitted by infusions of pasteurized plasma protein solution or albumin.

Table 3. *Comparison of the clinically most important side-effects and disadvantages of transfusions with blood or plasma preparations*

| | Blood | Fresh plasma | Stored pooled plasma | HDP | PPS | Albumin |
|---|---|---|---|---|---|---|
| Mortality | + | (+) * | (+) * | (+) * | — | — |
| Hepatitis risk | +++ | +++ * | +++ | ++ | — | — |
| Transfer of other diseases | + | (+) * | — | — | — | — |
| Bacterial contamination | + | + | (+) | — | — | — |
| Allergic Reactions | + | + | (+) | (+) | (+) | (+) |
| Incompatibility | + | (+) | — | — | — | — |
| Hemolytic reactions | + | (+) | — | — | — | — |
| Volume effect | sometimes unreliable | sometimes unreliable | good | good | good | good |

* definite data lacking.

3. The volume effect after infusion of 4—5% PPS or albumin solutio into hypovolemic individuals corresponds to the amount infused.

4. The water binding capacity for every gram of albumin in the vascula system is approximately 18 ml.

5. PPS and albumin have proved useful in the management of hemor rhagic shock conditions. Their effectiveness is limited like that of a erythrocyte-free solutions, because they are unable to carry oxygen. A expressed in Part One, one can not assume that a reduced tissue perfusio with oxygen occurs as long as the Hct does not fall much below 30% afte volume replacement.

6. The disadvantages of PPS and albumin are as follows:

They are available only in limited supply since their manufactu depends upon blood donors,

They are extraordinarily expensive,

They are not a complete plasma replacement since they do not contai any globulins (PPS only traces), especially $\gamma$-globulins.

7. *Table 3* shows a comparison of the clinically important side effec and the disadvantages of transfusing blood or plasma preparations.

## C. Volume Replacement with Artificial Colloid-Containin Infusion Solutions

### I. Introduction

The world-wide demand for colloids free from the risk of hepatitis ca not even be filled in times of peace by means of PPS and albumin solution This situation will hardly change very much in the forseeable future. Becau of this, and also for military considerations, there is a real need for infusio solutions containing artificial colloids.

The use of artificial colloids in place of PPS or albumin is justified ev more when they show definite advantages over the plasma derivative HÄSSIG [*674*] feels that plasma replacement substances generally differ fro blood and plasma in that the artificial colloids must be broken down by t organism and excreted. However, the same is true for blood and plasm A really essential difference is that plasma replacement substances can manufactured in unlimited quantities at a much lower price.

### II. Terminology

A great number of names appear in the literature which refer to arti cially manufactured solutions which contain crystalloids and colloids:

| | |
|---|---|
| Replacement fluids | Blood volume expanders |
| Blood replacement substances | Blood expanders |
| Blood substitutes | Blood volume replenishers |

| | |
|---|---|
| Blood volume restorers | Plasma expanders |
| Blood fluid replacement substances | Plasma replacement substances |
| Plasma substitutes | Plasma extenders |
| Plasma volume expanders | Volume replacement substances |

Most authors use the various terms alternately as synonyms. Others [*14, 1038*] reserve the expression "expander" for substances which lead to a volume effect which exceeds the amount infused. Thus they keep to the meaning of the word "expanding" in the narrower sense. However since this expansion is a temporary phenomenon, word play in this sphere is hardly of value. Then there are authors [*200*] who object to the name "substitute", since certain artificial colloids, e. g. dextrans, sometimes have advantages over plasma.

It is unequivocal that there are still no *blood* replacement solutions as such, for nothing can replace the oxygen carrying capacity of the erythrocytes. All substances to be discussed below are thus *plasma* replacement substances [*928*]. It goes without saying that even today there is no artificial plasma. It is of course conceivable that chemistry may some day succeed in finding a formula for artificial proteins or even such substances which could reversibly bind oxygen [*1483 a*]. Until then we must be satisfied with the knowledge that the ideal plasma replacement substance which gives us all of the characteristics and functions of human plasma does not exist.

*Plasma replacement substances are solutions which are able to normalize reduced blood volume for some time after i. v. infusion,* as is the case with homologous plasma.

The expressions *colloid-containing or colloid-free infusion solutions* characterize the *properties* rather than denote the function. For this reason they are used here as major terms.

## III. The Requirements for Artificial Colloid-Containing Infusion Solutions

For about 50 years blood replacement fluids have been sought. During this time emerged the major problem of finding colloids which for the most part correspond to the physico-chemical properties of plasma proteins and which can be broken down by the organism without being antigenic.

In 1957 GRÖNWALL [*575*] required the following properties of an artificial colloidal infusion solution:

1. The colloid should have *molecular dimensions* which guarantee an adequate colloid osmotic effect.

2. The solution should have a *colloid osmotic pressure* and *viscosity* of the same order of magnitude as blood plasma.

3. The colloidal substance should be as little foreign to the body as possible and have *no toxic properties.* It should cause no injury by being

stored up in the body tissues and organs, but should be *eliminated* from the body *through metabolism and/or excretion.*

4. The colloidal substance should *remain in the blood* during a *sufficiently long* time, and at a concentration adequate to warrant a therapeutic effect.

5. The solution should not develop *pyrogenic or allergic reactions.* It should not develop sensitivity through *antigenic properties.*

6. The solution must stand *sterilization* by autoclaving and be free from virus contamination.

7. It should be possible to *produce* the solution *with constant and clearly defined properties.*

8. The solution should be stable enough to be *stored for long periods* of time under varying temperatures.

Similar programs have since been set up by various health authorities and have been taken as a standard for the manufacture of plasma replacement substances. They are included in the pharmacopeias of these countries [*461*].

Today points 1, 2 and 4 of GRÖNWALL's requirements are again in the foreground of discussion. It is partly the task of this work to find out whether and to what extent one can still keep to these criteria.

In 1963 the American *National Research Council* determined the following more specifically [*1074*] (we reproduce those points which contain changes or additions to the requirements of GRÖNWALL; italics by the author):

1. A satisfactory plasma volume expander should be capable of being administered at such a concentration that its colloidal osmotic pressure is equivalent to that of normal blood plasma. *This does not exclude the use of higher or lower concentrations.*

2. *When employed to increase plasma volume after blood loss it should be retained to the extent of 50% of the infused volume for at least 6, and preferably for 12 hours.*

7. The *viscosity* of the expander solution should be sufficiently low to permit easy intravenous administration and to cause no added work to the heart in maintaining circulation.

8. It should not interfere with *hemostasis* or blood coagulation, *at the levels employed in transfusion.*

10. *It should have no tendency to cause agglutination or lysis* of erythrocytes or damage to leucocytes. It should not interfere seriously with *blood grouping.*

11. It should be metabolized or ultimately eliminated from the body in such a way as to cause *no delayed interference with the function of any of the organs,* even after repeated administration.

12. It should not interfere with the mechanism involved in *resistance to infection.*

13. It should not interfere with *hemopoiesis* or with the formation of plasma proteins.

14. It should not interfere with *renal function or cardiac output, nor create metabolic acidosis.*

According to this the highest requirements are placed on an artificial colloid. It will be difficult to find a substance which will satisfy these points in an ideal manner. Even if this were possible, one must still consider that even the best artifical preparation replaces only the colloid osmotic properties of human plasma, but can not take over the specific protein functions. On the other hand it has not yet been shown that functions of the proteins other than colloid osmotic functions play an important part in initial management of shock.

*The following practical advantages should promote the use of an artificial colloidal solution:*

1. The product could be produced industrially in unlimited quantities.

2. The cost of such a production would be lower than the actual cost of blood and plasma derivatives.

3. Large-scale storage would be possible for long periods of time, no attention having to be paid, within reasonable limits, to changes in temperature.

4. Blood serology need not be considered. The solutions can be given to all irrespective of blood groups.

5. Such solutions could be kept available at places where emergency administration may be necessary, e. g. in ambulances.

6. The risk of virus or other kinds of infection would be eliminated.

7. The frequency of pyrogenic reactions and other undesirable secondary effects could be reduced to a minimum.

8. There would be good possibilities for effective chemical and biological control.

9. They would help to save blood.

The following substances have been tested for their usefulness as plasma replacement substances [*1227, 1430, 1522*]:

*Human Products:*

Cadaver blood
Placentary blood (Amniokrovin USSR)
Ascitic fluid
Hemoglobin solutions
Plasma and plasma fractions (see Chapter B)

*Animal Products:*

Animal sera
unmodified
despecified (heat denatured, formaldehyde treated)
from horses and cattle
Plasma hétérologue déspécifié (PHD)
Plasma bovin déspécifié (PBD)
Isoplasma (Spain)
Heteroplasma (Portugal)
Hémoplasme (France)
Anaplasma (Italy)
Adaequan (Germany)
Plasmonal (Japan)
VK 8 (USSR)
L 103 (USSR)
Amniol (USSR)
fractionated:
Cattle albumin [*705*]
Cattle globulin
Isinglass [*636, 1421*]
Casein
Gelatin (see Chapter C, p. 140 f.)

*Plant Products:*

Gum arabic [*111, 769*]
Cellulose methylether
Pectin [*660, 769*] (e. g. Graplasmoid, made by Life, Quito, Ecuador)
Glykoalgin [*1418*] (see Chapter C, p. 146)
Starch (see Chapter C, p. 140 f.)
Levan (see Chapter C, p. 146)
Dextran (see Chapter C, p. 55 f.)

*Synthetic Products:*

Polyvinyl alcohol [*636*] (see Chapter C, p. 136)
Polyvinyl pyrrolidone (=PVP) (see Chapter C, p. 135 f.)
Pluronic F-68 (A. C. Hymes, 1968) a nonionic surfactant (MW 8350) 0.4% in 0.9% NaCl for priming the heart lung machine.

*Crystalloid Solutions:*

Electrolyte solutions (see Chapter D, p. 146 f.)
e. g. with additions such as rutin
Sugar solutions

Most of the substances named had to be abandoned soon after use since they did not satisfy in one, or usually more, of the requirements (especially breakdown and antigenicity).

Today dextran, gelatin, PVP and Alginon are in use, the first much more so than the others. South America has introduced a pectin solution (Graplasmoid).

In the USA a new plasma replacement substance with a starch base is being developed (see p. 140 f.) but this is not yet available commercially. Along with these colloid-containing solutions the use of large amounts of electrolyte solutions has again recently been recommended, especially in America (see p. 146 f.).

The types of solution to be discussed will be examined more closely below.

## IV. Physico-Chemical Characterization of Artificial Colloids

First some remarks about the physico-chemical characterization which are valid for all artificial colloidal solutions.

### 1. Molecular Weight

Number average and weight average values of the molecular weight, the molecular weight distribution of a polymer [*699 a*], and the structure (e. g. branching, substitution) of a monomer are some of the basic parameters which must be known for the characterization of macromolecular substances.

For the *number average of the molecular weight* ($\overline{M}_n$ = "average number") the following equation is valid:

$$\overline{M}_n = \frac{\Sigma\, n_i\, M_i}{\Sigma\, n_i}, \quad \text{or} \quad \frac{\text{total weight of all molecules}}{\text{total number of molecules}}$$

($n_i$ = number of molecules with the molecular weight $M_i$).

The number average is obtained by measurements which determine the number of molecules present (e. g. by osmometry, cryoscopy, ebullioscopy, and chemical end-group analysis).

For the *weight average of the molecular weight* ($\overline{M}_w$ = "average weight") the following formula is valid:

$$\overline{M}_w = \frac{\Sigma\, n_i\, M_i^2}{\Sigma\, n_i\, M_i},$$

$$\frac{\text{Sum (weight of all molecules of every size} \times \text{their mol. weight)}}{\text{Total weight of all molecules}}$$

This average weight is obtained from measurements in an ultracentrifuge or by means of light scattering. According to the American specification [*47*] for clinical dextran, $\overline{M}_w$ must be determined by light scattering, which is an absolute method.

It can be concluded from the formulas for $\overline{M}_w$ or $\overline{M}_n$ that $\overline{M}_w$ is larger than $\overline{M}_n$ for all polydisperse substances. The ratio $\overline{M}_w/\overline{M}_n$ provides a measure of the polydispersity of a polymer sample [*159 a*].

One can also conclude from this that at least the number average *and* the weight average values must be known for the approximate description of the molecular weight distribution of a polymer. Thus $\overline{M}_n$ is not enlightening concerning the size of the upper and lower fractions, while $\overline{M}_w$ provides the best clues for the behavior of the preparation in vivo (see [*357*]).

The meaning of $\overline{M}_n$ and $\overline{M}_w$ is obvious in the following example [*699 a*]:

Two piles of stones, representing different polymers (A and B), are compared. Each stone represents a molecule. Both piles have a total weight of 1000 g and contain stones of various sizes:

| Pile A | | Pile B | |
|---|---|---|---|
| 500 stones at 1 g = | 500 g | 400 stones at 1 g = | 400 g |
| 2 stones at 250 g = | 500 g | 100 stones at 6 g = | 600 g |
| Total = | 1000 g | Total = | 1000 g |

$$\overline{M}_n = \frac{1000\text{ g}}{502} = 1.99 \qquad \overline{M}_n = \frac{1000\text{ g}}{500} = 2.00$$

Although the size distribution of the individual stones (molecules) in both piles (polymers) differs vastly, this important fact can not be recognized from $\overline{M}_n$.

$\overline{M}_w$ for the two piles reveals

$$A = \frac{(500 \times 1) + (500 \times 250)}{1000} = 125.5$$

$$B = \frac{(400 \times 1) + (600 \times 6)}{1000} = 4$$

A: $\frac{\overline{M}_w}{\overline{M}_n} = \frac{125.5}{1.99} = 63$, i. e. *broad* molecular weight distribution

B: $\frac{\overline{M}_w}{\overline{M}_n} = \frac{4.0}{2.0} = 2$, i. e. *narrow* molecular weight distribution

It becomes clear that $\overline{M}_w$ is much better suited than $\overline{M}_n$ for discovering differences in the molecular weight distribution of the two substances.

With regard to the molecular weight determinations of Nitschmann, the reader should refer to the chapter on gelatin, p. 108 f.

## 2. Viscosity

Terms for various concepts in viscosity [*1368*]:

| Symbol | Name | Formula |
|---|---|---|
| $\eta$ | Viscosity of the solution | |
| $\eta_0$ | Viscosity of the solvent * | |
| $\eta_{rel}$ | relative viscosity | $\eta/\eta_0$ |
| $\eta_{sp}$ | specific viscosity | $(\eta-\eta_0)/\eta_0=\eta_{rel}{}^{-1}$ |
| $\eta_{sp/c}$ | reduced specific viscosity | $\frac{(\eta-\eta_0)/\eta_0}{c}=\frac{\eta_{rel}{}^{-1}}{c}$ |
| $\lvert\eta\rvert$ | intrinsic viscosity = limiting viscosity | $\lim_{c\to 0}\frac{\eta-\eta_0}{\eta_0\cdot c}$ where $c$ designates the concentration of the dissolved substance in g/100 ml |

* $\eta_0$ distilled water = 1.0.

The viscosity is measured in poise (or centipoise). 1 centipoise is the viscosity of water at 20° C.

Other important expressions which occur in connection with viscosity measurement are [*1180 a*]:

shear stress: force/surface, measured in dyn/cm²

shear rate: (= velocity gradient), measured in $\frac{cm}{sec}\times\frac{1}{cm}=sec^{-1}$

$$\text{viscosity} = \frac{\text{shear stress}}{\text{shear rate}}.$$

# V. The Various Artificial Colloids

## 1. Dextran

### *a) Definition*

Dextrans, like starch and glycogen, are high molecular polysaccharides built up from glucose molecules. They are produced by the action of an enzyme, dextran sucrase, during the growth of various strains of the bacteria Leuconostoc in media containing sucrose (survey of literature concerning dextan chemistry and production see [*214, 575, 766, 784, 1192, 1376, 1653, 1654, 1741,* regarding British dextran see *1676*]). Raw dextran with a molecular weight of $10^7$—$10^8$ million is developed in sugar refineries by means of the bacterial effects mentioned above as a byproduct of sugar beet juice. Sucrose is converted into dextran according to the formula.

$$n \text{ Sucrose} \xrightarrow{\text{Enzyme}} (\text{Glucose} - H_2O)\, n + n \text{ Fructose}$$

$$\uparrow$$

$$\text{Dextran}$$

$$\downarrow$$

$$n\, C_{12}H_{22}O_{11} = (C_6H_{12}O_5)\, n + n\, C_6H_{12}O_6\,.$$

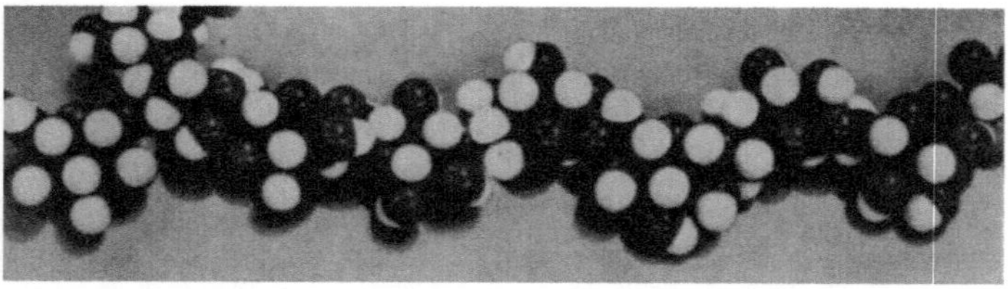

Fig. 7. Model of a dextran molecule (portion). Chain with about 9 glucose molecules and branching (Knoll AG, Ludwigshafen a. Rh.)

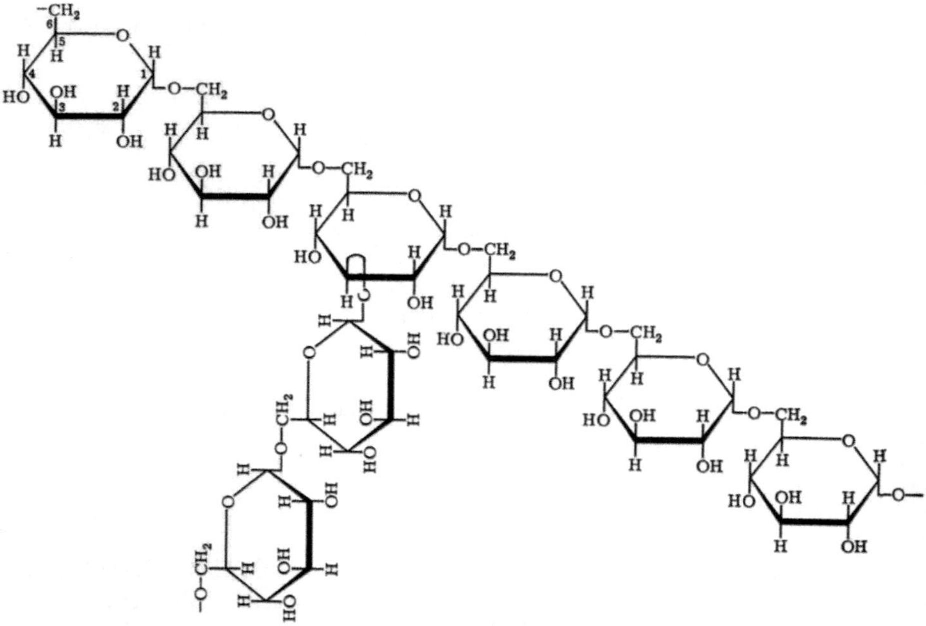

Fig. 8. Structural formula of dextran: fragment of a molecule (from GRÖNWALL [*577*], INGELMANN [*766*])

GRÖNWALL and INGELMAN [*570, 571*] were the first to recognize the possibility of using dextran as a plasma replacement substance. By means of partial hydrolytic fractionation of raw dextran and fractionation with alcohol or acetone, they obtained a dextran with an average molecular weight of about 75,000. They introduced this into clinical use in 1947 under the name Macrodex (for the history of the first dextran experiments, see [*1442*]).

In aqueous solution the threadlike dextran molecules *(Fig. 7)* form random coils. The bacteria strain Leuconostoc mesenteroides B 512 has been used in Sweden since 1953 for the manufacture of dextran. They have used this because it became evident that other strains, e. g. VII E, lead to preparations which often cause secondary reactions due to formation of different and stronger degrees of branching in the molecules [*805*].

More than 90% of the molecules contained in the commonly used dextran preparations, possess $\alpha$ 1,6 glucosidic linkages. Such dextrans thus demonstrate a relatively low degree of branching, i. e. with few side chains *(Fig. 8)*. By combining with approximately 450 units of glucose [*577*] a dextran molecule is formed in the $\overline{M}_w$ size of an albumin molecule which has about 30 branching points. Dextran molecules are neutral; in solution they are hydrated and the chains are very flexible [*762, 763*].

## *b) General Preliminary Remarks for Evaluating Literature on Dextran*

In evaluating the results of research on dextran, great difficulty arises because various dextran preparations are manufactured in several countries by differing methods and with different properties. Unfortunately very few investigators indicate the characteristics of the dextran they use, and the manufacturer's data (lot number) are mentioned only in the rarest instances. Even worse, many authors of survey articles — as WILLENEGGER stated in 1950 [*1522*] — do not place sufficient importance on these facts and use the results which were obtained with one particular preparation to draw conclusions about all other dextran preparations [*158, 829, 929, 1014, 1460, 1463, 1465*].

The situation is further complicated in that the oldest and most often used preparation, Macrodex, has likewise gone through certain changes over the years. The most important of these concerns an alteration of the Leuconostoc strain used in manufacturing dextran (since 1953) and the repeated reduction of the average molecular weight by narrowing the molecular weight distribution. As a rule the older preparations have higher average molecular weights and higher top fractions [*377*].

The physico-chemical and biological properties of a dextran solution depend upon the following factors:

average molecular weight,
molecular weight distribution *(Fig. 9)*,
concentration,
molecular structure.

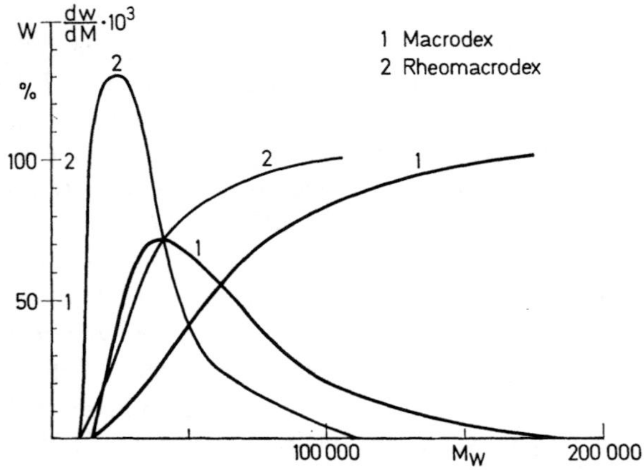


Fig. 9. Differential molecular weight distribution of Macrodex (1) and Rheomacrodex (2). On the abscissa are the molecular weights; on the ordinate are the proportion of weight (*dW*) of the polymer within a molecular weight interval (*dM*) or the cumulative weight per cent (*W*%) of the 2 preparations (Pharmacia AB, Uppsala)

The last of these is determined mainly by the type of Leuconostoc strain used. With the exception of concentration, these factors are responsible for the side-effects attributed to the older forms of dextran. Some side-effects are: allergic reactions, influence on blood coagulation and blood group determination. As a simplification, one can say that the complications increase with higher average molecular weight, broader molecular weight distribution and more pronounced degree of branching of the molecule.

It is extremely difficult to evaluate articles critically which do not contain the above information nor the name of the preparation used. Only when one knows which product was used and in which year the publication appeared can one make any retrospective judgment concerning the validity of the information given for the dextrans used clinically today.

We have tried to obtain from the manufacturers the most important information concerning molecular weight distribution, etc.; Table 4 is a compilation of data available concerning most of the dextran preparation on the world market, and for comparison, the older preparations most often quoted in the literature. In the dextran literature the following simple *terminology* has become standard: *dextran 70 signifies a dextran with an* *average $\overline{M}_w$ of about 70,000, dextran 40 a dextran with an $\overline{M}_w$ of about 40,000, etc.*

## c) The Various Dextran Preparations +

Only the most important of the preparations currently used are described here in detail; see Table 4 for other products.

*Macrodex®* * (synonyms: Clinical dextran, Swedish-American dextran). Dextran DRI ** in 0.9% NaCl or 5% glucose solution.

| Conc. | Na | Cl | mosm/l | cal/l | |
|---|---|---|---|---|---|
| | mval/l | | | | |
| 6% | 154 | 154 | 308 | almost 0 | in normal saline |
| | glucose | | | | |
| 6% | 50 g/l | | 277 | 200 | in glucose |

* Trade mark by Pharmacia, Uppsala (Sweden).
** DRI = quality code for dextran 70 by Pharmacia.

$\overline{M}_w$ = approx. 70,000 (Macrodex "Knoll": approx. 60,000)

$\overline{M}_w$ = approx. 39,000

Molecular weight distribution $\overline{M}_w$ for more than 90% of the molecules is between 25,000 and 125,000 (determined according to A.D.M.P.D., [*47*]).

$$\eta_{rel} = \text{approx. } 3.4 \text{ (at } 37^\circ \text{ C)}; \quad |\eta| = \text{approx. } 0.260 \quad \frac{\overline{M}_w}{\overline{M}_n} = 1.85.$$

As well as this, a 10% Macrodex in 5% glucose is on the market. This is indicated for reduction of edema in nephrotic syndrome. 10% Macrodex "Knoll" contains no additional crystalloids.

*Contraindications:* Pronounced bleeding tendency, e. g., in thrombopenia; severe myocardial insufficiency.

*Rheomacrodex* Pharmacia (synonyms: LMWD = low molecular weight dextran, LVD = low viscous dextran).

Dextran RMI * in 9.9% NaCl or 5% glucose solution.

| Conc. | Na | Cl | mosm/l | cal/l |
|---|---|---|---|---|
| | mval/l | | | |
| 10% | 154 | 154 | 308 | almost 0 |
| | glucose | | | |
| 10% | 50 g/l | | 277 | 200 |

* Quality code for dextran 40 by Pharmacia.

$\overline{M}_w$ = approx. 40,000; $\overline{M}_n$ = approx. 25,000.

+ Dextrans in 5% glucose, like other glucose containing solutions should not be given through the same infusion tube as blood. Globulin precipitation and spontaneous erythrocyte aggregation can occur in the tube if preserved blood is mixed with glucose solutions containing no electrolytes. This rule does not apply to dextrans in electrolyte solutions.

Molecular weight distribution: $\overline{M}_w$ for more than 90% of the molecules is between 10,000 and 80,000.

$$\eta_{rel} = \text{ca. } 5.4$$

$$|\eta| = \text{ca. } 0.190 \quad \frac{\overline{M}_w}{\overline{M}_n} = 1.6.$$

In addition there are "*Rheomacrodex Knoll*" preparations: the properties of the dextran used in these differ from those of "Rheomacrodex Pharmacia" in that the $\overline{M}_w$ of the 10% top fraction of "Knoll" is less than 70,000. "Knoll" also uses 5% and 20% Sorbit as well as NaCl as a vehicle.

There is now also a Polish LMWD called Fluidex K.Z.F. [*1794*]. The preparation used in Czechoslovakia is named Rheodextran. For these preparations detailed physico-chemical data is not available.

*Contraindications:* The same as with Macrodex, also: hypofibrinogenemia and organic renal diseases with pronounced oliguria or anuria.

*English Dextran:* (synonyms: Dextran BP, Intradex, Dextraven) Dextran in 0.9% NaCl.

| Conc. | Na mval/l | Cl | mosm/l | cal/l |
|---|---|---|---|---|
| 6% | 154 | 154 | 308 | 0 |

$\overline{M}_w = 110{,}000$ (not measured directly, but assumed on the basis of $|\eta| = 0.27$—$0.32$ determinations).

This preparation has only been available since 1966 [*213, 1193, 1676*].

There is also the old English dextran with an $\overline{M}_w$ of 150,000—200,000 (assumed on the basis of $|\eta| = 0.20$—$0.35$ determinations), with top fractions of up to 500,000 ($|\eta|$ smaller than 0.5) [*979*].

More recently there is also a dextran BP 40 (see Table 4). Here again the molecular weight is only estimated on the basis of $|\eta|$ measurements, which is unreliable [*141 a, 1677*].

## Dextran Preparations not Used for Volume Therapy

Dextrans are also used for other purposes in biology and medicine. To avoid recurring misunderstanding and confusion in the following, the names of a few preparations which are not used as infusion fluids are explained.

*Sephadex:* Dextran types which form a three-dimensional network by cross-linking of the linear dextran molecules. They are used for gel filtration, i. e. separation of substances with various molecular sizes.

*DEAE-Sephadex:* By introducing ionized groups in Sephadex, substances with ion exchange properties are obtained. These can be used, for example, for separating sensitive plasma proteins.

*Dextran Fractions:* Especially sharp fractions with various molecular weights differing from those in commercial preparations, used for biclogical and medical research purposes.

*Dextran sulfate:* A polysaccharide with sulfate groups like heparin which influences blood coagulation. Rarely in clinical use because of its side-effects, but sometimes used for purification and concentration of viruses (see [*1203, 1482*]).

### d) Compatibility of Macrodex and Rheomacrodex with Medications

Whether precipitation or incompatibility phenomena occur depends among other things on pH, buffer capacity, electrolyte content and concentration of the solutions to be mixed.

*pH levels of Macrodex and Rheomacrodex infusion solutions in bottles:*

| | |
|---|---|
| Macrodex 6% in 0.9% NaCl | approx. 5.1—5.7 |
| Macrodex 6% in 5% glucose | approx. 4.5—4.9 |
| Rheomacrodex 10% in 0.9% NaCl | approx. 4.5—5.6 |
| Rheomacrodex 10% in 5% glucose | approx. 4.4—5.6. |

The buffer capacity for Macrodex and Rheomacrodex solutions is less than 2 mval/l [cp. *1590*].

The acid pH of dextran solutions in bottles places no burden on the acid-base balance of the organism. It is due to the sterilization process, whereby the pH decreases as with other carbohydrate solutions. The blood pH is not lowered after infusion of dextran into the organism [*116*]. This places only a very slight strain on the body's own buffer capacity, in contrast to liquid gelatin ([*1341*], cf. also [*951, 1382*]).

*The following drugs can be mixed with Macrodex and Rheomacrodex:*

sympathomimetics: adrenalin, noradrenalin, metaraminol, angiotensin,

analeptics: nikethamide,

anticoagulants: heparin,

chemotherapeutics: D-Doctacillin, Ekvacillin (these only with Macrodex), chloramphenicol succinate, tetracycline chloride, oxytetracycline chloride,

vitamins: vitamin B-complex, vitamin C,

steroids: hydrocortisone,

insulins,

muscle relaxants: succinyl choline chloride,

local anesthetics: procaine hydrochloride (only with Macrodex),

proteins: human albumin.

Table 4. *Physico-chemical data on the most important dextran preparations discussed in the literature*

| *Generic name* Trade name | Concen-tration | $\overline{M}_w$ [1] | Molecular weight distribution Low mol. fr. 10% | peak fraction 10% | Electrolyte content Additions | Manufacturer |
|---|---|---|---|---|---|---|
| *Dextran 70* | | | | | | |
| Macrodex | 6% or 10% | 70,000 [2] | > 25,000 [2] | < 125,000 [2] | 0.9% NaCl or 5% Glucose | Pharmacia AB, Uppsala Poviet, Amsterdam |
| *Detran 60* | | | | | | |
| Macrodex | 6% or 10% * | 60,000 [2] | > 25,000 | < 110,000 | 0.9% NaCl or 5% Glucose | Knoll AG, Ludwigshafen |
| Macrodex | 6% | 60,000 [2] | > 25,000 | < 110,000 | Na 140 mval/l<br>K 10 mval/l<br>Ca 5 mval/l<br>Mg 3 mval/l<br>Cl 103 mval/l<br>Lactate 55 mval/l | Knoll AG, Ludwigshafen |
| *Dextran 70* [3] | | | | | | |
| Dexran Cutter | 6% | 70,000 [2] | > 25,000 [2] | < 125,000 [2] | 0.9% NaCl or 5% Glucose | Cutter, Berkeley |
| Dextran Don Baxter | 6% | 70,000 [2] | > 25,000 [2] | < 125,000 [2] | 0.9% NaCl or 5% Glucose | Don Baxter, Glendale |
| Gentran | 6% | 70,000 [2] | > 25,000 [2] | < 125,000 [2] | 0.9% NaCl or 5% Glucose | Travenol, Morton Grove |
| Dextran 70 | 6% | 70,000 | — | — | 0.9% NaCl or 5% Glucose | Vifor S.A., Geneva |

[1] As given by the manufacturer or in the literature.

[2] Before 1960, $\overline{M}_w$=75,000—80,000 with a molecular distribution between 25,000 and 200,000, before 1955, $\overline{M}_w$=80,000 (25,000 to 200,000).

[3] Often called "clinical dextran". (Formerly there was another preparation, "Plasran", Mead Johnson, Evansville.)

Table 4. (continued)

| *Generic name* Trade name | Concen-tration | $\overline{M}_w$ [1] | Molecular weight distribution Low mol. fr. 10% | peak fraction 10% | Electrolyte content Additions | Manufacturer |
|---|---|---|---|---|---|---|
| *Dextran 75* [5] | | | | | | |
| Dextran Abbott | 6% | 75,000 | > 25,000 | < 200,000 | 0.9% NaCl or 5% Glucose | Abbott, Chicago |
| Injection Dextran | 6% | 75,000 | > 25,000 | < 200,000 | 0.9% NaCl | Pharmachem Corp., USA |
| *Dextran 40* [6] | | | | | | |
| Rheomacrodex | 10% | 40,000 | > 15,000 | < 80,000<br>< 80 000<br>< 70,000 | 0.9% NaCl or 5% Glucose | Pharmacia AB, Uppsala<br>L'Equilibre Biologique, Paris<br>Knoll AG, Ludwigshafen |
| Rheomacrodex | 10% | 40,000 | > 15,000 | < 70,000<br>< 80,000 | 5% Sorbit | Knoll AG, Ludwigshafen<br>L'Equilibre Biologique, Paris |
| Rheomacrodex | 10% | 40,000 | > 15,000 | < 70,000 | 20% Sorbit | Knoll AG, Ludwigshafen |
| Dextran 40 LMD | 10% | 40,000 | > 15,000 | < 80,000 | 0.9% NaCl or 5% Glucose | Abbott, Chicago |
| *Dextran 40 Inj.* BP | | | | | | |
| Intraflodex | 10% | 40,000 [4] | $\vert\eta\vert \geqq 0.08$ | $\vert\eta\vert \leqq 0.27$ | 0.9% NaCl or 5% Glucose | Glaxo Ltd, England |
| Lomodex | 10% | 40,000 [4] | $\vert\eta\vert \geqq 0.08$ | $\vert\eta\vert \leqq 0.27$ | 0.9% NaCl or 5% Glucose | Fisons Pharm. Ldt, England |
| Dextran 40 | 10% | 40,000 | — | — | 0.9% NaCl or 5% Glucose | Vifor S. A., Genf |
| *Dextran 45* | | | | | | |
| Rheotran | 15% | 45,000 | — | — | 0.9% NaCl | Pharmachem Corp., USA |

[4] Not determined. Only the limiting numbers of the internal viscosity $|\eta|$ are given; these permit only an indirect evaluation of the molecular weight.

[5] No longer available.

[6] Often called low molecular weight dextran (LMWD) or low viscous dextran (LVD).

Table 4. (continued)

| Trade name<br>*Generic name* | Concen-<br>tration | $\overline{M}_w$ [1] | Molecular weight distribution<br>Low mol. fr.<br>10% | <br>peak fraction<br>10% | Electrolyte content<br>Additions | Manufacturer |
|---|---|---|---|---|---|---|
| *Dextran 150 Inj.* BP | | | | | | |
| Dextraven | 6% | 150,000 [4] | — | $\|\eta\| < 0.50$ | 0.9% NaCl or<br>5% Glucose | Fisons Pharm. Ltd<br>(formerly Benger, England) |
| Intradex | 6% | 150,000 [4] | — | $\|\eta\| < 0.50$ | 0.9% NaCl or<br>5% Glucose | Glaxo Ltd, England |
| *Dextran 110 Inj.* BP | | | | | | |
| Dextraven 110 | 6% | 110,000 [4] | — | $\|\eta\| < 0.40$ | 0.9% NaCl or<br>5% Glucose | Fisons Pharm. Ltd, England |
| Intradex | 6% | 110,000 [4] | — | $\|\eta\| < 0.40$ | 0.9% NaCl or<br>5% Glucose | Glaxo Ltd, England<br>Nyco, Oslo |
| Plasmodex [5] (Dextran-Glycerin-Glucosid) | 6% | 75,000 | — | — | — | Roskilde Med., Denmark |
| Neo-Subsidal | 4% | 45,000 | — | — | Sorbit 20 g/l<br>Rutin 0.3 g/l<br>Ascorbic acid 0.3 g/l<br>NaCl 4.62 g/l<br>Na acetate · 3 $H_2O$:6.12 g/l<br>KCl 0.30 g/l<br>$CaCl_2 \cdot 2\,H_2O$: 0,29 g/l<br>$MgCl_2 \cdot 6\,H_2O$:0.31 g/l | Pfrimmer, Erlangen |
| Longasteril 75<br>with electrolytes | 6% | 75,000 | — | — | $Na^+$ 140, $K^+$ 10<br>$Ca^{++}$ 5<br>$Mg^{++}$ 3<br>$Cl^-$ 103<br>Lactat —55 mval/l | Dr. Fresenius, Bad Homburg |
| or with NaCl | | | | | in 0.9% NaCl | |
| Longasteril 40<br>with NaCl | 10% | 40,000 | — | — | 0.9% NaCl | Dr. Fresenius, Bad Homburg |

Table 4. (continued)

| *Generic name* Trade name | Concen- tration | $\overline{M}_w$ [1] | Molecular weight distribution Low mol. fr. 10% | peak fraction 10% | Electrolyte content Additions | Manufacturer |
|---|---|---|---|---|---|---|
| Parenteral D | 5.5% | 85,000 | — | — | $Na^+$ 140 $Mg^{++}$ 3,6 mval/l $K^+$ 23.5 $Cl^-$ 120 $Ca^{++}$ 4 $Acetate^-$ 33 | Serag-Wiessner, Neila/Bavaria |
| Onkovertin | 3% | 75,000 | — | — | 2.5% Levulose + 2.5% Glucose $Cl^-$ 10 mval/l $K^+$ 10 mval/l | Braun, Melsungen |
| Dextran Spofa | 6% | 70,000—80,000 | — | — | 0.9% NaCl | Leceiva, Prague |
| Dextran Polfa | 6% | 60,000—80,000 | — | — | 0.9% NaCl cf. MIODUZEWSKI 1966 [*1023*] | Kutnowskie Zaklady Farmaceutycne, Polfa, Poland |
| Plasmodex | 6% | — | — | — | 0.9% NaCl | Human, Budapest [*1802*] |
| Polyglucin | 6% | 60,000—90,000 | — | — | — | USSR (ROZENBERG [*1200*]) |
| Synkol | — | — | — | — | — | USSR |
| Infukoll M 40 | — | — | — | — | — | VEB Serumwerke Bernburg, DDR |
| Osmodex Choque | 10% | — | — | — | 0.9% NaCl | Zimaia, Portugal |
| Osmodex | 6% | — | — | — | 0.9% NaCl | Zimaia, Portugal |
| Infudex | 6% | — | — | — | 0.9% NaCl | Roskilde Med., Denmark |
| Rheodextran | 10% | 40,000 | — | — | 0.9% NaCl | Leceiva, Prague [*1341*] |
| Rheopolyglucine | 10% | — | — | — | 0.9% NaCl | USSR (Shtykhno [*1813 a*] |
| Fluidex | 10% | 40,000 | — | — | | K.Z.F., Poland [*1794*] |

In [*1362*] is a list of 65 medications compatible with dextran. A carefully checked brochure about many other substances which can be mixed with Macrodex and Rheomacrodex is available from Pharmacia Great Britain, Paramount House, 75 Uxbridge Rd., London, W 5. See also [*1773*].

### *e) Colloid Osmotic Pressure and Effect, Water Retaining Capacity*

A pure solvent possesses a higher chemical potential than a solution. Every system of solution and solvent strives to obtain a balance by means of concentration equalization. If a semipermeable membrane is placed in between, permeable only to the molecules of the solvent, pressure must be applied on the solution side in order to prevent flow of the solvent through the membrane. The pressure difference between the two sides is the

*colloid osmotic (=oncotic) pressure.*

The volume of solvent (in ml/g), which is retained by the non-diffusing polymer at a certain colloid osmotic pressure, is called

*osmotic effect or water retaining capacity* [*1249*].

This water retaining capability of colloids is a hydrodynamic property. It has nothing to do with the hygroscopic properties (e. g. of magnesium sulfate) since the latter exist even when no membrane is present.

The following formula is valid for calculating the colloid osmotic pressure ($\pi$) of high molecular solutions:

$$\pi = \frac{R \cdot T}{M_2} \cdot c_2 + B c_2^2 + C c_2^2 + \cdots$$

where $R$ = gas constant (see below)
$T$ = temperature (see below)
$M_2$ = molecular weight ($\overline{M}_n$) of the polymer
$c_2$ = concentration of the polymer.

The first term of this equation corresponds to van't Hoff's law, which is only valid for ideal solutions. For polymer solutions in finite concentrations the higher deviation terms caused by intermolecular interference add considerably to colloid osmotic pressure [*1249*]. See Fig. 9 a!

The size of the higher virial coefficients B, C, etc. depends upon the polymer structure and upon the system of polymer and solvent. For dextran in water, B is about 14, for plasma about 2—3 [*850*]. The higher coefficients can usually be disregarded in lower concentrations. It is generally accepted that linear molecules show a much stronger concentration dependency than spherical molecules do.

*For calculating the colloid osmotic pressure* $\pi$ (in mm $H_2O$) *of a dextran solution, the following equation is valid:*

$$\pi = \frac{R \cdot T}{\overline{M}_n} \cdot c + 14\, c^2 + \cdots$$

where $R$ = gas constant = 8480 (if one is using the dimensions $c$ in g/100 ml and $\pi$ in mm $H_2O$, $R$ by definition = 0.08205 liter-atm./degrees, mol.)

$T$ = absolute temperature: 310° K

$c$ = dextran concentration in g/100 ml.

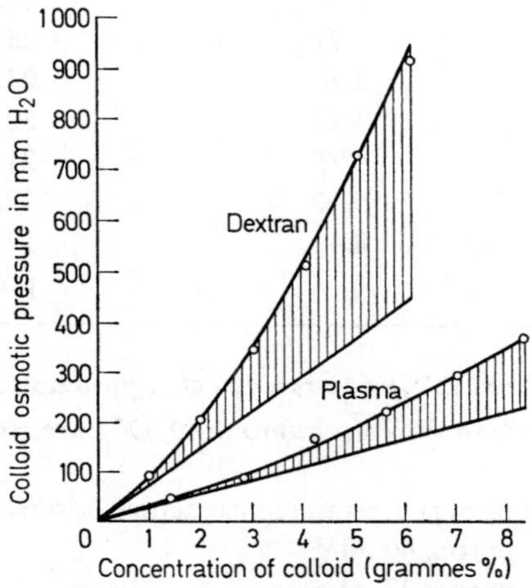


Fig. 9 a. The relationship between the colloid concentration and colloid osmotic pressure for a dextran with an average molecular weight of 70,000 is graphically depicted. The corresponding values for normal plasma are given as a comparison. The straight lines represent the osmotic pressure, calculated from VAN'T HOFF's law, while the shaded areas signify the osmotic pressure contribution from molecular interaction (after HINT [714]).

In the second half of the equation $c$ is squared and is next to a relatively large constant $B$ which is practically independent of the molecular weight. Because of this it is obvious that the colloid osmotic pressure of a dextran solution is much more dependent upon the concentration [*1219*] than on $\overline{M}_n$, as is often assumed.

One can calculate with the following simpler formulas:

for dextran 40: $\pi = 120 \cdot c + 14\, c^2$ (at 37° C)

for dextran 70: $\pi = 70 \cdot c + 14\, c^2$ (at 37° C).

The following compilation by HINT [*713*] (p. 68) provides the values of blood iso-oncotic concentrations and the water retaining capacities calculated from them for various dextran fractions.

The higher the molecular weight is, the larger the concentration has to be, so that the colloid osmotic pressure corresponds to that of blood. The ratio is by no means linear; with 50 times increase of $\overline{M}_n$, the concentration must only be somewhat more than doubled to achieve the same colloid osmotic pressure.

| Dextran fraction $\overline{M}_n$ | Blood iso-oncotic conc. (376 mm $H_2O$) | Water binding capacity in ml/g dextran |
|---|---|---|
| 20 000 | 2.37 | 42.2 |
| 40 000 | 3.42 | 29.2 |
| 60 000 | 3.91 | 25.6 |
| 80 000 | 4.20 | 23.8 |
| 100 000 | 4.38 | 22.8 |
| 200 000 | 4.75 | 21.0 |
| 1 000 000 | 5.10 | 19.6 |
| Plasma proteins | 8.4 | 12 ml/g protein |

*A solution of about 2.5% dextran 40 ($\overline{M}_n$ approx. 25,000) and a solution of about 3.5% dextran 70 ($\overline{M}_n$ approx. 40,000) are approximately blood iso-oncotic.*

The corresponding water retaining capacities *in vitro* are:
for dextran 40 approx. 40 ml/g
for dextran 70 approx. 27 ml/g.

If, however, one considers the excretion of the low molecular weight portion in vivo, *then one can count on a water retaining capacity of approx. 20—25 ml $H_2O$ per g dextran in circulation for the clinically used dextrans (Fig. 9 b).*

This figure is not influenced by the amount of water added; thus it depends only on the amount of dextran in the blood. In vivo it is also practically independent of $\overline{M}_w$ (for the molecular weights which are encountered clinically), so long as the molecules are large enough to remain in circulation at all. On the other hand, it *is* influenced by the existing colloid osmotic pressure [*713*].

A 6% solution of *dextran 70* (Macrodex) accordingly exerts a higher colloid osmotic pressure than blood does. This makes up for the quickly eliminated low molecular fractions.

The colloid osmotic pressure of 10% *dextran 40* corresponds in vitro to that of an approx. 17% albumin solution [*137*]. The smaller dextran molecules are quickly excreted in vivo. Thus the colloid osmotic effect produced by Rheomacrodex in vivo drops more quickly than that of a corresponding albumin solution. The permeability of the membranes in the glomeruli is most important for the effect in vivo. For dextran the renal threshold is about MW = 50 000 (see metabolism). Solutions of molecules whose size is below this can thus only have a temporary volume effect. In other tissues as well, the colloid osmotic effect depends upon the permeability of the respective capillary membranes. This can be subject to considerable local fluctuations which must be taken into consideration with in vitro organ perfusions.

As a result of the exchange effects between plasma and dextran a mixture of plasma and dextran exerts a colloid osmotic pressure which is greater than the sum of the effects of the colloid components [*1219*].

According to HINT [*715*] *colloid osmotic effect* is understood as the fluid transport through capillary membranes, which occurs due to changes

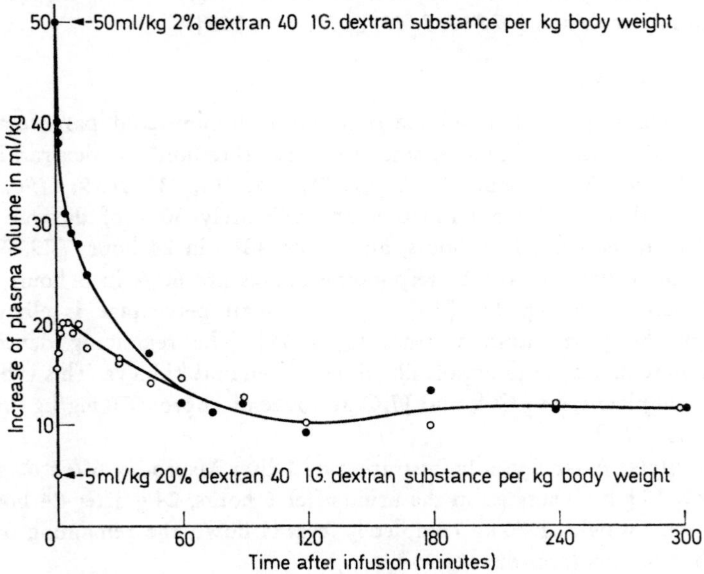


Fig. 9 b. The in vivo water-binding capacity of dextran is shown to be relatively independent of the concentration of infused dextran solution. Two groups of rabbits received identical amounts of dextran ($\overline{M}_w$ 40,000) in a dosage of 1 g of dextran substance per kg body weight. One group received 50 ml/kg of a 2% solution and another 5 ml/kg of a 20% solution. The 2% solution was colloid hypotonic (colloid oncotic pressure 245 mm $H_2O$), while the 20% solution was strongly colloid hypertonic (7,500 mm $H_2O$). The expected initial plasma volume increase for the group of rabbits receiving the dilute solution was 50 ml/kg body weight (i. e. the injected volume). However, because 1 g of dextran 40 is capable of retaining only 20—25 ml of water in circulation, the excess of water was rapidly filtered out into the tissues or excreted and the plasma volume decreased until the maximum water-retaining capacity of the circulating dextran was reached. For the other group the injected volume was only 5 ml/kg body weight. It can be seen, however, that, only a few minutes after the injection was finished, the plasma expansion amounted to about 20 ml/kg and therefore water must have been rapidly absorbed from the tissues into the circulation. This experiment shows that the colloid osmotic effects of colloid hypertonic and colloid hypotonic solutions are quite different. A hypertonic solution absorbs water from the extravascular space, while a hypotonic solution has the opposite effect (HINT in [*447 b*]).

of the intravascular colloid osmotic pressure. Thus it depends upon th colloid osmotic *pressure*, which a dextran solution can exert *in vivo*. Sinc every gram of dextran in the circulation retains approx. 20—25 ml water one can roughly calculate the pressure in a relatively simple manner at an time. If a highly concentrated dextran solution, with a colloid osmoti pressure greater than that of blood, is given intravenously then the capil laries take up water from the extravascular space. The opposite effect occur with administration of diluted solutions: the excess water leaves the circu latory system quickly, but approx. 20—25 ml water per g dextran wil remain in circulation [*378, 638, 639, 808, 809, 838*].

### *f) Metabolism*

The major part of a volume of dextran administered parenterally i excreted through the kidneys, since the renal threshold for dextran is at molecular weight of about 50,000 [*67, 75, 175, 578, 732, 1099, 1190, 1220 1479*]. With normal renal function approximately 30% of dextran 70 i excreted in the urine in 6 hours, and about 40% in 24 hours [*73, 74, 75 638*]. For dextran 40 the corresponding figures are 60% in 6 hours, 70% in 24 hours (see Fig. 11; [*73*]). A very small percentage is eliminate through the gastrointestinal tract [*1, 1266*]. The remaining dextran i taken up temporarily in organs like liver, spleen and kidneys. This is broke down completely into $CO_2$ and $H_2O$ at a rate of approx. 70 mg/kg b.w. pe 24 hours [*383*].

*Example:* After i. v. administration of 1 liter Macrodex 6% = *60 g dex tran 70*, 18 g are excreted in the urine after 6 hours, 24 g after 24 hours.

A man weighing 70 kg completely breaks down the remaining 36 g i less than 8 days (approx. 5 g/24 hours).

From 1 liter Rheomacrodex = *100 g dextran 40*, 60 g are excreted in th urine after 6 hours, 70 g after 24 hours.

A man weighing 70 kg breaks down the remaining 30 g in approximatel 6 days.

If fasting *dogs* receive $^{14}C$ marked dextran, the glucose-nitroge quotient in the urine rises, i. e. dextran is broken down to glucose [*554*] It has also been shown that $^{14}CO_2$ appears in the breath [*262, 1422*], an marked atoms are combined into other substances such as amino acids. Mor than 90% of radioactively marked dextran is excreted in approx. 10 days 64% of it in urine, 26% as $^{14}CO_2$. Practically all of the radioactive materia is eliminated within 2 weeks, 30% of it in the form of $^{14}CO_2$ [*383, 554 575, 1225, 1422, 1423, 1424, 1766*].

The presence of a *dextranase* (dextran-1-6-glucosidase) was first dem onstrated in animals in spleen, liver, lungs, kidneys, brain and muscle tissue [*1221, 1222, 1223, 1224*]. Later, similar evidence was found in human [*52*].

The *capillary permeability for dextran* has been tested variously [*72, 76, 341 a, 471, 472, 588, 665 a, 1132, 1194, 1300*]. It was shown that dextran molecules with an $\overline{M}_w$ of approx. 50,000 behaved like albumin; this was judged from studies of *heart lymph* [*65*]. ARTURSON [*72, 76, 1594*] has shown a slightly raised capillary permeability for dextran, depending upon the extent of trauma, after burns, x-ray radiation and freezing damage.

Dextran does not pass the *placenta* ([*432 a, 826, 1194 a*]; see also [*388*]). On the other hand dextran molecules with an MW of up to 15,300 can pass slowly through rabbit and human *skin* [*1455*].

After rapid infusion of dextran 40 no dextran could be found in *cerebrospinal fluid* [*337*]. Regarding *renal peritubular permeability* see [*1725*].

## *g) Plasma Concentration, Excretion in Urine, Renal Function*

*Fig. 10* shows the plasma concentration of normovolemic individuals 1 hour after infusion of 500 ml 6% Macrodex or 10% Rheomacrodex in 0.9% NaCl. For normal adults plasma concentrations of 0.5—1.5 g/100 ml plasma are reached after infusion of dextran 40 and dextran 70 with the usual clinical dosages of approx. 1/2 to 1 1/2 liters in several hours [*67, 73, 74, 179, 378, 638, 732, 1099, 1220, 1432*]. With regard to other dextrans see [*1516, 1802*].

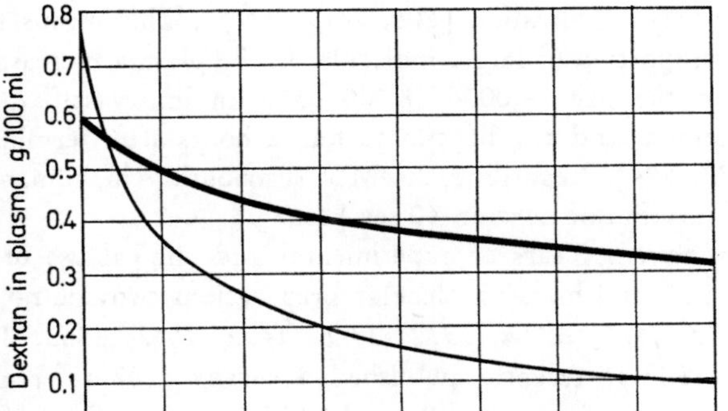


Fig. 10. Plasma dextran concentration after infusion of 500 ml 10% dextran 40 (Rheomacrodex in 0.9% NaCl solution = thin curve) or 500 ml 6% dextran 75 (Macrodex in 0.9% NaCl solution = thick curve) in healthy volunteers (infusion duration = 1 hr) (according to ARTURSON [*73*])

Plasma concentration and excretion through the kidneys depend upon several factors: The molecular weight distribution of the dextran preparation used, the amount infused, the rate of infusion, and the condition of the patient (hypo- or hypervolemia, colloid osmotic pressure of the plasma). After infusion of dextran 40, the plasma dextran concentration declines more rapidly than after infusion of the same amount o dextran 70 *(Fig. 11).*

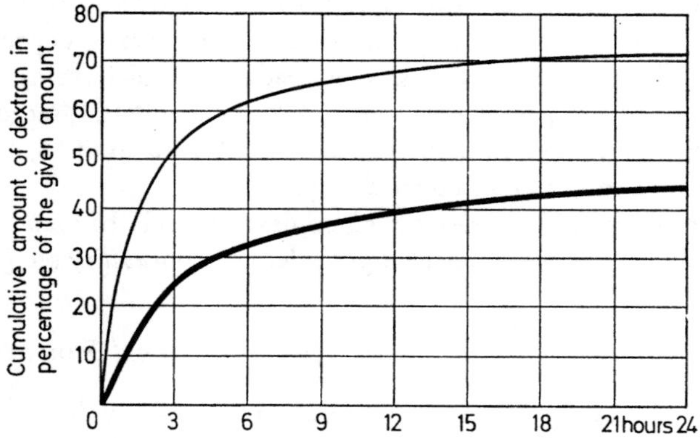


Fig. 11. Excretion of dextran in the urine in percent of the amount infused Experimental procedure, see Fig. 10 (Rheomacrodex = thin curve, Macrodex = thic curve) (according to ARTURSON [*73*])

Smaller molecules leak through the capillary membranes and return i part to the vascular system by way of the lymphatic system; in this wa molecules with an MW below 50,000 are quickly excreted in the urin through glomerular filtration [*208, 1479, 1755*]. This means that as tim passes, the proportion of larger molecules in the plasma increases relatively Molecules of the size 14,000—18,000 have an intravascular half-like o about 15 minutes and are difficult to find 2 hours after termination of th infusion [*77, 524*]. Regarding the MW distribution in human serum an urine after infusion of dextran 40 see [*1687*].

*Renal function:* Years of experimental and clinical use of dextran 4 and dextran 70 and higher molecular preparations provide no evidence o renal toxicity [*575, 692 a, 1312, 1376, 1433, 1657, 1663, 1732, 1763*] MATHESON [*967 a*] recently published a survey (182 references) dealin with the influence of dextran 40 on the kidneys; the effects of dextran 7 and older preparations are also considered here. GOLDENBERG et al. [*534* found no changes in urea clearance, non-protein nitrogen and alkalin phosphatase in the rabbit and dog after infusion of very large amounts o dextran. Animal experiments to study the toxicity of dextran 40 likewis revealed no evidence that this preparation in clinical dosage could lead t any kind of renal damage (see [*966, 1561 a*]).

Creatinin and inulin clearance do not change in humans with infusio of 500—1500 ml dextran 70; the PAH clearance increases ([*143, 299, 44 830, 1478*]; cf. also [*1066*]). Burn patients who often receive large amount of dextran show no signs of toxic renal damage [*422, 575, 682, 1376*].

Two authors have provided data concerning infusion of excessive amounts of *dextran 40* in humans. One individual was given 30 (!) liters of 10% dextran 40 in 10 days in an investigation of its influence upon the sedimentation rate [*1324*]. Although it is not clear in the article, these infusions were in fact given to one and the same patient (personal information). The patient felt poorly as a result of the overtransfusion, but otherwise no adverse effects were noted! — An older woman was given 44 (!) liters 10% dextran 40 in 44 days [*1072*]; here as well, apparently no side-effects occurred which could point to toxicity. On the basis of the data mentioned above, this patient excreted approx. 3 kg dextran through kidneys during that period!

As regards the clearance level of low molecular dextran, it can be easily calculated that temporary dextran concentrations of 30—50% can occur in the urine with rapid infusion of large amounts of dextran 40 [*1829, 1830*]. Arturson [*73*] shows how the kidney can compensate for the rise in urine viscosity by dilatation of the tubules. Mailloux [*1743*] makes the hypothesis that a reduction in filtration pressure combined with a marked increase in urinary viscosity generated by dextran 40 may lead to tubular stasis and subsequent blockade.

Clinical experience shows that such highly viscous urine is not observed with normal renal function, since the first highly concentrated urine is diluted immediately by the urine which follows. Sometimes, however, severely dehydrated individuals without need of a colloid are at the same time under the strong influence of antidiuretic hormone (ADH). This is for example the case postoperatively. Should these patients be given large amounts of dextran 40, then in certain cases a highly viscous urine with reduction in urine volume can be observed [*138*]. This phenomenon was also investigated carefully in experiments with dehydrated cats [*1384*]. The findings showed that in animals and in humans [*138*] the phenomenon is fully reversible by means of adequate hydration and introduction of an osmotic diuresis, e. g. by giving small amounts of mannitol.

In his original report Gelin [*506, 508*] described a slightly increased diuresis in the postoperative phase after infusion of dextran 40. We, however, found no significant difference in diuresis in healthy volunteers after removal of 450 ml blood and rapid infusion of 500 ml Rheomacrodex, compared with plasma, gelatin, electrolyte solutions or no therapy at all [*600*]. Matheson et al. [*964*] observed a slight but definite increase in diuresis after larger abdominal operations and infusion of 1000 ml 10% dextran 40 in normal saline or glucose solution. This was thought due to an increase in free water clearance as a result of reduced ADH secretion, which in turn was due to the increase in plasma volume (cf. [*962, 963*]).

Extensive toxicological investigations [*1091*] and a large number of clinical and experimental articles report on the use of dextran 40 in various circumstances [*1699*]. These investigations reveal no disturbance of the renal function; often the good urinary excretion was particularly emphasized [*3, 4, 93, 94, 125, 192, 289 a, 337, 505, 508, 537, 750, 945, 1152, 1570, 1572, 1573, 1686*].

Some authors [*1366*] see pronounced protective properties in dextran 40 for kidney function and recommend using it for the prophylaxis and treatment of ischemic damage and management of transfusion complications [*84, 85, 86, 87*]. Atik [*88*] used Rheomacrodex in 150 patients, all of whom were candidates for the development of acute renal failure, and some of whom were already anuric. He observed no complications.

Other investigators sometimes using smaller doses [*1338*] observed no protective renal effect of dextran 40 [*701, 807, 1826*]. Trede [*1454*] observed a damaging influence with massive overdosage (more than 6 g/kg bw) in dogs. An improvement of renal perfusion and a rise in oxygen supply [*712*] seem now confirmed, after infusion of dextran 40 and dextran 75 [*137, 402, 790, 794, 830, 958, 967, 1257, 1340, 1839, 1840*]. It is assumed that there is a redistribution of flow [*1065*].

Originally it was assumed that administration of dextran 40 led to an osmotic diuresis. However several careful investigations have revealed that the slight osmotic diuresis depends on the crystalloid content of the dextran solutions [*138, 964, 1151*].

More recently, several reports have been published [*1670, 1677 a, 1743, 1829, 1830*] incriminating dextran 40 as the causal factor in renal insufficiency, anuria, and in one case [*1047*] death of a patient. In view of the importance of this problem, these articles are to be discussed in greater detail below.

In the 6 cases mentioned by Gracy [*547*], Wilkinson [*1518*] and Daniel [*332*] several factors are present, which alone could explain the occurrence of anuria. These causes are narcosis, surgical trauma plus hypotensive phase, preexisting renal diseases, use of vasopressors and dehydration. Certainly these articles do not prove dextran 40 to be the factor injurious to renal function.

The burn cases reported by Almgård [*43*] and by Birke and Liljedahl [*161*] belong in the same category. These cases were not initially treated by the authors. In a reply to the latter article it was pointed out that serious mistakes were made in the water and electrolyte therapy used in the treatment of these patients [*39*]. The authors were not able to refute these arguments in their answer [*161 a*]. In a comprehensive questionnaire given to 107 surgical clinics in Sweden, Gelin [*518*] received word of 12 cases in which oliguria occurred. In not one of these cases could the complication definitely be traced to the administration of dextran 40. A careful study of the case histories revealed that usually serious untreated dehydration was present.

Morgan, Little and Evans [*1047*] report on 3 patients who became oliguric in the course of a serious disease while receiving dextran 40 (cf. also [*89 a*]). At the same time Evans and Wong [*425*] published the histological findings of the same cases. A comparison of the data given in the two articles reveals various contradictions. Case 1 (in both articles) suffered a hypotensive phase during the amputation according to Evans though Morgan in his summary states that no blood pressure drop occurred.

In the sections on histological findings there are again conflicting reports regarding the presence of renal pathology, for although Morgan reports "No glomerular, arterial or interstitial pathology was found" there were in fact hypertensive changes in the arterioles and a congenital malformation with cystic changes in the region of the collecting tubules. This patient's pre-operative blood pressure was 270/110. Furthermore, this patient received 14 liters of Rheomacrodex *in 5%/o glucose* in 12 days preceding his operation, a considerable overdose for which no explanation was given.

Because of the absence of electrolyte data it is difficult to form an accurate picture of the terminal course. However since dextran was administered in glucose, one can easily suspect that severe hyponatriemia existed. It is certainly possible that in these as in other cases [*539, 1082, 1670, 1683*] patients were overdosed and the principles of water and electrolyte therapy ignored. Matheson [*966*] has published a commentary concerning the histological changes reported; this commentary agrees with the statements in the next chapter (cf. also [*1047 a*]).

Hulme and Lawson [*751*] comment on the report by Matheson [*966*]. They mention 12 further cases from the literature [*859, 944*] and 3 of their own patients who developed renal insufficiency after infusion of dextran 40. Here again proof is lacking that this occurred as a direct result of the administration of dextran. Common to all of these cases is that overdosage of Rheomacrodex was given to patients who already had renal insufficiency due to other causes and whose water and electrolyte balance was not normal [*408, 1670, 1683*]. In most of the articles, data concerning serum-electrolyte values is lacking [*1670*]; where such data was given, extremely severe degrees of hyponatriemia were present [*539, 1082*].

On the basis of the existing results it seems that one may assume that dextran 40 has no renal-toxic properties in itself [*967 a, 1677 a*]. It can also be assumed that its improper use (in 5%/o glucose without addition of sodium!) can aggravate early renal insufficiency [*965*], particularly with extremely high dosage [*1561 a, 1670, 1683*] and preexisting dehydration [*1561* a].

*For this reason one must remember the following points which are to be considered in therapy with dextran 40:*

1. 10% dextran 40 is a highly hyperoncotic solution and should be given to dehydrated patients only with simultaneous correction of the water and electrolyte deficit. This point was already stressed in 1963 [*591*].

2. Only cases of prerenal kidney insufficiency are an indication for dextran 40. Organic renal insufficiency with anuria is a contraindication.

3. In patients with chronic kidney disease 6% dextran 70 should be used in emergencies, since it is excreted more slowly.

4. With severe hypovolemia (loss of more than 20% of the BV) the volume should not be refilled exclusively with dextran 40 [*1564*]. The initial volume therapy *can* be started with dextran 40 but must be augmented by the same amount of balanced electrolyte solution as well as blood when necessary [*518*].

### *h) Histological Investigations*

6 weeks after administration of dextran 70 in very high doses not common in clinical use, the substance could no longer be demonstrated in histological preparations [*897*]. According to another article no more dextran was to be found after the same period in the liver nor after 12 weeks in the kidney (animal expt.) [*477*].

Other workers showed with the help of an acid fuchsin dye, that dextran could be found temporarily in the kidneys and spleen, but not in the liver, lungs and heart. These authors determined also that temporary deposition in individual organs is not accompanied by pathological changes [*473, 1053*]. Comparative investigations showed formation of foam cells in the spleen, lymph nodes, bone marrow, medulla of the suprarenal gland, liver, lungs and thymus after infusion of 3½% PVP but not after 6% dextran [*232, 765, 1079*].

Other authors as well conclude from their experiments that dextran is depolymerized in the body [*1452*]. In 31 patients who had received dextran infusions from 1 hour to 4 months before death, deposits of dextran could not be found in liver, spleen, kidneys, lungs, nor in the lymph nodes ([*1515*]; see also [*53, 657*]).

WILLENEGGER [*1522*] was unable to find any definite cell damage in parenchymatous organs after infusion of dextran. TURNER [*1462*] observed a moderate hyperplasia of the reticuloendothelial system (RES) and in 2 out of 5 dogs small liver necroses after administration of a very high molecular preparation.

In 1947 GOLDENBERG et al. [*534*] first reported on the occurrence of a so-called osmotic nephrosis (tubular vacuolization) after dextran infusion. With clinical doses such symptoms were not to be found [*232, 473, 701*]. These renal findings were confirmed in a few cases (after infusion of 500—3000 ml) in the autopsy of soldiers who fell during the Korean War [*1467*]. The amounts of dextran found in the RES were not significant, and in no case could it be linked with dextran toxicity.

Gloor [*530*] has exposed the problem of osmotic nephrosis very well in an excellent article. He was able to show that the histological changes depend upon the dose but not upon the concentration, i. e. that the term, osmotic nephrosis, appears not to be justified (Kief proposes the term "reabsorptive vacuolisation" [*1712*]). The presence of shock had no influence on the symptoms. On the basis of investigations made by the same school of investigators it is probable that the vacuole formation is related to the specificity of cellular enzymes. For that reason it is more pronounced after infusion of substances like inulin [*712*], mannitol and PVP, for which no enzymes are present [*1677 a*]. Apparently these vacuoles represent a temporary functional condition and are an expression of the transport of reabsorbed material [*331, 969, 1657*], which does not lead to impairment of renal function [*1658, 1663, 1712*].

On the basis of kidney biopsies, Lampe [*847*] recently showed that these changes after administration of mannitol are also temporary in humans. (Further data concerning histological changes after dextran infusion can be found in [*379, 894, 895, 896, 898, 899, 900, 901, 902, 903, 1657, 1663, 1670, 1821*].)

### *i) Immunological Investigations*

Opinions differ concerning the question whether dextran is an antigen [*800, 801, 802, 803*] or whether it first must be combined with a protein or another prosthetic group before it can act as an antigen [*531, 1579*]. Various authors [*424, 1026, 1486*] assume that dextran acts like a haptene and for this reason it comes under suspicion as a cause for allergic reactions. Many articles discuss the role of dextran as a haptene in cross reactions with various bacterial antisera [*687, 688, 689, 690, 691, 692, 775, 776, 801, 971, 1075, 1076, 1077, 1078, 1397, 1578, 1807*]. Apparently species-specific differences play a part in this respect. In guinea pigs, for example, no antibody formation could be produced with dextran [*974*].

Reports of an antigenic effect of dextran in humans deal with studies using older preparations of higher average molecular weight and different molecular weight distribution [*691, 773, 801, 805, 806, 971*] and/or ones with molecules with a greater degree of branching [*30, 774, 801, 802, 804, 805, 806, 971*] compared with the solutions available today (cp. [*1651*]).

*Grönwall [576] and Kabat and Bezer [806] have shown that infusions of dextran 40 and 75 in humans are not able to cause any significant antibody formation.*

### *k) Allergic Reactions*

When Grönwall and Ingelman [*570, 571, 572, 764*] introduced dextran as a plasma expander, they assumed that it was serologically indifferent and that only few patients would react to it with side-effects such as urticaria and fever [*1438*]. Thus at the beginning it could not be decided whether the rarely observed side-effects were due to contamination of the dextran or to antigenic properties [*184*].

Later, however, reports appeared concerning relatively frequent allergic reactions after dextran infusion [*67, 382, 695, 838, 926, 978, 1147, 1419, 1462, 1516*]. From an analysis of these articles it can be seen that the preparations used generally came from a different bacterial strain than the one used today for the manufacture of dextran [*805*]. In addition great differences existed with regard to the average MW, the MW distribution and the molecular structure [*1441, 1517, 1743 a*].

Various explanations are presented for the origin of the possibly specific and rarely occurring dextran antibodies: dextran occurs, as has been shown, in sugar and other foods [*687, 1076*]. In addition the human gastrointestinal tract contains dextran-producing micro-organisms. TERRY and YUILE [*1422, 1423*] assume that dextran is naturally present in various tissues. 24 of 28 streptococcus strains isolated from the blood of patients with subacute endocarditis showed serologically active dextran production [*688*]. However rare reactions have been reported after administration of the modern products [*1754*]. Perhaps they appear more often in normovolemic patients who are not anesthetized [*1261 a, 1824*].

Although it is clear that until 1953 much higher molecular preparations were used, allergic reactions even at that time were extremely rare, after dextran infusions [*784*]. In one series no complications of any kind were observed [*1501*]. From other statistics one can see that during 4 years of using dextran 75 in 2000 patients, 4 cases of chills were observed in the first two years; later, however, no further side-effects were confirmed [*920*]. In 256 burn cases in which dextran 75 was infused in amounts up to 6 liters in 48 hours, no allergic reactions occurred ([*682*]; see also [*79*]). *The absence of important allergic reactions has since been confirmed many times for the preparations now on the market* ([*14, 589, 601, 612, 759, 1272*]; see also [*53, 1181, 1370*]).

### *l) Influence on Sedimentation Rate, Aggregating and Disaggregating Properties*

The normal sedimentation rate is the expression of a constantly present tendency of the erythrocytes to aggregate (rouleaux formation). The SR increases when relatively more high molecular weight proteins (globulins and fibrinogen) or other colloids are present in the plasma. The significance of the SR is limited in that increased erythrocyte aggregation and plasma viscosity partially compensate for each other.

HINT [*714*] has shown that the *aggregating tendency* of plasma can be quantified by the determination of those plasma colloid concentrations which cause a SR of 1 mm/hr *(critical concentration).*

The following figures are approximately valid:

Plasma * 3.44% ± 0.05% (mean ± SE),
Dextran 70 approx. 1%,
Gelatin 40 approx. 1%,
Dextran 93 approx. 0.6%,
Gelatin 58 approx. 0.6%.

The *relative erythrocyte aggregating capacity (REAC)* reflects the aggregation tendency of a particular solution with respect to normal human plasma [*714*].

This figure is 0 for a dextran fraction with a $\overline{M}_w$ of 50,000, and 1 for a dextran fraction with a $\overline{M}_w$ of 60,000, (this corresponds to that of normal plasma).

With increasing MW of the dextran solution, the REAC climbs sharply, and is approximately 10 for $\overline{M}_w$ 100,000.

Plasma from patients with an SR of over 100 mm/hr has a REAC of approx. 2.

The figure for fibrinogen is 17.

A modified liquid gelatin with a MW of 40,000 has a REAC of 4. A normal gelatin solution of the same MW has a REAC of approx. 14. If the MW of such normal gelatin rises a little to 45,000, figures comparable to those of fibrinogen are reached!

These statements show that the REAC is raised many times by the presence of artificial colloids, compared with pathological proteins.

The MW distribution in dextran 70 is such that a slight rise in the SR occurs after infusion. The SR is not affected by dextran 60 and is lowered by dextran 40 [*510, 582, 781, 1324, 1569*].

DHALL et al. [*350, 1647, 1649*] described the changes in the aggregating tendency of *thrombocytes* in vitro. The authors show that clinical dextran solutions cause platelet aggregation *in vitro* when used in concentrations as they occur in blood. SAKAI [*1239*] observed a reduction in platelet aggregation. DHALL made his experiments at room temperature (see also [*1308 a*]); clinical dextrans do not lead to thrombocyte aggregation at body temperature (personal information from G. THORSÉN; see also [*1504*]). DHALL has confirmed this now in vivo [*1646, 1648*].

With dextrans of very high $\overline{M}_w$ (over 150,000) intravascular aggregation of formed blood elements ("sludging") can be caused [*1619, 1820, 1821*]. This corresponds to that caused by pathological plasma or gelatin [*509, 1403*]; STALKER [*1378, 1820, 1821*] reports on hypoxic changes in organs which result from aggregation of formed elements.

---

* Average figures for more than 100 normal individuals (personal information from H. HINT, Uppsala, 1967).

RICHTER [*1186, 1189*] and ELIASSON [*407*] have pointed out the species differences existing with regard to the erythrocyte aggregating tendency. It is marked in horses and cats, moderate in humans, pigs and dogs, slight in guinea pigs, rats and mice, and very weak in sheep, chickens and cattle. Rabbit erythrocytes behave atypically, since a low SR accompanies a raised erythrocyte aggregating tendency.

The *disaggregating tendency of dextran* can be measured quantitatively in vitro [*1656*]. Unfortunately simple, good methods for quantitative measurement of this phenomenon in vivo do not yet exist. In vitro the disaggregating effect for dextran is strongest with an $\overline{M}_w$ between 30,000 and 40,000 [*586, 1187, 1188, 1569*].

This fact was first proved clearly by THORSÉN and HINT [*1440*] in vitro and in vivo, and it led to the development of low molecular dextran by GELIN and INGELMAN ([*502*]; see also [*500*]). A 2.5% solution of a dextran fraction with a $\overline{M}_w$ between 20,000 and 40,000 causes an 80% reduction of the SR [*1188*].

ENGESET et al. [*416, 416 a, 1659, 1660, 1661*] have shown that this specific effect for humans and dogs can not depend upon a dilution phenomenon (see also the corresponding section in "Gelatin").

## *m) Influence on Viscosity*

The reader is referred to the corresponding chapter in Part One concerning the importance of viscosity for flow conditions in the microcirculation (see p. 12 f.; for nomenclature see p. 55); survey in [*875*]. The influence of dextran solutions on viscosity has been studied in detail in vitro [*563*] and in vivo.

The clinical dextran solutions (6%, or 10%!) have a much higher relative viscosity than normal plasma in vitro ($\eta_{rel} = 1.72$—$1.96$; [*582 864*]). The $\eta_{rel}$ for:

6% dextran 70 is approx. 3.4—3.99
10% dextran 40 is approx. 5.1—5.4 [*502, 580, 581*].

This fact, however, is without clinical importance, since after all we are concerned with the viscosity conditions after infusion into the organism. For the same reason viscosity measurements *in vitro* (with variation of the proportions of plasma and plasma replacement substance) are *not* very *conclusive* [e. g. *1601, 1602, 1656, 1751, 1752, 1791, 1848*].

It has long been known that additions of various dextran fractions increase the *plasma* viscosity, depending on concentration and molecular weight, with various shear rates — increasing MW and concentration = higher viscosity [*561, 562, 563, 999 a*]. WELLS [*1506*] found a reduction of blood viscosity in vitro due to dextran 40 and 75.

The decisive factor for improvement of the flow characteristics of a plasma replacement substance is whether it is able to reduce a pathologically raised whole blood viscosity at low flow rates, i. e. at low shear rates (cf. [*1507 a*]). GROTH [*582*] has shown that infusions of 500 ml dextran 40 are able to reduce a high plasma viscosity in humans. A slight rise occurs with a normal initial value as well as after infusion of dextran 70 (cf. [*1294*]). GROTH [*586*] investigated the levels of blood viscosity which are of clinical interest; in his article he compares dextran 40 with albumin 10%. Raised blood viscosity is lowered by both substances to the same degree. Normal blood viscosity levels, on the other hand, do not change with infusion of dextran 40 and 70 [*199*].

Several careful investigations show that raised blood viscosity from various causes (trauma, blood loss, endotoxin, experimentally used high molecular dextran) can be reduced by infusion of dextran 40 in animals and humans [*127, 393, 501, 502, 511, 745, 1258, 1308, 1337, 1562, 1607, 1613, 1748*]. See Fig. 11 a.

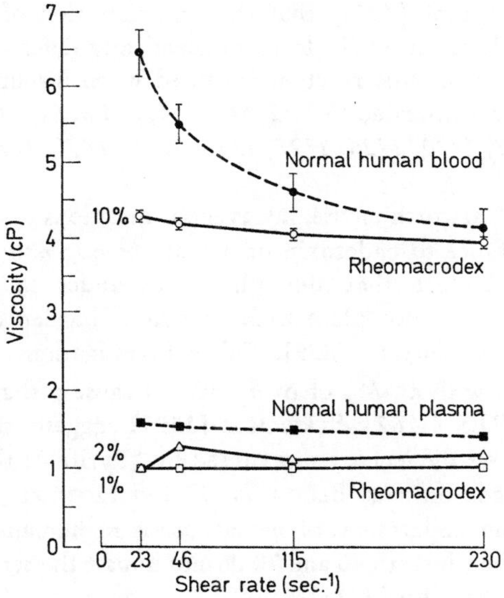


Fig. 11 a. Rheomacrodex, as supplied in 10% solution, is fairly viscous. At low shear rates however its viscosity is less than that of normal blood. The viscosity of the Rheomacrodex solution in the bottle anyway is quite irrelevant to its in vivo effects, because the circulating dextran is diluted. Rheomacrodex 10% is a hyperoncotic solution. Almost immediately after infusion it draws water from the extravascular space. Therefore the circulating dextran concentration in clinical use is around 1% and rarely exceeds 2%. The viscosity of a 1% and even a 2% Rheomacrodex solution is well below that of normal plasma so that a specific viscosity-lowering effect is to be expected. (Adapted from GROTH [*586*], and personal communication from O. TANGEN, Uppsala)

## n) *Influence upon Blood Group Determination*

For some time it has been known that the presence of "British" dextran or of other high molecular dextran preparations can lead to pseudoagglutination of erythrocytes (rouleaux formation) [*232, 370, 384, 959, 1477, 1799*] (see p. 78).

For this reason these authors recommend taking blood for cross-matching before every dextran infusion. *Under normal investigation conditions, however, dextran 40 and 70 have no influence on blood group determination* [*53, 70, 175, 176, 194, 1128, 1153, 1204, 1371, 1462, 1501, 1731, 1799*].

## o) *Influence upon Defence against Infection and Non-specific Resistance*

On the basis of poisoning experiments in rats with allyl alcohol, Eger [*391, 392*] believes he has proved that dextran leads to a lowering in general resistance. But since he gives no attention to the specific sensitivity of the rat to dextran, these experiments are not convincing. It has been known for a long time [*1471*] that the administration of dextran in *rats* and certain breeds of mice [*57*] leads to genetically determined generalized edema. This species-specific reaction is caused when histamine [*426 a*] and several enzymes are liberated [*5, 532, 543, 555, 655 a, 845, 1588, 1630, 1635, 1636, 1675, 1708, 1720, 1726, 1727, 1728, 1729, 1733, 1776, 1808, 1812 a, 1831, 1846*].

In the white Carworth mouse, intravenous injections of dextran 70 cause no reduced resistance to endotoxin or a toxic *homogenate* of burned skin. This suggests therefore that this plasma expander in amounts up to 2.5% of the bw does not place a demonstrable burden on the RES nor does it impare its function [*239*]. Other investigations show that only dextran fractions with an $\overline{M}_w$ of over 150,000 cause a slight and transient blocking of the RES [*1262*]. Streicher [1395] suggests that injections of dextran 70 suppress the leucocytosis caused by "Pyrifer"; these experiments were likewise made on rats. Bloom [*176*] and Howard [*732*] found no leucopenia and no impairment of hematopoesis in humans. In addition it has been shown that dextran 40 and 70 do not impair the serum bacteriocidal properties [*155*]. See also [*1718*].

## p) *Carcinogenicity*

Lusky and Nelson [*930*] could show no carcinogenicity 73 weeks after repeated injections of 6% dextran. In all other histological investigations as well (see p. 76 f.) and in autopsy material from patients, some of whom had received large doses of dextran, no traces of carcinogenicity were found.

Recently work has been done with regard to the microcirculation in tumors [*129, 1666*] and the influence of dextran on metastasis formation from experimental tumors. FISHER and FISHER [*447*] believe that administration of dextran in rats increases the metastasis of "Walker" cells. However their experimental procedure does not permit these conclusions. The control animals were subjected to drastic blood removal with inadequate volume replacement, while some dextran animals received massive overtransfusions. In addition there is the question of the species-specific dextran sensitivity of rats and the particular type of tumor used. GRIFFIN and AUST [*568*] found fewer but larger metastases in mice which received dextran 40. GORDON's experiments are not conclusive because of overdosage [*1685*].

In extended studies C. M. RUDENSTAM [*1226 a*] found that metastasis formation of various types of tumors in various species is influenced in many ways by dextran 40. The number of metastases is sometimes greater, sometimes less; at times no effect is found (personal information; [*514, 517*], see also [*1730*]).

ARMSTRONG and COHN [*68*] were able to show that i. p. administration of dextran 40 significantly reduced the spread of tumor cells in rabbits. These authors recommend rinsing the abdomen with dextran 40 following operations for cancer.

### *q) Influence upon Blood Coagulation*

The influence of dextran on hemostasis has been investigated extensively, because the first preparations gave rise to blood coagulation disturbances in a few cases. The most important articles are briefly summarized below. However this is not an easy task, since many authors do not mention the type and amount of dextran used.

**Dextran 70 and Older Dextran Preparations.** *In vitro experiments:* LAURELL [*867*] assumes that a fibrinoplastic activity of dextran and a retardation of thrombin formation compensate for each other; for this reason no bleeding tendency can be determined when clinical doses are used. JACOBAEUS [*771*] later confirmed the fibrinoplastic activity of dextran. ABILDGAARD [2], however, showed that the enzymatic activity of thrombin on fibrinogen is not influenced by the presence of dextran 40, 110 and 500 nor of Ficoll (synthetic sucrose polymer). In plasma dextran is said to have only a slight fibrinoplastic effect. RICKETTS [*1191*] and WEIL and WEBSTER [*1503*] were able to show a dextran-fibrinogen complex under certain conditions, but this was later doubted [*1138*]. FLETCHER et al. [*451*] produced such complexes with PVP also; but they attach no significance to this since only 10% of the fibrinogen present was involved in formation of the complex. VIERECK and KÖHLER [*1468*] conclude from their studies that dextran neutralizes heparin present in plasma. Another theory [*6, 9, 1215*] maintains that dextran inhibits the release of thrombocyte factors; this could also be measured quantitatively [*1217*]. SEEGERS et al. [*1310*] suggest that dextran with an average MW of 91,700 reduces the threon activity (threon =

product of the reaction between platelet co-factor 1 (factor VIII) and platelet factor 3, necessary for converting prothrombin to thrombin).

*Animal experiments:* HUMMEL and HALSE [*753*] found a hemostatic effect after i. v. injection of 2.5 ml 6% dextran per kg b.w. in rabbits. MONKHOUSE [*1035*] and SEMPLE [*1313, 1314*] carried out exchange transfusions with dextran; in the course of these transfusions a 20% decline in fibrinogen as well as occasional blood oozing were noticed. HORVATH [*728*] and BLOOM [*179*] found a prolonged bleeding time after repeated administration of dextran in normovolemic dogs and rabbits. ADELSON et al. [*8*] confirmed these results and made additional infusions in irradiated dogs. They were unable to explain the prolonged bleeding time by the thrombopenia and hemodilution alone (cp. [*1719*]). MICHAELSEN and HOWLAND [*1015*] studied the effect of dextran infusions after administration of bishydroxycumarin, acetyl biscoum acetate, heparin and phenindion. From their results the authors conclude that the bleeding tendency observed after dextran infusions is not based upon influence on coagulation factors but on injury of the vessel integrity. SWANK [*1403*] likewise assumes that a dextran-fibrinogen complex is formed, which could cause filtration of thrombocytes out of the circulation (cf. [*535 a, 1433*]).

*Clinical investigations:* Observation of a total of several thousand patients is the object of articles by various authors who have found no evidence of a raised bleeding tendency after dextran infusion [*79, 174, 307, 682, 733, 1501, 1824*]. Exceptions sometimes occurred with transfusion of very large amounts [*732, 770, 771, 1089, 1488, 1503*]. After extrapleural pneumolysis there was even a reduction in bleeding complications [*1468*].

The following articles discuss a raised bleeding tendency after administration of dextran: CARBONE [*257*] and ADELSON [*8*]attempt to explain the increase in bleeding time as being due to disturbances of hemostasis at the points of vascular lesions. Impairment of thrombocyte function was also considered [*9, 853, 1403*].

In 1955 BRONWELL et al. [*218*] concluded from their experiments that the bleeding complications observed after administration of dextran depend on the amount and molecular weight of the preparation used.

Of 85,000 births, 8 cases of hypofibrinogenemia were observed and attributed to administration of dextran. The molecular weight of 63% of the dextran molecules was between 130,000 and 150,000 [*1306*]. This hypothesis is not confirmed by any of the articles quoted (see also [*1129*]), and it is known today that hypofibrinogenemia also occurs spontaneously post partum. Prolonged bleeding times with normal coagulation times could not be explained by the slight decline in prothrombin concentration [*779*]. On the basis of prothrombin consumption tests, JACOBAEUS [*771*] believes he has shown that dextrans have an inhibitory effect on coagulation. However, it seems doubtful to him that this effect is sufficient to raise the bleeding tendency, particularly since dextran has a fibrinoplastic effect which can make up for the reduced thrombin formation.

Dextrans of higher molecular weight ($\overline{M}_w$ over 80,000) in clinical dosage can thus retard normal blood coagulation [*1589*]. The volume expanding effect, i. e. the dilution of the coagulation factors as well as species differences must be taken into account.

**Dextran 40.** LONG [*919*] has shown that Rheomacrodex in doses of more than 4—6 g/kg bw prolongs the bleeding time in dogs. He also showed that identical changes occur with equal doses of 10% albumin. The author assumes that the prolongation of the bleeding time after these massive doses is non-specific and is caused by overloading of the vascular system. In clinical doses dextran is said not to cause changes in the bleeding time.

These findings are supported by the careful investigations of BERGENTZ, EIKEN and NILSSON [*124*]. They measured the bleeding time as well as coagulation time, number of thrombocytes, prothrombin consumption, fibrinogen level, and factors V and VII. This study was extended and also confirmed in humans by NILSSON and EIKEN [*1084*] and by CRONBERG et al. [*316*].

A large number of experimental and clinical investigations show that dextran 40 in doses up to 2.0 g/kg bw does not influence the coagulation mechanism in the pathological sense [*3, 90, 174, 201, 254, 503, 862, 865 a, 890, 916, 961, 1081, 1153, 1824*].

MELROSE et al. later published results of 306 patients who had had surgery with cardiopulmonary bypass [*121, 1354*]. These showed that administration of 2 g Rheomacrodex/kg bw raises postoperative bleeding by 258 ml/m$^2$. However no disturbances of blood coagulation were found. On the contrary, among the patients of the Rheomacrodex group, postoperative coagulation conditions were more often normal than in the control group. Serious postoperative complications were less frequent in the Rheomacrodex group (3.6%) than in the control group (7.5%).

DUGDALE et al. [*368*] observed increased prothrombin consumption and unfavorable influence on the fibrin thrombus in dogs with hypothermia and extracorporeal circulation; at the same time, however, dextran 40 had a protective function. This led to a longer survival time.

HELLSTRÖM and BJÖRK [*700*] observed a slight increase in postoperative bleeding with use of Rheomacrodex in the cardiopulmonary bypass. According to Fig. 2 in their article, increased bleeding occurred only when the perfusion lasted longer than 90 minutes. Because of the lack of uniformity in their material and the figures which sometimes contradict each other (tables and text!) this article is hard to evaluate. The differences between the various groups appear to be insignificant. The article by DYBKJAER et al. [*373*] is also hard to interpret, for it is not clear whether correction factors were used for the blood dilution or not. Evaluation of the study by GOLLUB [*535 a*] is also difficult; the blood losses were measured only by estimation.

LUNDSGAARD [*924*] quotes an article by GARZON et al. According to the latter, dextran 40 is said to cause pronounced disturbances in the coagulation mechanism. These authors observed an increase of 562% in blood loss after bleeding and infusion of large amounts of dextran 40 in rather unphysiological experiments (deep unsutured skin incisions). This increased blood loss shows an improvement in capillary circulation, as stated by the authors themselves. These findings are without great clinical importance since the situation seldom arises where plasma replacement substances are given as therapy for untreated skin lacerations. With other injuries the extrinsic system of blood coagulation always takes over. Many years of clinical experience confirm that increased capillary bleeding rarely occurs.

MULDER et al. [*1057*] observed no increase in bleeding with the recommended doses of 15—20 ml/kg bw; on the other hand bleeding increased with higher doses [*207, 365, 641 a, 885, 891, 1416, 1847*]. RAISON [*1154*] assumes that bleeding with use of higher doses is due to hemodilution. He also shows that the entire postoperative blood loss after the use of Rheomacrodex is smaller. ROE et al. [*1207*] also found a somewhat lower blood loss in groups whose infused blood was diluted with dextran 40 than in groups which received only whole blood. CUELLO and LILLEHEI [*324*] observed a slightly increased volume in thoracic drainage after dextran 40 compared to 5% glucose; at the same time they stated: "Rheomacrodex has a definite place in extracorporeal circulation, especially for longer perfusions and for acquired valvular surgery where a low postoperative cardiac output and a high plasma hemoglobin may lead to oliguria or anuria." See also [*1736*].

PERKINS [*1123*], DYBKJAER [*372*] and KRØLL [*840*] used large amounts of dextran 40 (sometimes 15% solution) in 5% glucose in their in vitro experiments. The precipitation caused by this was probably due to dilution of the electrolyte concentration and the "water excluding effect". The latter phenomenon is common to all colloids and was studied in detail [*868*].

*Fibrinolytic activity.* DEUTSCH [*347*] and FISCHER et al. [*445, 445 a*] believe that dextran can activate the fibrinolytic system. This view is contrary to the results of NILSSON [*1084*] and CRONBERG [*316*]. O'NEILL [*1104*] has shown that increased fibrinolysis occurs in all patients on bypass; this fibrinolysis is increased by the presence of dextran 40, but his experiments were all made under hypothermia.

### *r) Pharmacological Properties*

The pharmacological effects of dextran depend upon a series of physicochemical properties of the dextran fraction used, the most important of which are colloid osmotic pressure, viscosity, adsorption on vascular surfaces and blood cells, influence on the electric charge of blood cells and vascular surfaces, interaction with plasma proteins and interaction with colloidal reactions. This means that molecular weight, molecular weight distribution and molecular shape play a decisive part. Together with the colloid osmotic effect, the antithrombotic and disaggregating effects (see p. 79) are the most important pharmacological properties of dextran.

*The Antithrombotic Effect.* When dextran was introduced as a plasma expander it was regarded as a pharmacologically inert colloid. Only later did it become known that it also possesses pharmacological properties of clinical interest. Thus many articles in recent years confirm that dextran is able to reduce the frequency of thrombosis under various experimental conditions [*82, 143, 146, 186, 221, 223, 224, 225, 251, 270, 278, 279, 398, 417, 430, 430 a, 450, 608, 614, 753 a, 797, 798, 1003, 1004, 1032, 1033, 1198, 1231, 1232, 1244, 1420, 1541, 1542, 1586, 1633, 1699, 1852*]. For extensive excellent *reviews see* [*1626, 1627*].

The first *clinical* paper in this area was written by KOEKENBERG [*834*]. The incidence of postoperative thrombo-embolic complications was reduced by 80% when Macrodex was infused, rather than blood, during surgery. Also in thrombotic diseases good results were obtained with dextran 70 and 40 ([*88 a, 125, 128, 225, 307, 308, 452, 758 a, 758 b, 799, 1032, 1219 a, 1242, 1243, 1469, 1664*]; see also [*907*]).

*Mode of Action.* Naturally the antithrombotic effect of dextran is closely connected to its influence on blood coagulation; many of the articles mentioned with regard to that are also applicable here.

The following possibilities may help to explain this mode of action:

1. Dextran coats the vascular endothelia and the formed blood elements with a thin film ("coating"). It thus reduces the activation of contact factors which normally trigger the coagulation mechanism [*178, 180, 885, 1217, 1575, 1600*].

2. The dextran shell neutralizes the positive potential which occurs at the site of an intima lesion. Thus the aggregation of blood cells is reduced at this point ([*149, 266, 1215*]; cf. also [*300*]).

3. The adsorption of dextran onto the external surfaces of thrombocytes reduces their aggregation [*1600, 1628*], the release of platelet factor 3 [*429, 771, 841, 1847*], and the viscous metamorphosis at the site of vascular lesion ([*146, 209, 342, 348, 1139, 1310, 1620*], cf. also [*874, 1504*]).

4. Dextran improves the flow rate and thus hinders the growth of an already existing thrombus [*189*].

Recently we showed that the antithrombotic effect can not be based upon the volume expanding and flow-improving effects of dextran, since albumin with the same colloid osmotic effect does not prevent the occurrence of experimental thrombi (Figs. 12 and 13; [*599, 608, 614, 618 a*]).

Formation of vein thrombi

| Number of veins | Therapy | Absence of thrombus in |
|---|---|---|
| 10 | Control | 10% |
| 10 | Saline | 10% |
| 20 | Albumin | 10% |
| 20 | Dextran | 60% |

Difference A/D: $p < 0.05$

Fig. 12. Thrombus frequency after administration of iso-oncotic solutions of dextran and albumin in rabbits (GRUBER [*614, 618 a*]).

We have investigated the *thrombo-prophylactic effect* of equal amounts of two colloids having the same volume-expanding effect in 30 rabbits. First a micro-hematocrit determination was made on blood taken from the ear of the animal. Under general anesthesia contusions were made in the tissue of the thighs by means of 50 light padded hammer blows made in a standardized manner. 48 hours later the animals were again anesthetized, and a second Hct determination was made. The animals were then given alternately 12 mg/kg bw of one of the following solutions intravenously: 1. 0.9% normal saline, 2. 5.8% human albumin (Kabi AB, Stockholm), 2. 4.1% dextran, fraction DRT 776, $\overline{M}_w$ 77,500 (Pharmacia AB, Uppsala), 4. A control group received no therapy.

The albumin and dextran solutions are approximately blood iso-oncotic, i. e. they have a colloid osmotic pressure of 400 mm $H_2O$. Immediately after i.v. injection of the first dose of one of the solutions mentioned, we ligated both femoral veins with 0000 silk. 2 hours later we made another Hct determination and administered the same amount of the same solution as before. 6 hours after the first injection, the Hct was again determined, the femoral veins were clamped off and excised. These veins were opened and examined for the presence of thrombi (see also Fig. 13).

Hematocrit changes

| n of animals | 5 | 5 | 10 | 10 |
|---|---|---|---|---|
| Therapy | **C** | **S** | **A** | **D** |
| before trauma | 33.9 | 34.9 | 36.1 | 35.5 |
| 48 hrs later (ligature) | 34.0 | 33.3 | 35.5 | 33.4 |
| 6 hrs after ligature | 33.0 | 35.0 | 33.6 | 31.9 |
| end of experiment | 34.5 | 32.2 | 29.4 | 28.3 |

**C** = Control **S** = Saline
**A** = Albumin **D** = Dextran

Difference A/D: not significant

Fig. 13. Hematocrit changes after administration of iso-oncotic solutions of dextran and albumin in normovolemic rabbits

The plasma volume expansion is the same after giving both solutions. Thus flow should be improved to the same degree. It is known that following administration of dextran 40 and albumin in dosages which cause an identical increase in plasma volume (GRUBER [*614, 618 a*]), flow increases (as measured in the kidney with the aid of PAH clearance) correspondingly.

The results available at this time indicate that much importance should be attached to the effect of dextran on platelet aggregation. BENNETT et al. [*120, 1605*], BYGDEMAN et al. [*249, 250, 1625*] and CRONBERG et al. [*316*] used the methods of BORN (see [*409*]) and HELLEM [*698, 699*] to show that reduced platelet adhesiveness occurs after infusion of dextran in humans. This is probably the result of changes in plasma factors. It seems improbable that the reduced platelet adhesiveness in vivo is due to an effect of dextran on the ADP reactive receptors on the surface of the platelets [*248, 1600, 1629, 1648, 1649*].

The antithrombotic properties of dextran are not doubted today. Their effect is used in clinical dosage where no abnormal shift of the coagulation factors is seen apart from normal variations. Good results have been observed after i. v. infusion of 500 ml dextran 75 or dextran 40 for 3 days in humans [*308, 1168*]. In several studies concerning the antithrombotic effect of dextran, the coagulation mechanism was tested at the same time which as a rule was normal [*398, 452, 1542*].

At this time it is still unclear why the biologically interesting phenomenon of the antithrombotic effect is not connected to a measurable influence on coagulation. The studies of SEEGERS and co-workers [*1310*] provide a possible explanation: dextran impairs viscous metamorphosis if thrombin formation is caused by the "intrinsic system" alone, as in a thrombosis. On the other hand, the "extrinsic system" is also involved in hemostasis; tissue thromboplastin is released and thrombin is formed, which completely eliminates the inhibitory effect of dextran on threon activity. In spite of the presence of dextran, the viscous metamorphosis can occur.

It has not yet been decided which form of dextran offers a better antithrombotic effect [*1699*]. With equal doses, dextran 70 appears to be more effective [*1625*], while dextran 40 is excreted more quickly. There are no comparative studies where identical plasma concentrations were maintained for a long period in vivo with various dextran fractions [*1244*]. Proof is also lacking that the antithrombotic effect depends on the dextran concentration. Various findings favor dextran 70 for the best antithrombotic effect. For this reason Macrodex is clinically more often used for prophylaxis and management of thrombo-embolic complications. Where flow improvement is desired at the same time, as in vascular surgery, use of dextran 40 is recommended.

*The following doses are recommended for prophylaxis and management of thrombo-embolic complications:*

Initially 10—20 ml/kg bw,

i. e. 500—1000 ml dextran 70 or 40 in 4—6 hours, then 500 ml i. v. in

4 hours or more slowly every other day until symptoms disappear, at most for 2 weeks.

Allowance should be made for the type of solvent used (5% glucose or 0.9% NaCl).

Certain experimental and clinical data indicate that *low molecular weight dextran* can improve the course after *myocardial infarction* [*169, 170, 171, 350 a, 623, 631, 842, 854, 855, 856, 857, 858, 860, 892, 918, 1127, 1541, 1702, 1721, 1721 a, 1761, 1786*].

Definite conclusions can not yet be made in this field [*892 a*]. Even so, the results might be traced back, at least in part, to the antithrombotic effect of dextran.

This property also accounts for at least part of the success in treating impaired circulation of the extremities [*62, 122, 123, 125, 157, 455 a, 480, 788, 844, 960, 1045 a, 1142, 1158, 1233, 1348, 1612, 1639, 1709*] and in *vascular surgery* [*128, 131, 222, 301, 457, 863, 1650, 1709*]. In the same category, we find the results which were obtained with dextran 40 in *cerebral ischemia* [*191, 1789, 1842*], *cerebral infarctions* [*325, 390, 456, 560, 1011 a, 1397 a, 1526*], *mesenterial infarctions* ([*56, 60, 332, 878, 879*], cf. [*1673*] and *cold injury* [*58, 1061, 1062, 1493*]. See Fig. 13 a!

For reviews regarding LMWD see [*401, 922, 1312, 1411, 1611, 1668*].

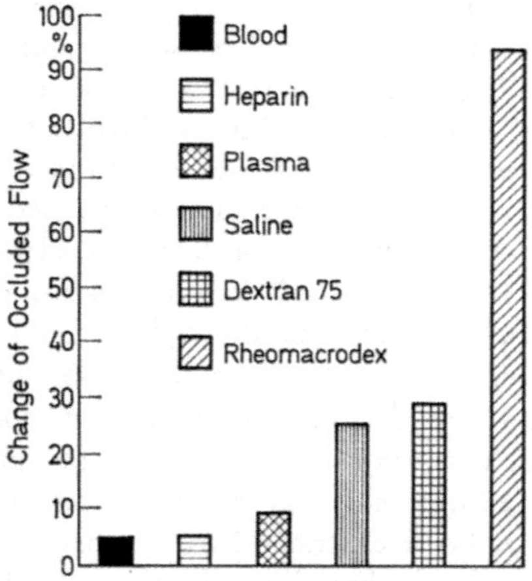


Fig. 13 a. Increase in collateral blood flow around an acute arterial obstruction after administration of 6 different agents (Adapted from Moraes [*1045 a*]).

*Influence on Blood Lipids.* Some interest has been aroused recently by the findings of Flotte [*453, 454*] concerning the reduction of pathologically raised *cholesterol* levels and atheromatous plaques after administration of dextran in rabbits and man. The role of cholesterol in the genesis of arteriosclerosis remains contested. No conclusion may be drawn in this matter at present. A connection with the antithrombotic effect is possible (see also [*1609, 1618, 1735, 1772, 1800*]).

For several years many articles have dealt with the effect of dextran on blood *lipids in general* [*23, 24, 323, 404, 453, 706, 791, 792, 793, 814, 815, 816, 827, 845 a, 883, 931, 932, 933, 947, 1029, 1049, 1118, 1119, 1124, 1146, 1218, 1238, 1308, 1367, 1456, 1480, 1491, 1547 a, 1610, 1674, 1800, 1827*].

### *s) Influence on Laboratory Investigations*

W. Appel and co-workers [*61 a*] have investigated the influence of dextran 40 and 70 (Rheomacrodex and Macrodex) on 50 laboratory tests; they checked 86 methods in 3800 analyses (cf. also [*71*]):

*The following determination methods are not affected by the presence of dextran:*

Enzymes:

- GOT after Reitman-Frankel and after Karmen,
- GPT after Reitman-Frankel and after Karmen,
- LDH after Wroblewski-LaDue,
- IDH after Taylor-Friedmann,
- aldolase after Racker,
- creatinin-phosphokinase after Tanzer-Gilvarg,
- alkaline and acid phosphatase after Bessey-Lowry and rapid test,
- alpha-amylase after Smith-Roe,
- lipase after Cherry-Crandall,
- amino acid arylamidases after Schön et al. modified,
- leucinamino-peptidase after Greenbaum-Fruton, Smith mod.,
- gly-gly-dipeptidase after Smith mod.,
- aminotripeptidase after Smith mod.,
- carboxypeptidase A after Schön et al. mod.,
- trypsin and cathepsin after Anson mod., Nelson et al. mod., Riedel and Wünsch mod., Russler and Schön mod., Hummel,
- chymotrypsin A after Hummel,
- pepsin after Fruton et al. mod., Anson mod., Nelson et al. mod.

Organic substances:

- glucose after Stein, Keston-Teller, Fehling-Trommer, Benedict, Rédei-Nagy, rapid tests (see [*1615*]),
- fructose after Bang,
- lactose after Wöhlk, Rubner-Bucher,
- pentoses after Bial,
- acetone after Lange,
- acetic acid after Arnold,

ketone bodies rapid test,
phenyl pyruvate rapid tests,
protein rapid test,
electrophoresis,
serum instability reactions,
urea N after Berthelot-Stegemann, rapid tests,
creatinin after Clark and Thompson,
cholestrol after Searey-Bergquist, Pearson-Stern, Zak, Schmidt-Thomé,
non-esterified fatty acid after Novak,
bilirubin after Malloy-Evelyn, With,
hemoglobin after Bethke-Savelsberg,
blood quick test,
ethanol after Bücher-Redetzki.

Inorganic substances:

$Na^+$, $K^+$ flame-photometry,
$Ca^{++}$ after Diehl-Ellingboe,
$Fe^{++}$ after Zak,
$Cl^-$ after Schales-Schales,
$HCO_3^-$ after Van Slyke,
Pi after Fiske-Subbarow,
Hct after McGovern-Jones.

In certain circumstances the presence of dextran can have a slight influence (1.5—7%) on the methods mentioned for lipase, chloride, hemoglobin, and cholesterol (after Pearson) (for details, see [*61 a*]).

*The following determination methods are disturbed by the presence of dextran:*

glucose (see [*1615*]): after Hagedorn-Jensen, Crecelius, Hultmann, Nylander (urine), polarimetrically (urine),
protein: refractometrically, Biuret (useful with precipitation of the proteins with trichloracetic acid),
fatty acid esters,
cholesterol (after Sperry-Webb),
fructose (after Seliwanoff),
sorbit dehydrogenase.

In each case the results are elevated or false positive.

Concerning determination of the inulin clearance in the presence of dextran see [*1070 a*].

Appel and Wirmer [*61 b*] also describe accurate new macro- and micromethods for examination of dextran in blood, urine, cerebro-spinal fluid, gastric juice, intestinal fluid, and saliva.

### *t) Stability during Storage*

MAYCOCK and RICKETTS [*980, 982*] have shown that storage for 5 and 10 years [*1954—1959—1965*] at 4° C does not change the physico-chemical and biological properties of British and American dextran. A limitation can be placed on storage capability only by obvious defects in the containers (lid, rubber cork, glass) but not by instability of the dextran solution as such.

Due to temperature fluctuations (when the upper half of the bottle is warmer than the lower half) flake formation can occur [*428*]. These flakes are aggregates of dextran molecules which dissolve again when the solution is heated for 10 minutes in an autoclave at 100—110° C ([*1362*]; see also [*356*]).

### *u) The Volume Effect of Dextran*

**Animal Experiments.** HILDEBRANDT [*708*] removed $^1/_5$—$^1/_4$ of the BV from dogs and then infused dextran 70. The colloid-osmotic pressure remained practically unchanged (confirmed in [*378*]); the viscosity showed only a slight degree of fluctuation. The Hct and the red cell count dropped until the 6th day and then climbed sharply until the 14th day. BOLLMANN et al. [*185*] proved the good volume effect of dextran 70 and 120 compared with dextran 24 and normal saline solution in rabbits.

RIEGER and LILJEDAHL [*1195*] observed a restitution of volume in dogs 4 hours after 30% blood loss and infusion of dextran 40 and 70 in *glucose;* this corresponded to the effect of dog albumin and dog plasma. 24 and 48 hours later the plasma volume in the dextran animals was less; this is probably due to the absence of sodium. The authors believe that the smaller plasma volume is explained by a *raised diuresis* and binding of interstitial water in the extravascular space. There is no basis for the latter assumption since the colloid-osmotic effect depends upon the presence of a semipermeable membrane.

An identical or initially somewhat greater volume effect after equal amounts of 6% and 10% dextran 40 or 75 in 0.9% NaCl, compared with plasma or blood, as well as the superiority over gelatin and PVP, is described in several articles with various types of animals [*179, 337, 341 a, 344, 396, 578, 703, 745, 761, 808, 809, 837, 923, 937, 953, 1257, 1313, 1347, 1488, 1593, 1739, 1748, 1787*].

DRAKE [*362*] has measured the volume effect of dextran 40 in *hypothermic* dogs. After 10% dextran 40 the initial rise in volume is more pronounced due to the strong colloid-osmotic effect, but it does not last as long as after dextran 75 (see human experiments).

The volume restitution after infusion of dextran 70 is complete even with large blood losses and continues until body mechanisms have refilled the plasma volume.

**Human Experiments.** In principle the relationships are the same as in animals. The duration of the volume effect of a dextran solution depends on the initial volume here as well. In hypovolemic individuals and those who have reduced colloid-osmotic pressure, the effect lasts longer than in healthy normovolemic individuals ([*639, 754*]; see also [*1313, 1488*]).

*Tables 5 and 6* provide a survey of the results of blood volume determinations by various authors using dextran 40 and 70 in hypo- and normovolemic individuals (cf. also Figs. 6 and 16).

Several other investigations confirm that the infusion of dextran 40 and 70 in hypo- and normovolemic individuals leads to an increase in plasma volume of long duration; this increase corresponds to the amount infused or is a little more:

Dextran 70 and older preparations: [*67, 175, 177, 194, 334, 376, 433, 574, 620, 681, 693, 759, 838, 853, 927, 1012, 1099, 1106, 1159, 1299, 1537, 1538, 1546, 1643, 1707, 1713*]. The temperature of the infusion solution between 4° C and 20° C probably does not influence its volume effect [*1690*].

Dextran 40: [*505, 958, 1265 a, 1416, 1604, 1662, 1713, 1794*].

Grünert [*619*] worked with a 6% dextran 40. Furthermore, Baumgartl [*109, 110*], tried to test various blood replacement substances by means of plasma volume measurement. But his method does not provide any reliable data (BV fluctuations of 3—4 liters!); for this reason the results and conclusions are not convincing. It is clear though that the normalization of the blood pressure in the shock experiments was achieved more quickly with Macrodex than with PVP or electrolyte solutions.

### *v) Hemodynamics*

It can be seen on the basis of a large number of exact measurements in dogs and humans under normal conditions and in shock that

cardiac output is raised,
venous return is increased,
blood pressure is raised,
pulse and peripheral resistance are lowered,
pulse pressure amplitude is enlarged, and
circulation time is shortened

by *dextran 40* [*93, 94, 258, 288, 289, 289 a, 455, 518, 790, 1196, 1257, 1265, 1265 a, 1298, 1416, 1496, 1543, 1612, 1614, 1662, 1669, 1686, 1702, 1709, 1710, 1734, 1744, 1789, 1839, 1840, 1850*], *dextran 70 and older dextran preparations* dissolved in 5% glucose or 0.9% NaCl [*63, 112, 232, 289 a, 459, 460, 572, 573, 656 a, 1059, 1060, 1068, 1152 a, 1229 c, 1269, 1360, 1546, 1596, 1624, 1644, 1678, 1715, 1716, 1739, 1785*].

Table 5. *Volume effect of dextran preparations in normovolemic individuals*

| Author | Year | Ref. | Preparation | Method | *n* | Amount in ml | Infusion duration in min | Volume increase in ml hrs after infusion 0 | 1 | 6 | 24 |
|---|---|---|---|---|---|---|---|---|---|---|---|
| Hammarsten, J. F. | 1953 | [*639*] | 6% dextran (80?) | T 1824 | 10 | 1000 | 50 | — | 755 | 534 | — |
| Metcalf, W. | 1954 | [*1009*] | 6% dextran Laros $\overline{M}_n$: 66,000 (?) | T 1824 | 12 | 1000 | ? | 1000 | — | 550 | 260 |
| | | | 6% dextran CSC $\overline{M}_n$: 56,000 (?) | T 1824 | 12 | 1000 | ? | 1000 | — | 610 | 340 |
| Harrison, J. H. | 1954 | [*657*] | 6% dextran $\bar{M}_n$: 60,000 | T 1824 | 29 | 1000 | 120 | — | — | 909 | — |
| | | | *with dextran 40 (Rheomacrodex)* | | | | | | | | |
| Hume, R. | 1964 | [*752*] | 10% dextran 40 | $Cr^{51}$ + RIHSA (?) | ? | 500 | 30 | 960 | — | — | — |
| | | | | | | | 120 | 750 | — | — | — |
| | | | | | | | 180 | 585 | — | — | — |
| | | | | | | | 240 | 350 | — | — | — |
| Schneider, K. W. | 1965 | [*1274*] | 10% dextran 40 | T 1824 | 29 | 1000 | ? | 985 | — | — | — |
| | | | | $Cr^{51}$ | 29 | 1000 | ? | 876 | | | |

Table 6. *Volume effect of dextran preparations in hypovolemic individuals*

| Author | Year | Ref. | Preparation | Method | *n* | Amount in ml | Infusion duration in min | Volume increase in ml hrs after infusion 0 | 1 | 2—4 | 6 | 12 | 24 |
|---|---|---|---|---|---|---|---|---|---|---|---|---|---|
| Hammarsten, J. F. | 1953 | [*639*] | 6% dextran (80?) | T 1824 | 8 | 1000 | 40 | — | 1020 | — | 820 | 700 | 860 |
| Gruber, U. F. | 1962 | [*589*] | 6% dextran 75 | RIHSA | 10 | 500 | 30 | 550 | — | 520 | — | — | — |
| Ahnefeld, W. F. | 1965 | [*14*] | 6% dextran 60 | RIHSA | 30 | 500 | 15 | 562 | 495 | 493 | — | — | — |
| | | | *with dextran 40 (Rheomacrodex)* | | | | | | | | | | |
| Gruber, U. F. | 1965 | [*601*] * | 10% dextran 40 | RIHSA | 8 | 500 | 30 | 1140 ** | — | 650 | — | — | — |
| Ahnefeld, W. F. | 1965 | [*14*] | 10% dextran 40 | RIHSA | 30 | 500 | 15 | 666 | 442 | 421 | — | — | — |

* In this work only the percentages of increase, based on the initial volume, are given.

** In fully hydrated individuals.

In addition, GIANELLI et al. [*521*] have investigated acid-base balance in humans after infusion of dextran 40 (see also [*1382*]) and pulmonary function (see also [*455, 1180*]).

CAREY [*261*] observed a more rapid improvement of the circulation after dextran 40 compared with blood in shocked patients ($n=23$); he showed that a definite rise in cardiac output continues for about 4 hours [*260*]. KHO [*1710*] has shown that at the same time $O_2$-consumption and $pO_2$ are increased. In view of the fact that the most important hemodynamic effect is an increase in cardiac output, it is not surprising that dextran 40 is not able to improve peripheral flow where normal conditions are present from the beginning, or when an increase of cardiac output is prevented experimentally [*292, 820, 820 a*].

The *flow-improving properties of dextran 40* were discovered and extensively investigated by GELIN and his co-workers [*501, 502*]. These properties are based on the fact that the largest portion of the molecules in this preparation have a $\overline{M}_w$ of less than 60,000. They show a definite disaggregating effect (see also [*1295*]) which is enhanced by the fact that Rheomacrodex is a 10% solution. Because of the strong colloid-osmotic effect, interstitial fluid is drawn into the vascular tree, thus lowering Hct and viscosity. It is possible that a passive dilation of the capillaries occurs due to this influx of fluid, which in turn contributes to a rise in cardiac output (cf. [*1662*]). ENERSON [*412, 413, 414*] has shown in vitro that dextran 40 counteracts the swelling of cells which results from hypoxia and hypothermia (see also [*1820*]).

SCHJELDERUP [*1260*] observed a flow improvement in skin flaps, and GOULIAN [*541 a*] has demonstrated a prolonged survival time for pedicled skin flaps (cf. [*1623, 1749*]). BURRI and MATTER [*242*] have measured the perfusion of lip plasties after infusion of dextran 40 or gelatin. Gelatin solution was not able to change the temperature, whereas dextran 40 raised it. The authors attribute this to an improvement in capillary circulation. ONEAL [*1770*] did not see a significant increase in survival of skin flaps after treatment with dextran 40 (see also [*1780*]).

Mucosal lesions in the stomach, occurring in hemorrhagic shock in rabbits [*651*], are prevented by dextran 40, which effect is also attributed to its rheological properties [*652*, cf. *1673*].

GROTH and LÖFSTRÖM [*585*] have shown that the infusion of dextran 40 raises the *oxygen partial pressure* in rabbit skin due to improved perfusion. Another article demonstrates the superiority of dextran 40 and albumin over blood and dextran 70 for raising the $pO_2$ in the muscles [*587, 1850*]. The increased oxygen consumption which occurs after infusion of low molecular dextran also points to an improvement in capillary perfusion [*820, 820 a, 1669, 1753, 1789, 1806*]. (Cf. also [*123 a, 1666, 1700*]). The rat experiments of Evonuk [*426 a*] are inconclusive because of the species-specific hypersensitivity.

Various authors assume that circulation of erythrocytes can be retarded significantly after trauma and serious blood loss [*92, 133*]; Shoemaker [*1334*] and Suzuki [*1398, 1399, 1400*] speak of a slowly circulating red cell mass. Although these results could not be confirmed by others [*327, 774*], and the clinical importance of this phenomenon is still unclear, Sherman et al. [*1325*] have recently shown that infusion of dextran 40 in endotoxin shock causes a more rapid equilibration of $^{51}Cr$-marked erythrocytes. The same phenomenon was recently demonstrated in fracture patients [*215 a*]. Dextran 40 treatment seems to be favorable in preventing edema secondary to tourniquet ischemia [*1642*].

With regard to the influence of plasma expanders on hemodynamics see also p. 12 f., 78 f., 80 f., and 86 f.

## *w) Therapeutic Results*

**Dextran 70 and Older Preparations.** *Animal experiments:* Grönwall and Ingelman [*572, 573*] showed that the blood pressure in animals can be normalized quickly and completely after blood loss by dextran infusions. Subsequently, several research groups [*185, 232, 476, 708, 1313, 1439, 1462*] have often demonstrated the effectivity of dextran in shock experiments and in massive exchange transfusions [*1229 c*].

In various trials with several species, numerous investigators found a 6% dextran solution little worse, just as effective, or better than albumin, plasma, blood, or other expanders [*100, 237, 240, 352, 494, 578, 579, 703, 925, 925 a, 1048, 1117, 1133, 1155, 1313, 1345, 1347, 1352, 1433, 1466, 1538, 1696*] or clearly better than the same amount of an electrolyte solution.

In an excellent article Drucker [*363*] has shown that in irreversible shock in dogs refilling the BV with dextran 40 or 150 is just as effective for restoration of erobic metabolism as retransfusion of the autologous blood. The survival times in both groups were the same, although the Hct in the dextran group was only 19%. On the other hand, the results were definitely worse when twice the amount of a physiological saline solution was infused.

Influence of the vehicle solution:

Agersborg et al. [*11*] recommend using balanced electrolyte solutions as vehicles for dextran. They base their recommendations on shock experiments in dogs. Pathological plasma- or erythrocyte-electrolyte values were shown neither with physiological saline solution nor with 5% dextrose. The survival rate was greater when dextran was given in Gey's solution; however, the number of animals involved in the experiment is too small ($n = 4$/group) for definite conclusions. Motion picture studies of *cell cultures* confirm the superiority of balanced electrolyte solutions [*1137*].

In their shock experiments in dogs Stěrba et al. [*1385*] were able to prolong the survival times by an average of 50% by adding 40 mg glutathion/100 ml infusion solution. They compared blood, cattle serum and 2 dextran preparations without indicating the molecular weight. The authors assume that the favorable effect of glutathion is based on better use of the oxygen bound to hemoglobin.

Triner et al. [*1457*] showed that addition of 5% glucose and insulin to dextran in 0.9% NaCl solution significantly prolongs the survival of rabbits in hemorrhagic shock.

*Clinical results:* The first clinical results concerning the use of dextran for treatment of shock were published in 1946 by Bohmansson et al. [*184*]. Shortly afterward, Thorsén [*1438*] also confirmed the superiority of dextran over equal amounts of electrolyte solution in the management of shock in humans. Since then a large number of clinical studies have appeared concerning the effectivity of dextran in the management of shock. Several articles quoted under "Hemodynamics" and "Volume effect" also contain information on this topic. All of these studies show that infusion of a 6% dextran solution in hypovolemic shock leads to therapeutic results which correspond to those after treatment with plasma [*90, 118, 232, 289 a, 620, 681, 927, 1149, 1501, 1707, 1777*].

In the early 1950's Craig et al. [*309*] and Bowman [*194*] reported on successful treatment of 2500 cases in the USA; Fayot [*433*] published his results on 350 patients in France.

The article by Amspacher [*53*] provides proof of the clinical effectivity of dextran 75 in the management of shock, this article deals with seriously injured patients in the Korean War. It is interesting to note that many batallion surgeons always complained when the dextran supplies were exhausted, since they found that dextran was superior to plasma. In all cases the diuresis was good, although the Hct dropped to 20 in several patients after volume was restored (see also [*79, 232*]).

Likewise, there are many reports about the successful prophylactic administration of dextran 70 during anesthesia and surgery, and as a replacement for intraoperative blood loss [*118, 184, 200, 232, 309, 433, 825, 926, 957, 958, 1515, 1538*].

In all of these situations the reduction of the circulating erythrocyte mass is of course the limiting factor for the maximum volume of dextran which can be given. The same applies to plasma. We know of no clinical studies which prove the superiority of plasma preparations over a 6% solution of dextran 70.

In *shock due to burns,* plasma loss is most important. Thus this is an ideal application of plasma replacement substances, since in contrast to hemorrhagic shock oxygen transport is not jeopardized, even with infusion of larger amounts. There is no doubt that equally good initial results can be obtained with dextran as with plasma in this area [*79, 135, 232, 421, 422, 497, 578, 682, 789, 978, 1034, 1056, 1170, 1210, 1211, 1326, 1376, 1616, 1819*]. Administration of gamma globulins is recommended, since they are very important later in combatting infection [*888*].

In 1962 METCALF et al. [*1011*] reported on a *new type of dextran, called S-50*. This dextran is said to be synthesized directly into the desired molecular weight distribution ($\overline{M}_w = 65{,}000$) through streptococcus DS-50. It was tested in 34 patients; its characteristics correspond for the most part with dextran 70. The authors assume that the manufacturing costs for dextran S-50 would be lower than for the dextran available today. There have been no further reports on this subject.

**Dextran 40.** *Animal experiments:* In a shock experiment with loss of 40% of the BV in 40 dogs, LEPLEY [*880*] found that only 1 of 10 animals died which had been previously treated with dextran 40 (15%). In the dextran 75 (15%) group, 5 animals did not survive, and in the control group the number was 7. Before the shock period he had removed 1.5% of the bw in blood and replaced this with autologous blood, dextran 40 or 75. The experiments are not conclusive with regard to the superiority of dextran 40 over blood, since the infusion of 15% dextran creates a hypervolemic situation at the start. On the other hand, the experiments point out a superiority of dextran 40 over dextran 75 which is not fully explained on the basis of the volume effect (cf. also [*1470*]).

SCHENK et al. [*1257*] observed a mortality of 27% in the control group in a shock experiment with dogs; there were no fatalities after infusion of dextran 40 or 75. They observed "dramatic improvement in flow and blood pressure after a small volume of dextran had been infused. This response was never observed after blood or saline infusion". After loss of 50% of the BV, treatment with dextran 40 plus fibrinolysin (mortality 10%) proved to be more effective than infusions of 0.9% normal saline solution or dextran 40 (mortality 80%) or of fibrinolysin in physiological saline solution (mortality 50%). These experiments dealt with exchange transfusions rather than with actual shock experiments [*1261*].

EINHEBER and CARTER [*399*] tested the effect of equal amounts of blood and 10% dextran in hemorrhagic shock lasting for 8 hours. 4 monkeys received blood, 4 others dextran. Compared with those in the blood group, the 4 dextran animals were overtransfused by exactly 100%. Thus it is not astounding that all 4 animals died, compared with 2 in the blood group.

Blood pressure behavior shows that massive overtransfusion was present for after infusion of 57% of the total amount, the blood pressure no longer rose but fell continuously. 30 minutes after infusion the dextran animals had a Hct of 10; that of the blood animals was 45! The animals were not ventilated, and the invisible water loss was not replaced. It therefore seems clear that survival after receiving dextran 40 was impossible.

In another irreversible shock model, an exchange transfusion was made initially. After the BP dropped to 30 mm Hg, autologous blood, dextran 40, or 0.9% NaCl solution were infused and then the BP was dropped to 30 mm again [*996*]. In the saline and dextran groups the hemodilution was the same (Hct below 20%). In spite of this the dextran animals sustained a (probably significantly) larger volume loss than the animals in the saline and blood groups. In addition, irreversibility occurred earlier in the latter two groups ($p < 0.05$). The authors conclude from their experiments that the favorable effect of dextran 40 was not due to the volume effect alone, since the hemodilution in the saline group was the same. Furthermore, these experiments showed that the presence of dextran 40 in the blood prolongs the time available for correction of shock and creates greater tolerance with regard to blood loss.

In a classical shock model with dogs (BP = 50 mm Hg for 3 hours), retransfusion of 10% dextran 40 ($n = 15$) instead of autologous blood ($n = 15$) proved to be slightly superior (mortality 33% and 53%). On the basis of these experiments, Greenfield and Blalock [*557*] recommend combined use of blood and dextran 40 for treating hemorrhagic shock (see also [*891*]). Schumer [*1295*] also arrives at the same conclusions. The studies of Navarro [*1764*] are not conclusive since he used a special dextran 31 preparation in 5% dextrose in water (see also [*1787*]).

*Clinical results:* Bergentz et al. [*125*] recommend the use of dextran 40 for management of shock conditions in burns, crush injuries, sepsis and fat-embolism, and in other situations where capillary circulation is impaired (thromboses, vascular insufficiency, extracorporeal circulation, application of large doses of x-ray contrast media). In the original publication these indications are documented with clinical examples. Because of the rapid restoration of blood volume and cardiac output in hypovolemic conditions we have also recommended using dextran 40 for initial treatment of hemorrhagic shock until tested blood is available [*605*]; we well know that the flow improvement is due to the strong colloid osmotic effect (see [*936*]). This means that the blood volume is increased temporarily at the expense of interstitial fluid. At this time there is no reason to believe that this procedure is accompanied by any dangers, if the intravascularly displaced fluid is replaced in the next phase of treatment by infusion of a balanced electrolyte solution [*1564*]. A 10% dextran 40 solution exerts a colloid-osmotic effect double that of plasma. Because of this, infusion of a quantity of electrolyte solution equal to that of the dextran 40 is sufficient. As yet there is no evidence that this method is any more advantageous in the clinic than primary replacement therapy with PPS, albumin, or dextran 70 [*1837*]. Such a procedure appears justified on the basis of the considerations mentioned above with regard to the importance of capillary circulation. Such an opinion is based on theoretical consideration and experimental data.

Carey et al. [*259, 260*] and Kho [*1710*] have compared the effects of blood, albumin, plasma, saline solution and dextran 40 in shock patients. The most pronounced improvement in cardiac output, circulation time, arterial and venous pressure, $O_2$ consumption, $pO_2$ and peripheral resistance resulted with dextran 40. In 70 patients Baker et al. [*93, 94*] observed equally good results without observing complications caused by the dextran 40 therapy (cf. [*261, 289 a*]; see also Sections r and v).

### *x) Summary and Conclusions: Volume Replacement with Dextran*

1. Dextrans are polysaccharides built up of glucose molecules.

2. Dextran was introduced into clinical use in 1944. Since then many preparations with diverse physico-chemical properties, average molecular weight, molecular weight distribution, molecular structure, and concentration have been produced. Because of this it is very difficult to evaluate data in literature. There are several thousand publications about dextran; dextran 40 was introduced in 1961, and there are now over 1000 articles which deal with it.

3. In the following only those results will be considered which are valid for the two dextran preparations used most often today, 6% dextran 70 (Macrodex) and 10% dextran 40 (Rheomacrodex).

4. The colloid-osmotic effectivity of dextran is based on the fact that every intravascular gram of dextran binds about 20—25 ml $H_2O$.

5. A 3.5% solution of dextran 70 and a 2.5% solution of dextran 40 are approximately blood iso-oncotic.

6. The renal threshold is at a MW of approx. 50,000.

7. In the human organism dextran is completely broken down or excreted at a rate of approx. 70 mg/kg bw/24 hours.

8. Clinically used dextrans do not pass the placenta.

9. In humans the dextran-plasma concentration after infusions of 0.5 to 1.5 liter is approx. 0.5—1.5 g-%.

10. There is no basis for believing that dextran infusions impair renal function. When infusing large amounts of dextran 40, one must assure normal conditions of water and electrolyte balance, since this highly colloid osmotically active solution displaces interstitial fluid into the vascular system.

11. Changes in the renal tubuli in the sense of "osmotic nephrosis" have been described after infusion of dextran. These are of functional and temporary nature and do not impair renal function.

12. The dextran preparations (Macrodex and Rheomacrodex) now available have no antigenic effect in clinical use.

13. Allergic side-effects occur much less often with these preparations than they do after blood or plasma transfusions.

14. The sedimentation rate rises slightly after infusion of dextran 70; infusion of dextran 40 lowers it.

15. The disaggregating effect is strongest with dextran fractions of a MW between 30,000—40,000.

16. Increased blood and plasma viscosity can be reduced by infusion of dextran 40.

17. Under standard conditions dextran 40 and 70 do not influence blood group determination in any way.

18. There is no basis for believing that infusion of dextran causes cancer or influences infection defense mechanisms and nonspecific resistance in humans.

19. With the molecular weight distributions of present dextran 40 and 70, no shifts in the status of coagulation to a pathological degree can be measured, when dosages of 1.5 or 1 g/kg bw respectively are used in humans [*316*, *1084*].

Dextran 40 and especially dextran 70 definitely *reduce platelet adhesiveness*. This probably contributes to a considerable degree to the *antithrombotic effect* of dextran.

20. The influence of dextran on blood lipids has been investigated intensively for several years; the clinical importance of available results is not yet clear.

21. The clinical laboratory investigations, which are disturbed by the presence of dextran, are summarized in Section s).

22. Dextran solutions can be *stored* safely for 10 years under constant storage conditions. Defects in the containers limit storage capabilities. Dextran substance can be stored indefinitely.

23. The *volume effect* of a *dextran 70* infusion in *hypovolemic individuals* is initially somewhat more than the amount infused. After replacement of a given loss with the same amount of dextran 70, the BV remains normal until the body's own regulation mechanisms have completely replaced the blood or plasma loss.

The initial volume effect of *dextran 40* is almost twice the amount infused, but it does not last as long. About 3—4 hours after infusion, the volume effect is still about the same as the amount infused.

24. In hypovolemic persons infusions of dextran 40 and 70 bring about normalization of blood pressure, increase in cardiac output and venous return, reduction of peripheral resistance, and decrease in circulation time.

Dextran 40 in particular improves capillary circulation and tissue oxygenation at the same time. This is caused by the volume effect and probably also by specific properties of low molecular weight dextran.

25. A large number of experimental and clinical studies confirm that the effect of dextran solutions is at least as good as that of the best plasma preparations. Several million bottles of dextran 70 and dextran 40 have

been administered to date. Evidence of a better effect of dextran 40 compared with dextran 70 is lacking in initial clinical shock management.

26. Table 7 compares the most important advantages and disadvantages of PPS (or albumin) and dextran 70.

Table 7. *Advantages and disadvantages of PPS (or albumin) and dextran 70 in clinical shock therapy*

| | PPS or albumin | Dextran 70 |
|---|---|---|
| Allergic reactions | rare | rare |
| Influence on blood group determination | none | none |
| Influence on blood coagulation | none | slight in doses over 1 g/kg bw |
| Influence on laboratory investigations | none | in certain cases |
| Production | limited | unlimited |
| Price | expensive | inexpensive |
| Antithrombotic effect | absent | present |

## 2. Gelatin

### *a) Definition*

Of the artificial colloids in use today, gelatin was the first to be tested for its clinical usefulness [*719*]. However the investigations were soon terminated because gelatin preparations were difficult to sterilize, caused allergic reactions, and at room temperature were not fluid. Only later could these disadvantages be eliminated.

Today three types of gelatin preparations are available which differ from each other both in the raw material used and in the manner of production (cf. [*1677*]. For reviews regarding collagen and gelatin chemistry and production see [*1768, 1812*].

### *b) General Remarks Concerning Evaluation of Gelatin Literature*

Generally speaking, what has been said for dextran is valid here. The situation is more difficult however, because most gelatin preparations are not fractionated (due to difficulty in manufacture?) as are the dextrans; thus most of them are available as mixtures of very small and large molecules. Only scanty data concerning molecular weight can be found and usually only $\overline{M}_n$ is determined. For this reason the physico-chemical characterization is not accurately known, and any comparison with dextran made difficult. In addition older forms have much higher concentrations than the preparations available today. Thus data of older authors can not be compared readily with more recent results.

### *c) The Various Gelatin Preparations*

One can distinguish the following 3 main types:

*Oxypolygelatin (OPG):*

Developed in 1951 by CAMPBELL [*255*].

Preparation: Gelifundol (Biotest).

*Modified fluid gelatin (MFG):*

Introduced later by TOURTELOTTE [*1446, 1447, 1448*].

Preparations: Plasmagel (Roger Bellon), Plasmagel (Braun), Physiogel (SRC).

*Gelatin crosslinked by means of urea bridges:*

First described in 1962 by SCHMIDT-THOMÉ et al. [*1267*].

Preparation: Haemaccel (Hoechst).

*Gelifundol* (Biotest-Serum Institut GmbH, Frankfurt a. M.).

OPG in 0.9% NaCl solution.

| Conc. | Na mval/l | Cl mval/l |
|---|---|---|
| 5.6% | 154 | 154 |

$\overline{M}_w$=30,000 (30,000 reviewed in [*551*]). See Fig. 14 b!

$\overline{M}_n$=20,000 (see [*654*]) (15,000, reviewed in [*551*])

$$\frac{\overline{M}_w}{\overline{M}_n} = 2.0$$

$\eta_{rel}$=2.1 at 20° C (see [*654*])

pH=7.0

Colloid-osmotic pressure = 39 mm Hg.

Manufactured after thermal depolymerization by means of crosslinking.

For chemistry of OPG see [*1790*].

*Plasmagel* (B. Braun, Melsungen; Roger Bellon, Paris).

MFG in electrolyte solution.

| Conc. | Na mval/l | Ca mval/l | Cl mval/l |
|---|---|---|---|
| 3% | 120 | 27.0 | 147.0 |

$\overline{M}_w$=35,000

$\eta_{rel}$=2.2 (see [*865*]).

Colloid-osmotic pressure = 28.5 mm Hg,

Isoelectric point = 2.65,

Gel point = 5° C,

pH = 5.8.

Molecular weight distribution 10,000—100,000, 60% between 20,000 and 60,000 (see [*795*, *1096*]).

Technique of manufacture: "First a 6% solution is produced from a special gelatin made from cattle bone by gradual thermal degradation. The solution thus obtained is treated with succinic acid and the derivative is then isolated and purified. The final 3% solution is manufactured from this solution".

*Contraindications:* Coronary infarction, pulmonary embolism, fat embolism.

*Physiogel* (Swiss Red Cross, Bern).

MFG in electrolyte solution.

| Conc. | mval/l | | | | |
|---|---|---|---|---|---|
| | Na | Ca | Cl | K | Mg |
| 4.2% | 120 *<br>122 +<br>146 *** | 24 ** | 125 *<br>155 +<br>156 ***<br>160 ++ | 0.4 | 3.4 |

MW: greatly varying data:
20,000 (BEUTL [*154*]: osmotic pressure measurement)
22,600 (NITSCHMANN [*1088*])
25,600 (NITSCHMANN [*1087*])
27,000 *
30,000 (old prospectus SRC)
15,000—40,000 (HÄSSIG [*668*])

* Swiss specialty catalogue,

** of which 14 mval are protein-bound, 10 mval ultra-filterable. These data have been valid since 1964; previously Physiogel contained 50 mvl Ca/l [*154*].

*** prospectus SRC.

\+ Brochure Steril Catgut Ges., Neuhausen a. Rheinfall, Switzerland,

++ Personal information from Dr. Kistler, SRC.

$\overline{M}_w = 35{,}000$ [*551*]

$\overline{M}_n = 16{,}000$ (GRANATH [*551*]) $\frac{\overline{M}_w}{\overline{M}_n} = 2.2$

$\eta_{rel} = 2.2$ (see [*154*])

$|\eta| = 0.208$

pH = 7.20

The raw material is calf skin; modification takes place by means of thermal degradation and succinylation [*154*]. STOLL [*1822*] has recently reported that oxidation of gelatin lowers its gel point.

The gelatin in Physiogel is not fractionated and contains a small number of low molecular breakdown products; the MW spectrum is said to be rather broad [*154*]. According to BEUTL (personal information) the molecular weight distribution is between 10,000 and 50,000; after precipitation with ethanol he found fractions with a $\overline{M}_n$ of 15,000—36,000. See Fig. 14 b!

*Haemaccel* (Farbwerke Hoechst AG, Abt. Behring-Präparate, Frankfurt a. M.).

Gelatin in electrolyte solution.

| Conc. | mval/l Na | K | Ca | Cl |
|---|---|---|---|---|
| 3.5% | 145 | 5.1 | 12.5 | 162.6 |

$\overline{M}_w$ = 35,000 (35,000—45,000, GRANATH [*551*]). See Fig. 14 a!

$\overline{M}_n$ = 15,000 [*551*] $\frac{\overline{M}_w}{\overline{M}_n} = 2.3$

$\eta_{rel} = 1.75$

colloid osmotic pressure = 350—390 mm $H_2O$,
pH = 7.2—7.3
isoelectric point = 4.7 ± 0.3

The raw material is cattle bone gelatin with a MW of approx. 100,000. By means of thermal degradation, polypeptides with a MW of 12,000 to 15,000 are formed. Then by means of diisocyanate these are crosslinked to form molecules with urea bridges; the molecules have an average MW of 35,000 [*1267*].

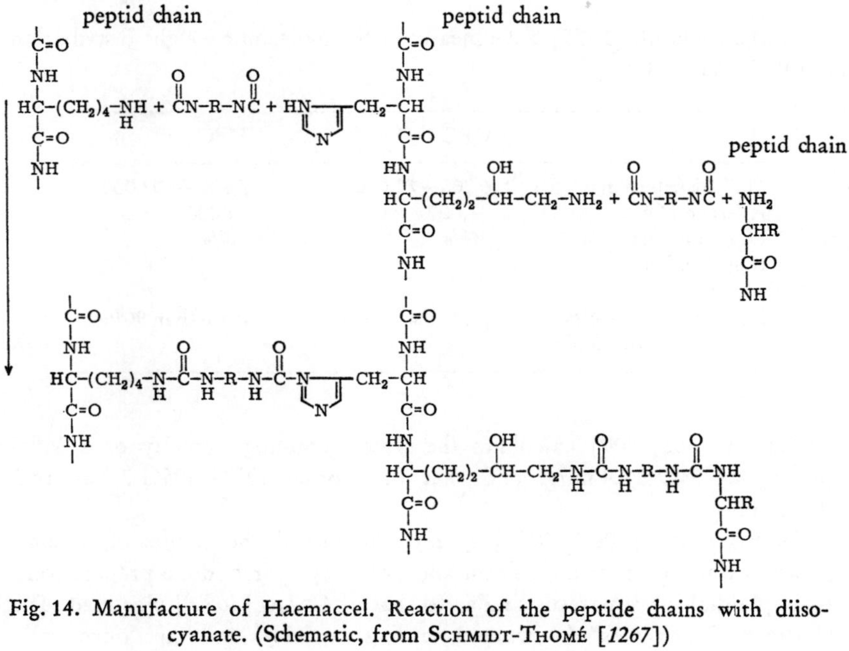


Fig. 14. Manufacture of Haemaccel. Reaction of the peptide chains with diisocyanate. (Schematic, from SCHMIDT-THOMÉ [*1267*])

*Contraindications:* Shock resulting from thrombo-embolism, coronary thrombosis, lung injury due to compression and massive fat embolism.

The best results regarding molecular weight distribution for the 3 types of gelatin available today are provided by GRANATH et al. [*551*]. See Table 7 a (p. 110).

## *d) Compatibility of Gelatin Preparations with Medications*

According to JULLIARD [*795*] *Plasmagel* can be *mixed* with phenobarbital, gallamine, piridosol, D-tubocurarin, procain and xylocain, though soluble precipitates form with chlorpromazine and promethazine.

*Haemaccel* can be *mixed* with normal saline, glucose and Ringer's solution, muscle relaxants, barbiturates, vasopressors, corticoids, vitamins, tetanus serum, penicillins and tetracyclines, so long as these are soluble in water (manufacturer's data, and [*183, 212, 549, 1216, 1322*]).

Because of the $Ca^{++}$ ion content, Plasmagel, Physiogel and Haemaccel should not be mixed with citrated blood and citrated plasma.

## *e) Colloid-Osmotic Pressure and Effect, Water Retaining Capacity (see also p. 66 f.)*

METCALF et al. [*1010*] have measured the molecular weight distribution of OPG and MFG:

| | OPG | MFG |
|---|---|---|
| MW distribution | 6,200—72,000 | 7,500—102,000 |
| Average MW | 31,000 | 34,000 |
| Low molecular portion, i. e. below 30,000 | 70% | 70% |
| Portion of molecules below renal threshold | more than 90% | more than 90% |

KALRA [*808, 809*] calculates the water retaining capacity of a MFG (Knox) as 39.0 ± 8.4 ml/g, and that of another MFG (MG-7) as 14.3 ± 1.12 ml/g.

NITSCHMANN [*1087, 1088*] recently published the results of a comparative study of dextran, gelatin and polyvinyl pyrrolidone preparations. A simple dialysis apparatus similar to that of CRAIG [*308 a*] was used. The "oncotic effectiveness" (= water retaining capacity) and the "oncotically active particle weight" of the preparation studied are provided by the balanced concentration between the plasma expander solution and a polyethylene glycol fraction. Ideal experimental conditions were by no means present (concentrations were too high!) and for this reason the results are unfortunately only of limited interest for characterization of these preparations. As the author himself states, the calculated particle weight may not be taken as the number-average molecular weight. Except for the well-fractionated dextran preparations the low molecular portions of the colloids studied leaked through the membrane and thus are not included. According to this the estimated $\overline{M}_n$ levels for gelatin are too high. See Table 7 a and Fig. 14 a, b!

Here as well only the conditions *in vivo* are of interest with regard to the "oncotic effectiveness". The results obtained must be correlated with the renal excretion and the water retaining capacity of the preparations (for

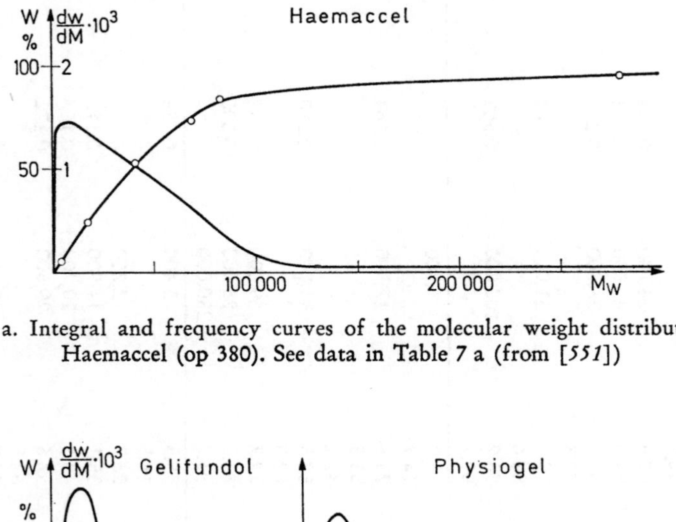


Fig. 14 a. Integral and frequency curves of the molecular weight distribution for Haemaccel (op 380). See data in Table 7 a (from [551])

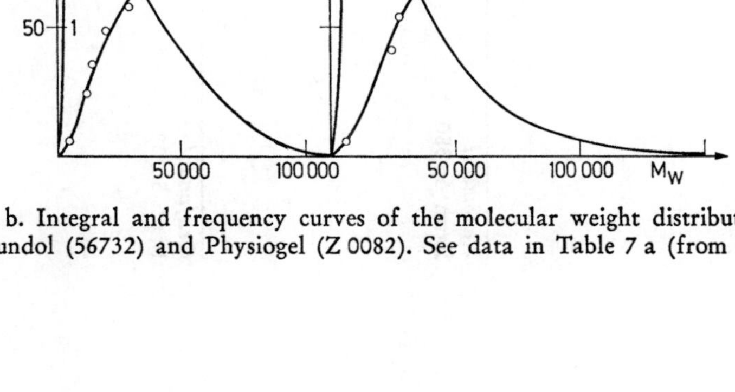


Fig. 14 b. Integral and frequency curves of the molecular weight distribution for Gelifundol (56732) and Physiogel (Z 0082). See data in Table 7 a (from [551])

Table 7 a. *Fractionation of Physiogel, Haemaccel and Gelifundol* (according to [*551*])

| Sample | Fraction size (%) | Cumulative weight fraction W % | $\overline{M}_w$ light scatt. | $\eta$, 20° dl/g | $\overline{M}_w$ calc. fr. distribution | $\overline{M}_n$ calc. fr. distribution | $\overline{M}_w/\overline{M}_n$ calc. |
|---|---|---|---|---|---|---|---|
| *Physiogel* | 11.5 | 5.7 | 6,200 | 0.082 | | | |
| Batch Z 0082 | 11.3 | 17.2 | | | | | |
| | 12.6 | 29.1 | | | | | |
| | 9.9 | 40.4 | 24,700 | 0.214 | | | |
| | 16.7 | 53.6 | 28,000 | 0.263 | | | |
| | 7.3 | 65.7 | 36,000 | 0.271 | | | |
| | 6.0 | 72.3 | | | 34,500 | 16,800 | 2.1 |
| | 8.9 | 79.8 | 51,000 | 0.364 | | | |
| | 8.9 | 88.6 | | | | | |
| | 6.3 | 96.2 | 100,000 | 0.502 | | | |
| | 0.6 | 99.7 | | | | | |
| *Haemaccel* | 11.5 | 5.8 | 4,300 | | | | |
| Batch op 380 | 6.5 | 14.7 | | | | | |
| | 11.6 | 23.8 | 17,500 | 0.144 | 66,500 * | 115,400 * | 4.3 |
| | 7.8 | 33.5 | | | | | |
| | 9.6 | 42.2 | | | | | |
| | 11.1 | 52.5 | 41,000 | 0.210 | | | |
| | 8.4 | 62.3 | | | | | |
| | 12.4 | 72.7 | 69,000 | 0.262 | | | |
| | 8.6 | 83.2 | 83,000 | 0.300 | | | |
| | 12.5 | 93.7 | 280,000 | | | | |
| *Gelifundol* | 10.7 | 5.3 | 5,400 | 0.056 | | | |
| Batch 56732 | 7.5 | 14.5 | | | | | |
| | 11.0 | 23.7 | 12,200 | | | | |
| | 11.8 | 35.1 | 14,500 | 0.117 | | | |
| | 14.3 | 48.1 | 20,200 | 0.167 | | | |
| | 4.5 | 57.6 | 29,600 | 0.172 | | | |
| | 6.2 | 62.9 | | | 28,700 | 15,100 | 1.9 |
| | 5.6 | 68.7 | 37,100 | | | | |
| | 8.9 | 76.0 | 41,500 | 0.217 | | | |
| | 9.5 | 85.3 | 52,300 | 0.261 | | | |
| | 8.1 | 94.0 | 66,000 | 0.296 | | | |
| | 1.9 | 99.0 | 100,000 | | | | |

* This batch of Haemaccel probably has, on account of the crosslinking process, a bimodal molecular weight distribution. A top fraction of 10% for Haemaccel op 300 gave $M_w$=140,000, thus indicating considerable variations between the batches studied.

Table 8. *Physico-chemical data of the most important gelatin preparations discussed in the literature*

| *Generic name* Trade name | Concen-tration | $\overline{M_w}$ | Molecular weight distribution Low mol. fr. 10% | peak fraction 10% | Electrolyte content in mval/l | Manufacturer |
|---|---|---|---|---|---|---|
| Gelifundol (OPG) | 5.6% | 30,000 | 5,400 [551] | 100,000 [551] | $Na^+$ 154<br>$Cl^-$ 154 | Biotest, Frankfurt |
| Plasmagel (MFG) | 3% | 35,000 to 40,000 | 10,000 | 100,000 | $Na^+$ 120<br>$Cl^-$ 147<br>$Ca^{++}$ 27 | Roger Bellon, Paris |
| Plasmagel (MFG) | 3% | 35,000 | — | — | $Na^+$ 120<br>$Cl^-$ 147<br>$Ca^{++}$ 27 | Braun, Melsungen |
| Physiogel (MFG) | 4.2% | 27,000 *<br>35,000 [551] | 10,000<br>6,200 [551] | 50,000<br>100,000 [551] | * | SRC, Bern |
| Haemaccel | 3.5% | 35,000 | 4,300 [551] | 280,000 | $Na^+$ 145<br>$K^+$ 5.1<br>$Ca^{++}$ 12.5<br>$Cl^-$ 162.5 | Hoechst-Behringwerke, Marburg/Lahn |

* see text.

dextran: 40 ml/g or 27 ml/g in vitro, 20—25 ml/g in vivo) in order to allow any predictions about the oncotic effect in vivo. This applies especially to gelatin and PVP preparations. Compared with Macrodex and Rheomacrodex their molecular weight distribution is very broad and they are excreted rapidly [*551*]. For example 75% of the Physiogel infused, 21% of the Macrodex and 54% of the Rheomacrodex was found in the urine of rabbits 5 hours after infusion. Thus it is evident that there is no justification for the conclusions drawn by LUNDSGAARD-HANSEN [*924, 925, 1738*] from the results of NITSCHMANN concerning the in vivo effect of gelatin. LUNDSGAARD [*925 a*] states that the results of NITSCHMANN for the dextran "were checked and confirmed *in the meantime* by the manufacturer" (which one?). However it will be noted that the figures for $\overline{M_n}$ of dextran preparations have been known for many years [*575, 1376*].

### *f) Metabolism*

About half of the OPG infused is found again in the urine [*1115*]. Nothing definite is known about breakdown in vivo [*808, 809*] since no one has yet been successful in tagging the individual amino acids in gelatin preparations [*654*]. An investigation with 42 patients [*718*] reveals that only small amounts are broken down during the first 72 hours (the gelatins had a $\overline{M}_w$ of 37,266—59,254). BRUNSCHWIG [*220*] attempted to use gelatin solutions for parenteral nutrition; assuming that at least a portion was broken down. Now, however gelatin preparations are not used for this purpose for the major portion is lost much too quickly through the kidneys, and there is no proof that gelatin can be directly utilized in the organism. Repeated infusion of OPG causes an increase of sulphthalein bromide retention [*1115*].

LEVINSON [*882 a*] believes that gelatin infusion retards protein synthesis.

According to CZOK [*326*] growth of rabbits, but not of rats, is retarded by weekly physiological doses of MFG. DETRICK [*1645*] too observed physical deterioration and illness of rabbits after long term administration of OPG.

Using hydroxyproline and radioactive gelatin [*1854*] determinations several investigators [*446, 479, 1006, 1027*] have demonstrated that the major portion of an infusion (500—1000 ml) of *Haemaccel* is excreted in the urine during the first 24 hours. 74% and 87% of the amount infused could be found after 4 and 10 days respectively [*679*].

### *g) Plasma Concentrations, Excretion in Urine, Renal Function*

ARDRY [*64*] has reported on a colorimetric determination method for gelatin (cf. [*882 a*]).

After infusion of 100 ml *5% gelatin* in normovolemic individuals HOFFMANN and KOZOLL [*718*] found a plasma concentration of 0.78 g-%

at the end of the infusion; 24 hours later it was 0.3 g-%. Only 55% of the gelatin infused was found in the vascular system at the end of the infusion, 23% had been excreted in urine, and 22% had filtered into the tissues (see also [*780*]).

Frawley [*464*], Gabor [*483*] and Metcalf et al. [*1009*] measured plasma concentrations of 20% and 25% of the initial level 6 hours after infusion of equal amounts of OPG or MFG in normovolemic individuals (cf. [*255*, *707*]. During the Korean War, dextran (probably with a $\overline{M}_w$ of 42,000) and MFG with an average MW of 34,500 were compared in 26 wounded soldiers. The plasma concentrations of the two plasma expanders were approximately the same (for clinical effectiveness, see p. 131 f.).

It seems important that the rate of excretion and the volume effect in hypovolemic individuals correspond to that of normovolemic individuals (cf. [*639*]). It has repeatedly been assumed that gelatin causes a better volume effect in seriously injured individuals than in slightly hypovolemic or normovolemic persons [*925*].

Muschaweck and Benoit [*1069*] determined the "half-life" of *Haemaccel* in 6 rats and 5 dogs. This is the time which has elapsed when only half of the original concentration remains. However, since Haemaccel can not be determined quantitatively in the blood [*1854*], the authors measure hydroxyproline [*1854*], which makes up 14.5% of the Haemaccel substance. There is, however, no data confirming that the hydroxyproline content and the Haemaccel concentration run parallel in the blood. For this reason, the results are not conclusive. 4 hours after infusion the hydroxyproline level was 50%, whereby pronounced scattering is evident in the dog experiments. Similar results were obtained in humans [*679*]; after 12 hours 27% of the hydroxyproline was still found, and after 48 hours, none (see also [*267*]). 74% of the Haemaccel infused was excreted in the urine in 4 days [*679*].

Little [*906*] has measured the capillary permeability for a *6—8% (Knox) gelatin* in the traumatized intestine of dogs. 35—60% of the plasma gelatin was found extravascularly, but the technical difficulties were great. Rieger [*1787*] has shown that the elimination of $^{131}$I-labelled Physiogel is extremely high. 30 min after injection into dogs only 30% and at 6 hours 6.5% remained in the blood (see also [*1811*]).

*Renal function:* After administration of gelatin expanders in rats, the phenolsulfonphthalein test showed significantly reduced renal function which returns to normal within 6 days. Control experiments with rat serum do not show impaired renal function [*564*, *565*, *566*, *567*].

Raisz [*1156*] and Gropper [*578*, *579*] have compared the renal function in normovolemic and hypovolemic dogs after infusion of *5% OPG* and 6% dextran. The excretion of both colloids was highly dependent on the state of hydration of the animals (cf. also [*833*]). From this work it would appear that dextran restores glomerular filtration and renal plasma flow more quickly, better, and for a longer period than gelatin does.

HOWARD [*731*], MICHIE [*1016*] and RAVDIN [*1160*] have observed no important disadvantages of gelatin infusions with regard to canine and human renal function (however for Gelifundol a decreased kidney function was observed [*692 a, 1713*], for Haemaccel cf. [*1027, 1069, 1713*]). A definite natriuresis occurs in normovolemic individuals after infusion of 500 to 1000 ml MFG or Haemaccel [*303, 446, 536, 1006, 1259, 1811*].

The excretion of gelatin is also proportional to its molecular weight [*718, 1680*]. Urine concentrations up to 15 g/ml were observed after infusion of a 5% preparation; the authors maintain that the urine viscosity reaches levels which could temporarily disturb renal function.

After chronic administration of *MFG*, water excretion in rats is clearly restricted in a high percentage of cases [*326*].

A noticeable increase in diuresis is often described in connection with all types of gelatin preparations [*44, 240, 303, 326, 395 a, 464, 808, 882 a, 1006, 1009, 1156*]. This increase is caused by the rapid excretion of a large part of the amount infused. In our studies on the volume effect of gelatin and dextran preparations we have determined that there is a marked increase in diuresis, especially after infusion of *Physiogel* [*589*] (see Fig. 15).

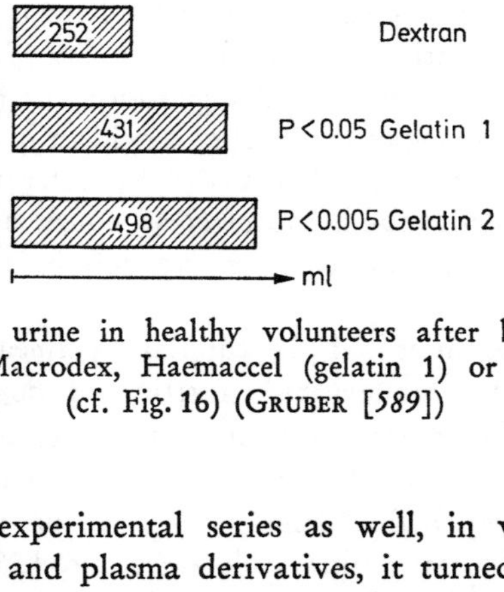


Fig. 15. Excretion of urine in healthy volunteers after bleeding (400 ml) and infusion of 500 ml Macrodex, Haemaccel (gelatin 1) or Physiogel (gelatin 2) (cf. Fig. 16) (GRUBER [*589*])

In our second experimental series as well, in which we compared gelatin, dextran 40 and plasma derivatives, it turned out that Physiogel caused the greatest diuresis. At the request of the Swiss Red Cross, similar studies were made with a larger group of volunteers [*600*]. Although the conditions for scientific investigations were difficult in a military situation, the result was the same. Every volunteer who received 500 ml Physiogel after removal of 400 ml blood showed excessive diuresis. LUNDSGAARD-HANSEN [*925*] would like to have our data interpretated with caution and thus stresses what we have stated in the discussion of our paper: "These studies confirm that only simultaneous, combined, direct measurement of the blood volume and urine excretion can provide information about the clinical usefulness of a plasma replacement substance when molecular size, and structure and concentration of the preparations used cause behavior different to that caused by human plasma." Later, the opinion was expressed [*303*] that the renal effect of Physiogel could be quite advantageous for protection of a shock kidney as long as fluid and saline supply are assured. This is pertinent, though in catastrophe and war situations, an adequate fluid supply is often impossible.

After infusion of Physiogel in normovolemic individuals, COTTIER and associates [*303*] observed no significant changes in glomerular filtration (inulin clearance) and in renal plasma flow (NaPAH clearance); on the other hand MERTZ [*1006*] found an increase in both figures for Haemaccel (see also [*1080, 1694*]).

## *h) Histological Studies*

In the cells of the convoluted tubules in rats, rabbits and mice, administration of *OPG, MFG* and *Haemaccel* causes reversible vacuolic change in the cytoplasm whilst OPG and Haemaccel cause a swelling and desquamation of the cells of the tubuli recti I. Furthermore, paraprotein particles were found after Haemaccel; these lead to cell destruction. Permanent injury could not be determined [*302, 567, 659 a, 660, 817, 1069*], however in DETRICK's study [*1645*] these changes were not reversible 14 days after administration.

MOREHEAD [*1046*] reports that repeated administration of gelatin in dogs causes atherosclerotic changes and interstitial nephritis. Renal swelling with changes in the tubuli was found in autopsy in 23 patients who had received gelatin [*1353*]. The renal changes observed are probably an osmotic nephrosis; this is similar to the situation after infusion of glucose, mannitol and dextran (see p. 77) where there are likewise no functional consequences. The other disturbances are unexplained. CZOK [*326*] has observed swelling of Kupffer's cells, deposit of fat in the liver, and beginning regeneration of the lobes of the liver in rats after gelatin administration (see also [*1115*]).

Many authors have noticed no morphological changes in liver, spleen and heart after administration of various gelatin preparations [*181, 302, 565, 566, 903, 1069, 1711*]. HÖLSCHER [*1694*] investigated a modified Haemaccel solution ($\overline{M}_n$ 30,000 instead of 24,000) and observed in rats a slight dilatation of the renal tubuli.

## *i) Immunological Studies*

In 6 rabbits no antibody formation could be caused with a 6—8% gelatin developed in India [*808*].

MAURER [*975, 976*] has shown that gelatins as well as *OPG* produce antibodies in humans, and that spontaneous gelatin antibodies occur in humans and in animals. HARRFELDT [*654*] never observed development of sensitivity after repeated s. c. injection in 50 patients; in 190 patients the compatibility was good.

*MFG* is not considered antigenic [*302, 326, 865, 973*]. In his survey on plasma replacement substances, however, THOMPSON [*1430*] writes that it is still important to consider that serum disease might occur with the use of gelatin solutions.

Whereas raw gelatin caused antibody formation in rabbits, the injection of Haemaccel in rabbits and guinea pigs had no such results. According to the method of MAURER gelatin antibodies could be demonstrated in the serum of healthy and ill individuals (especially with PCP), with raw gelatin and with Haemaccel. The latter caused a drop in the level of serum antibodies. The authors conclude that Haemaccel is similar to a hapten [*113, 1303*].

Other researchers have likewise found no antigenic properties in Haemaccel [*469, 479, 1130*]. Review in [*1812*].

### *k) Allergic Reactions*

After infusion of 500 ml *MFG* each in 10 individuals, 1 patient collapsed and developed an erythema which disappeared within 3 days [*303*]. TSCHIRREN [*1461*] used *Physiogel* in 29 cases and observed no side effects. Most of the patients were under anesthesia and in several cases were infused because massive hemorrhage could not be stopped. Thus these data on the compatibility of MFG can not reveal much. In another series, urticaria occurred in 2 of 68 patients [*1565*].

We ourselves observed side effects in 2 out of 10 slightly hypovolemic recruits who received Physiogel [*601*]; in another series with 10 volunteers there were no reactions [*589*]. On the other hand, the infusion of a 7.7% Physiogel solution which had been placed at our disposal by the SRC for experimental purposes, had such a bad effect on all volunteers that the experiment had to be stopped. Nausea, perspiration, sneezing, injected conjunctiva, paleness, coughing, urticaria, formication and acrocyanosis occurred. It could not be determined whether these symptoms were the expression of a pronounced erythrocyte aggregation. From animal experiments, however, it is known that similar symptoms occur after infusion of large amounts of colloids with strongly aggregating properties. In the chapter on the influence of dextran on the sedimentation rate (p. 78 f.), it has already been stated that the aggregating tendency is much greater for gelatin than for dextran.

Secondary reactions also occurred in a study by EBERLEIN [*375*] in 4 of 8 volunteers. They had received 500 ml *Haemaccel* in 10 minutes i. v. after bleeding. 2 persons complained of a sense of pressure, coughing or sneezing tendency respectively, difficulty in breathing, or tingling. With two others, spotty erythema with numerous wheals and moderate itching occurred after infusion of only 200 ml. 1 hour after termination of the infusion the symptoms had subsided without therapy.

FREUCHEN [*469*] observed temperature rise in 10% of the cases, and BARK [*105*] reports urticarial symptoms. The majority of authors recorded no side effects with several hundred infusions each (up to 6.5 l per patient) [*256, 268, 395 a, 420, 446, 479, 622, 679, 772, 818, 915, 1006, 1027, 1063*].

### *l) Influence on Sedimentation Rate, Aggregating and Disaggregating Properties*

As already explained in the chapter on dextran (p. 79), the *critical concentration* (that concentration of a certain colloid which causes a SR of 1 mm/h and causes microscopically visible rouleaux formation) is reached more quickly with gelatin fractions having a much lower molecular weight than dextran. The first thorough study in this field was made by THORSÉN and HINT [*1440*]. They showed that the *critical molecular weight*, i. e. the lowest MW of a colloid at which aggregation occurs, is 18,000 for gelatin, but 59,000 for dextran. Gelatins with a MW of about 35,000 (like Haemaccel) cause approximately the same acceleration of sedimentation [*183, 395, 469, 1080, 1120*] as dextran fractions of the *same* concentration with a MW of 75,000 (the gelatins on the market have a lower concentration!). Thus the conclusion is justified that gelatin preparations influence the suspension stability and in turn the blood sedimentation rate much more strongly than dextrans [*707, 714, 1569*].

The sedimentation accelerating effect of various gelatin preparations leads to rouleaux formation and is marked compared with other colloids; it has been described by many investigators in humans and animals, in vitro [*181, 632, 769, 882 a, 934, 1569*] and in vivo [*569, 1115*].

ZAHLER [*1566*] studied these relationships for *Physiogel* and arrived at the same results. On the other hand his comparative studies with dextran are hard to interpret for, as it often happens [*397*], he investigated unequal concentrations of unequal colloids in unequal solvents.

### *m) Influence on Viscosity (cf. p. 80 f.)*

The influence of Plasmagel, Physiogel and Haemaccel on plasma viscosity in vitro and in vivo was studied by LARCAN [*1722*], SCHÜLKE [*1294*], STOLL [*1823*] and ZAHLER [*1566*]. In vitro these preparations cause a slight increase in plasma and blood viscosity. The relationship for the plasma viscosity in vivo are documented with figures for Haemaccel only [*1294*]. Results with regard to the behavior of blood viscosity over a certain period after infusion of various amounts of gelatin preparations with various shear rates which occur in the organism (viscosimeter by Gregersen, Merrill-Wells, Dintenfass) are clinically important, but such results are not available.

The comparative studies by ZAHLER [*1566*] again offer little, for the reasons already mentioned (see p. 117), and the conclusions which the author draws from his in vitro experiments can not be accepted. He maintains, for example, that the infusion of 750 ml saline solution after blood loss of 1.5 l would reduce the viscosity better than colloidal infusion solutions, although this amount of normal saline would not even remain in the vascular system!

### *n) Influence on Blood Group Determination*

Pseudoagglutination with older gelatins has been described [*384, 1679*]. KOOP et al. [*836*] state that addition of a drop of glycine solution to the test system prevents difficulties in determining blood groups caused by infusion of gelatin solutions.

After infusion of Haemaccel, BÖHMERT [*183*] twice observed pseudo-agglutination. However the majority of authors are of the opinion that the gelatin solutions available do not make blood group determination difficult [*59, 469, 479, 549, 1371, 1825*].

### *o) Influence upon Defence against Infection and Nonspecific Resistance*

In amounts up to 2.5% of the bw in white mice, MFG causes no functional impairment of the RES [*239*]. The serum bactericidal activity is impaired by neither Physiogel nor Haemaccel [*155*] (cf. also p. 82 and [*391*]).

In dogs older preparations were administered i. v. for 1—2 weeks; toxic effects such as impairment of protein synthesis, loss of weight, and sometimes death were observed [*1203 a*].

### *p) Carcinogenicity*

There are no studies which suggest that gelatin solutions have a carcinogenic effect or influence metastasis formation (cf. also "Histological Studies", p. 115).

### *q) Influence on Blood Coagulation*

In older and one recent [*1739*] article prolongation of bleeding time, coagulation time and prothrombin time was observed in dogs after gelatin was used ([*633, 780, 882 a*], cf. also [*483*]).

Bludau [*181*] observed a prolonged coagulation time from 55 to 70 sec in 3 rabbits after infusion of Plasmagel.

Tschirren [*1461*] observed fibrinolysis in 3 patients who received Physiogel. After infusion of 500 ml (14 patients) or 1000 ml (1 patient) of Haemaccel, there was no great change in prothrombin and antithrombin times after 24 and 72 hours; on the other hand, a reduction of thrombocytes occurred immediately after infusion and lasted for 4 hours. This could not be explained by dilution [*679, 1847 a*].

Other authors observed no particular influence on blood coagulation after infusion of an Indian gelatin preparation [*808*] or after infusion of Plasmagel or Haemaccel [*97, 99, 113, 212, 267, 395, 395 a, 419, 445 b, 479, 1080, 1109, 1129, 1672, 1760, 1841 a*].

### *r) Pharmacological Properties*

Haimovici [*633*] created experimental thrombi in 12 dogs. In 2/3 of the cases he determined that gelatin has an antithrombotic effect when it is administered prophylactically, but not when it was infused after the thrombi had formed. The manufacturers provide no data about other specific pharmacological effects of gelatin preparations.

### *s) Stability during Storage*

The average MW of Physiogel remains unchanged after 4 years of storage at 10—15° C. Clouding or flake formation never occurred [*154, 1835*]. Haemaccel may be stored for 3 years [*1765*]. For Gelifundol data are available for 150 days [*1804*].

### *t) The Volume Effect of Gelatin*

**Animal Experiments.** Using the Evans blue method in dogs, Elder [*405*] observed a plasma volume increase after infusion of a *3% MFG* solution comparable to 5% human albumin. He does not provide precise figures.

Knutson [*833*] and Kalra [*809*] observed that a 6% gelatin solution or an MFG preparation was less effective than 6% dextran for maintaining the blood volume.

Steinbrunn [*1382*] has compared hemodilution of rabbits after exchange transfusions of 20 ml blood/kg b.w. with the same volume of Physiogel, dextran 40 and 70 and Ringer's solution. In contrast to dextran hemodilution immediately after infusion of Physiogel corresponded to the levels after infusion of Ringer's solution. 30 minutes after the exchange it was identical with that of the control animals which received no replacement. In addition there was a tendency toward metabolic acidosis with a simultaneous rise in creatinin. A drop in hematocrit from 42% (±5) to

35% (±2.7) was determined 2 hours after infusion of 10 ml of Haemaccel/kg bw in rabbits [*1069*].

Lutz [*937, 1739*] observed a clearly smaller volume effect with Haemaccel and Gelifundol than with dextran 75 and 60 in dogs. For OPG see [*1622, 1762*].

**Human Studies.** A survey of the volume effect of various gelatin preparations in normo- and hypovolemic individuals is found in *Tables 9 and 10*, p. 121 and 122.

In a comparative study with 26 normovolemic patients, *5% gelatin* produced a weaker initial volume effect of shorter duration than 6% dextran did [*761, 1012*].

45 minutes after infusion of 500 ml *OPG* (Gelifundol) in 12 normovolemic individuals, Heidland [*692 a*] observed an increase in volume which corresponded to the amount infused; the scattering, however, was quite large (see also [*1604*].

Elder [*405*] compared the volume effect of *3% MFG* with that of plasma. Precise information concerning the method and technique of the experiment are not provided; therefore one must regard the figures given with caution: i. e. continuing retention of MFG up to 91% after 4 hours and to 80% after 12 hours (levels for plasma 94% and 114%) (see also [*1160*]).

With 7 patients Julliard [*795*] measured a volume increase of 460 ml after termination of infusion of 500 ml Plasmagel (Roger Bellon); after 4—5 hours an increase of 300 ml was measured. He further states that s. c. infusion (with addition of hyaluronidase) produces practically the same results as i. v. application. This would mean that the effect of a 3% MFG solution corresponds for the most part to that of an electrolyte solution. The same authors also describe one of the few documented burn cases which have been treated with MFG. The patient suffered burns over 60% of his body surface. 48 hours after the accident, i. e. after the shock phase, the patient received therapy consisting of 1 bottle of MFG along with electrolyte and glucose infusion for 4 days; after 2 months the patient was discharged. No data is given concerning the degree of burn. The same authors report on the successful use of 500 bottles of MFG in French territory, but they do not provide data concerning its effectiveness.

Moeller [*1027*] has observed a Hct decline for 6 hours after infusion of *Haemaccel* in humans. Freuchen [*469*] was able to demonstrate a volume increase on the basis of erythrocyte counts in only 61% of the cases. The results of Giomini [*528*] are hard to evaluate; the data in the text and the curves (conflicting number of cases) only allow the conclusion that the volume effect of Haemaccel immediately after infusion of 1000 ml does not correspond to the amount infused (see also [*1110*]; for Physiogel cf. [*303*]).

Table 9. *Volume effect of gelatin preparations in normovolemic individuals*

| Author | Year | Ref. | Preparation | Method | *n* | Amount in ml | Duration of inf. in min | Volume increase in ml hrs after infusion 0 | 1 | 6 | 24 | |
|---|---|---|---|---|---|---|---|---|---|---|---|---|
| Hyde, G. M. | 1952 | [*761*] | 5% gelatin | $^{32}P$ | 7 | 500 | 60 | 960 | 935 | 647 | 152 | |
| Hunzinger, W. A. | 1954 | [*754*] | Oxypolyn (OPG) | single RIHSA inj. | 2 | 1000 | 20—30 | 970 | — | 0 | — | Zero level reached after 4 hrs |
| Metcalf, W. | 1954 | [*1009*] | OPG | T 1824 | 12 | 1000 | ? | 700 | — | 230 | 0 | |
| | | | MFG | T 1824 | 12 | 1000 | ? | 700 | — | 330 | 0 | |
| Lutz, J. | 1959 | [*934*] | 6% gelatin (E. Merck) | T 1824 | 16 | 1000 | 40—50 | 546 | — | 312 (4 hr level) | | |
| Froeschlin, W. | 1962 | [*479*] | Haemaccel | T 1824 | 22 | 500 | ? | 350 | — | 350 | (*n*=2) | These may have been hypovolemic patients |
| | | | | | 20 | 1000 | ? | 505 | — | 630 | (*n*=8) | |
| | | | | | 12 | 1500 | ? | — | — | 750 | | |
| Göltner, E. | 1964 | [*536*] | Plasmagel (Braun) | T 1824 | 15 | 500 | 30 | — | 394 | — | — | |
| | | | | | 15 | 1000 | 60 | — | 675 | — | — | |
| Schneider, K. W. | 1965 | [*1276*] | Haemaccel | T 182· | 14 | 1000 | ? | 499 | — | — | — | |
| | | | | $^{51}Cr$ | 12 | 1000 | ? | 355 | — | — | — | |

Table 10. *Volume effect of gelatin preparations in hypovolemic individuals*

| Author | Year | Ref. | Preparation | Method | *n* | Amount in ml | Duration of inf. in min | Volume increase in ml hrs after infusion 0 | 1 | 2—4 | 6 | 12 | 24 |
|---|---|---|---|---|---|---|---|---|---|---|---|---|---|
| Gruber, U. F. | 1962 | [*589*] | Haemaccel | RIHSA | 10 | 500 | 30 | 350 | — | 250 | — | — | — |
| Gruber, U. F. | 1962 | [*589*] | Physiogel | RIHSA | 10 | 500 | 30 | 360 | — | 180 | — | — | — |
| Havers, L. | 1964 | [*679*] | Haemaccel | RIHSA | 5 | 1000 | 30 | 920 | — | 840 | — | — | — |
| Ahnefeld, W. F. | 1965 | [*14*] | Haemaccel | RIHSA | 30 | 500 | 15 | 285 | 264 | 245 | — | — | — |
| Gruber, U. F. | 1965 | [*601*]* | Physiogel 4.2% | RIHSA | 9 | 500 | 30 | 480 ** | — | 390 | — | — | — |
| | | | Physiogel 7.7% (experimental preparation) | RIHSA | 4 | 500 | 30 | 710 ** | — | 350 | — | — | — |

* In this work only the percentages of increase, based on the initial volume, are given.
** In fully hydrated individuals.

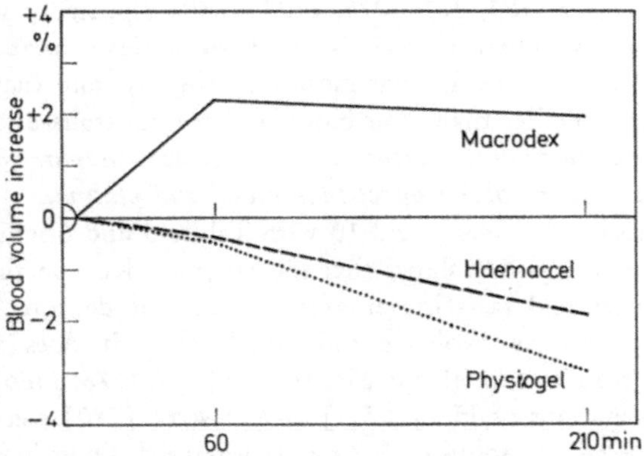


Fig. 16. Volume increase after bleeding (400 ml) and infusion of 500 ml of 6% dextran (Macrodex), Haemaccel or Physiogel. Difference between Macrodex and Physiogel after 210 min is statistically probably significant ($p$ less than 0.05). Same experimental protocol and means of demonstration as in Fig. 6 (GRUBER [*589*])

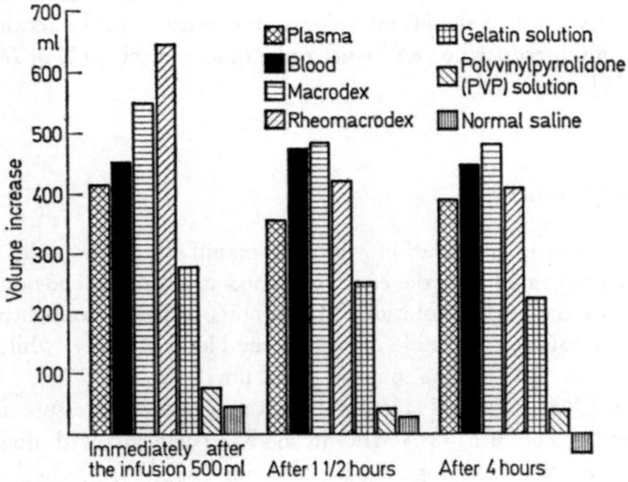


Fig. 16 a. AHNEFELD, HALMAGYI and ÜBERLA [*14*] conducted a series of experiments to compare the volume effects of four commercially available preparations currently offered as "plasma expanders" with autologous blood and plasma protein solution. 170 male volunteers of comparable size, age and weight were divided into five control groups and four test groups, the latter each consisting of 30 subjects. From every volunteer, with the exception of those in one control group, 400 ml of blood was withdrawn. Then, in the test groups, 500 ml of Rheomacrodex, Macrodex, Haemaccel or Polyvinylpyrrolidone solution was infused. The control groups received 500 ml of autologous blood, pasteurised plasma protein solution or normal saline. One control group was bled (400 ml) without any replacement. Blood volume determinations were performed prior to, immediately after as well as $1^1/_2$ and 4 hours after the infusion. (Diagram drawn after figures from AHNEFELD et al.)

Various authors [*183, 212, 1028, 1109, 1259*] repeatedly stress that an overtransfusion with Haemaccel is hard to achieve, that the venous pressure does not rise at all, or at most very slightly, and that the burden on circulation is smaller than after blood and plasma transfusions.

*All of these statements indicate that the gelatin preparations available today cause a smaller volume effect than blood and plasma.*

A comparison of Tables 9 and 10 with Tables 5 and 6 which deal with dextran (p. 95 and p. 96) shows that the volume effect, on the average, is initially stronger and lasts longer after infusion of dextran 40 or 70 in normovolemic and hypovolemic individuals than it does with gelatin preparations (see Fig. 6, p. 45 and Fig. 16, 16 a), (cf. [*578, 1466*]).

The investigations of Hyde [*761*] and Janota [*780*] were made with a 5% and 8% gelatin solution. $^{32}P$ tracer was used. Only in these experiments was there an excessive volume reaction which lasted for several hours. It is conceivable that with these high gelatin concentrations erythrocytes were "trapped" intravascularly and thus brought about high blood volume levels. Other technical problems (free $^{32}P$) must also be considered. In all other cases the volume at the end of the infusion barely reached or fell markedly short of the initial volume, and after a few hours the volume effect was much reduced or no longer to be observed (cf. [*523 a, 1682, 1684, 1713, 1811*]).

### *u) Hemodynamics*

Using a gelatin preparation which he manufactured himself, Wolfson [*1551*] demonstrated that the effect on blood pressure depends on the concentration of the gelatin solution. In 3 rabbits suffering from hemorrhagic shock, a 5% solution was able to restore the blood pressure, whilst a 2.5% solution and an 0.9% saline solution could not.

Kalra [*808*] observed a temporary rise in blood pressure in several cases after infusion of 6—8% MFG in shock experiments with dogs. In half of these splenectomized dogs the BP was only 68 ± 4% of the initial level 4 hours after the infusion; in all others the BP was maintained.

Gordon et al. [*540*] showed that an *8—10% gelatin* solution assumes an intermediate position between the effect of blood and glucose-saline solution with regard to restoration of BP. This is documented in further studies with other gelatin solutions [*81, 578, 661, 780, 927*] (cf. previous and following sections).

Some authors are unable to determine a difference in blood pressure after infusion of gelatin in shock, compared with other colloids [*240, 578, 925, 925 a*]. However one must realize that normalization of BP is not synonymous with restoration of volume. Lundsgaard [*925, 925 a*] argues that the difference in BV effect of 5—10% between dextran and gelatin has a detrimental effect on hemodynamics only when small quantities of expanders are used, i. e. with marked undertransfusion. It is known however that volume deficits up to 30% can be accompanied by normal blood pressure in humans. Such patients react with a drastic drop in BP when subjected to the slightest additional stress such as change of position during x-ray or on the operating table [*114*, *997*, *998*].

The influence of a plasma expander on cardiac output and the improvement of capillary circulation are important for evaluating the circulatory effect of that substance. There are only very few studies concerning this with regard to gelatin preparations in humans. (For venous pressure see previous section.)

After infusion of 500 ml Haemaccel in blood donors, Eberlein [*375*] recorded the pressure in the A. femoralis and in the V. mediana cubiti, as well as ECG, pulse pressure curve and blood pressure after RR. 10 minutes after infusion, BP amplitude and pulse frequency were identical with the initial levels.

Killian [*818*] has documented the effect of Haemaccel in 20 shock patients by means of BP levels and oscillograms.

After infusion of 20 ml/kg b.w. of *Plasmagel* in normovolemic patients, Staib [*1377*] found a significant rise in cardiac output which lasted for 1 hour. Careful circulatory analyses by K. Schmidt [*1265*] show that Haemaccel causes only an insignificant increase in cardiac output compared to dextran 40 and 70. No such studies have been published with regard to Physiogel.

There is no data concerning any specific flow-improving effect of the gelatin preparations available today. Nor do we know of any experiments under strictly controlled conditions which would show that gelatin solutions improve the impaired circulation in the capillaries caused by shock, apart from the transient volume effect. (Controlled conditions would entail comparison with other colloids of equal oncotic pressure, such as albumin.) Nor are there any measurements of the partial oxygen pressure in tissues. Since gelatin solutions exert no disaggregating effect but rather promote cell aggregation, a pronounced increase in tissue perfusion is not to be expected. Quantitative measurements of cell aggregation in vivo can only be made with great technical difficulty; the phenomenon hardly occurs in clinical experience because most of the gelatin is eliminated so quickly that the necessary concentrations scarcely occur in the organism.

### *v) Therapeutic Results*

**Animal Experiments.** Waters [*1490*] compared a 7% isinglass solution in 2 dogs with a *7% gelatin* in two others; the result was the same for both solutions. In a combined shock-exchange transfusion model in dogs, Parkins et al. [*1116, 1117*] obtained better results with 3% MFG than with 6% dextran (Commercial Solvents Corp., Lots 84,652 A and 84,686 A; MW unknown; it was probably dextran 80 with a peak fraction up to 200,000). For 1 hour the blood pressure was maintained at 30—35 mm Hg, whereupon the blood removed (initial bleeding volume = $H_1$) was replaced by an equal amount of the test substance. 3 hours ($H_2$) and 24 hours ($H_3$) later the animals were bled to a BP of 20 mm Hg; after the second bleeding, the blood removed was retransfused among with additional test substance. The additional amount of blood substitute corresponded to the difference between the first and second bleeding volumes ($H_1 - H_2$). For the animals in the dextran group this was an overtransfusion, which seems to be the weak point in this experimental program. The relationship of $H_2$ or $H_3$ to $H_1 \times 100$ is defined as the *bleeding index* (see below). The resulting figures show a scattering of more than 100% for the same replacement substance; there is no basis for assuming that significant importance can be attached to these figures concerning the effectiveness of an expander in shock management since too many uncontrollable factors (especially vasoconstriction) are involved. Furthermore, the number of animals involved in the experiments — 5 per group — was too small. After 24 hours the results were as follows:

| Test substance | Number of animals | Survivors |
|---|---|---|
| Heparinized blood | 5 | 4 |
| 0.9% NaCl solution | 5 | 2 |
| OPG 5% | 5 | 2 |
| dextran 6% | 5 | 3 |
| MFG 3% | 5 | 5 |

The results concerning the bleeding index are not listed here for the reasons mentioned.

Raisz and Pulaski [*1155*] arrived at similar results: Immediately after blood removal of 3% of the b.w., *rabbits* received infusion of the same amount of test substance.

Results:

| Test substance | Number of animals | Survivors |
|---|---|---|
| controls | 2 | 2 |
| pooled plasma | 17 | 15 |
| 0.9% NaCl solution | 16 | 8 |
| OPG 5% | 17 | 16 |
| dextran 80 6% (Pharmacia Lot No. 7574 A and No. Z 6932) | 15 | 12 |

The differences between the various colloids are insignificant.

Some authors have provided informative data concerning OPG and dextran; both substances caused intravascular erythrocyte aggregation. This observation indicates that these older dextran preparations contained a high molecular weight top fraction. It also confirms the report by THORSÉN and HINT [*1440*] that gelatin, even in relatively low concentration, causes aggregation phenomena.

In another model, MORRISON et al. [*1048*] determined the following in *guinea pigs*

| Test substance | Number of animals | Survivors |
|---|---|---|
| controls | 10 | 0 |
| 0.9% NaCl solution | 10 | 0 |
| dextran 6% | 10 | 5 |
| Periston 3.5% | 10 | 6 |
| Gelatin 5% (Plasmoid) | 10 | 8 |
| albumin | 10 | 10 |
| heparinized blood | 10 | 10 |

and in *rats*

| Test substance | Number of animals | Survivors |
|---|---|---|
| controls | 10 | 0 |
| 0.9% NaCl solution | 10 | 1 |
| dextran 6% | 10 | 7 |
| Periston 3.5% | 10 | 8 |
| gelatin 5% | 10 | 8 |
| albumin | 10 | 9 |
| heparinized blood | 10 | 10 |

The dextran results can not be used because of the species-specific sensitivity of rats.

MORRISON used an experimental procedure with *dogs* which was similar to that of PARKINS [*1117*], though he used a more complicated method of calculating the bleeding index: the animals were bled to a BP of 50 to 55 mm Hg and the amount removed was designated as $H_{1a}$. Immediately afterward the same amount of test substance was infused, and 4 hours later the animals were re-bled until death occurred (2 ml/kg bw/3 min). The amount of blood removed was designated as $H_2$, the remaining blood volume after removal of $H_{1a}$ is assumed to be 10.10 ml/kg bw and is designated as $H_{1e}$. Adding $H_{1a}$ and $H_{1e}$ results in $H_1$. This author defines the bleeding index as the ratio of $H_2$ to $H_1 \times 100$. This shows that these figures represent very hypothetical values and that various authors use different methods of calculation for the bleeding index. Therefore extreme caution must be used in interpreting such data, and we feel that much more importance should be placed on the survival figures. For the sake of completeness, the figures for the bleeding index calculated by MORRISON are listed here (ideal figure = 150) (cf. also [*882 a, 1074 a, 1473, 1474*]):

| | |
|---|---|
| heparinized blood | 94.6 ± 3.6 |
| human plasma | 78.4 ± 0.5 |
| dextran 6% | 77.1 ± 3.3 |
| gelatin 5% | 68.1 ± 3.8 |
| Periston 3.5% | 68.1 ± 4.3 |
| normal saline | 51.1 ± 7.3 |

The differences between dextran, gelatin and Periston are statistically insignificant.

It is interesting to note that gelatin solutions become contaminated much more readily than dextran and Periston, which have proved to be exceptionally resistant to bacterial contamination.

KALRA [*809*] also found the bleeding index of dextran superior to that of MFG and another gelatin. JANOTA et al. [*780*] tested 14 various gelatin in concentrations between 5.4—7.7% in 44 dogs. The effect was better than that of 0.9% saline solution. KALRA arrived at the same results [*809*] with *6—8% MFG* (cf. also [*872, 882 a*]. Only scattered studies on a small number of animals and with conditions of slight shock show the effect of *6% OPG* or *3% MFG* to be as good as plasma.

PARKINS [*1115*] found in *dogs*

| Test substance | Number of animals | Survivors |
|---|---|---|
| plasma | 3 | 3 |
| 6% gelatin | 5 | 5 |
| 0.9% NaCl | 5 | 2 |
| control | 3 | 0 |

The blood pressure was maintained between 30—40 mm Hg for 30 to 40 min, and the test substance was infused in an amount corresponding to that of the blood removed.

ELDER [*405*] used a model similar to that of PARKINS ([*1117*], see above) with dogs.

*The bleeding index was:*

| | after 3 hrs | after 24 hrs |
|---|---|---|
| blood | 96 | 94 |
| 0.9% NaCl solution | 54 | 68 |
| albumin 5% | 88 | — |
| MFG 3% | 83 | 75 |

When the BP was maintained at 30—35 mm Hg for 1 hour, the results were as follows:

| | after 3 hrs | after 24 hrs |
|---|---|---|
| blood | 72 | 63 |
| 0.9% NaCl solution | 12 | 15 |
| albumin 5% | 59 | — |
| MFG 3% | 67 | 68 |

Ivy et al. [*769*] found a poorer effect for gelatin than for plasma in hemorrhagic shock:

| | Mortality |
|---|---|
| heparinized plasma | 6% |
| gelatin U-17,578 (5% solution in 0.9% NaCl) | 40% |
| "Plasma gel" (5% solution in 0.9% NaCl) | 100% |
| 0.9% normal saline solution | 58% |
| control | 84% |

Gropper et al. [*578*] arrived at the following results:

| | Mortality |
|---|---|
| control | 85% |
| pooled plasma (frozen) | 22.2% |
| 0.9% normal saline solution | 55.5% |
| 5% OPG | 33% |
| 6% dextran (MW 40,000) | 22.2% |

The differences between the OPG and dextran groups are statistically significant.

The authors drew the following conclusions: "Dextran gives a greater and more prolonged expansion of blood volume than either dog plasma or OPG. Dextran restores glomerular filtration and renal blood flow more rapidly to greater levels and for a longer period of time than OPG. Dextran (6%) exhibits approximately twice the effect of withdrawing fluid from the interstitial compartment as does OPG (5%)". (See also [*542, 1466, 1739*]).

Results of studies on *Plasmagel* where 2% of the bw of 2 dogs was removed and replaced by the expander [*181*], show that 1 hr 20 min after infusion of Plasmagel the BP was 60 mm Hg; the initial level had been 120. After infusion of another 1.64% of the bw, the pressure was 100, and the pulse was still 180 (initial level was 100). The records of these 2 dog experiments were also published by Hascher [*661*].

NAHAS and ESTIME [*1071*] used the model of IVY [*769*] with dogs an obtained 80% survivors with Plasmagel and 50% with an equal amount c isotonic saline solution ($n = 10$ each) (cf. [*1762*]).

The first test of *Physiogel* in various hemorrhagic shock models in rabbi was made by BURRI and ALLGÖWER [*240*]. In severe shock of 90 minut duration the infusion of 1% of the bw produced the following surviv figures:

| | |
|---|---|
| animal's own blood | 80% |
| 6% dextran 75 | 60% |
| 4.2% Physiogel | 20% |

In light shock, the hemodilution caused by infusion of Physiogel wa about half that caused by infusion of Macrodex.

JANZARIK and LASCH [*782*] report on experiments with rabbits in newly developed experimental model for exchange transfusions. The autho speak of "short shock"; the animals are bled very quickly and drasticall and are then immediately infused with various solutions. 7 hours after th beginning of the experiment all investigations are terminated. Since 15% human albumin is a hyper-colloid-osmotic solution, only half the amount c this solution was administered, compared with the volumes used with th other groups. The 10% Rheomacrodex tested by the authors was given i the same dosages as the 3.5—5.6% gelatin solutions in spite of its greate initial oncotic effect. The authors state that dextran animals were ove transfused. Therefore it is not surprising that only few animals in thes groups survived. That these were not really shock experiments can b concluded from the fact that equal amounts of 0.9% saline solution an gelatin caused statistically insignificant differences in the mortality (c Electrolyte solutions, p. 147). In addition the authors confirm the results c BURRI and ALLGÖWER [*240*], that infusion of 1/3 of the amount remove as is usual under conditions in the field and other emergency situations, a 5 dextran animals survive, while the corresponding figures for gelati solutions are:

Physiogel 3/5, Gelifundol 2/5, Haemaccel 2/5.

LUNDSGAARD [*925*] has tested the effect of autologous blood, dextran 7 Physiogel, and Ringer's solution in 360 rabbits. All animals were treate beforehand with an adrenenergic blocking agent which drastically influenc the spontaneous regulation mechanisms which normally occur in shock. Th model is a situation which hardly corresponds to clinical conditions as ca be concluded from the fact that infusion of 1/10 or 10/10 of the amount o blood removed causes no significant difference in survival figures. On th other hand infusion of 1/10—1/3 Physiogel or Ringer's solution produces significantly poorer result than replacement of the entire amount remove with these solutions. Overtransfusion with Macrodex led to significantl poorer results which corresponded to the earlier results of JANZARIK and LASCH [*782*]. In confirmation of the studies of BURRI and ALLGÖWER [*240*], replacement of the blood volume removed by $^1/_{10}$—$^1/_3$ Macrodex was more effective than the same amount of Physiogel, although the differences here were not especially noticeable. LUNDSGAARD states that compared with dextran optimal effects are obtained with twice the amount of Physiogel or approximately 3× the amount of Ringer's solution. The conclusions from this article are discussed in Part 3, p. 177 f.

In another article [*925 a*] LUNDSGAARD retracts his opinion that the individual colloids must be given in different dosages to obtain an optimal effect. In a new rabbit model he was unable to show a differing effect with various plasma replacement substances with infusion of $^1/_3$ or $^2/_3$ of the amount of the blood volume removed (blood, Macrodex, Physiogel, Gelifundol, Haemaccel). The duration of shock in this model was 42 minutes on the average and depended upon the size of the "base excess". Thus these rabbit experiments were not actually shock experiments but rather a study of anoxia symptoms after hypovolemia of very short duration with subsequent exchange transfusion. Since the spontaneous refilling of the vascular system in rabbits occurs much more quickly than in larger animals and in humans, it would seem that this animal is poorly suited for testing plasma replacement substances, especially with an extremely short hypotensive phase, as in this case.

**Clinical Results.** There is no doubt that infusion of gelatin solutions after blood loss improves circulation as well as the general condition of the patient. On the other hand there are very few articles which permit an objective evaluation of the therapeutic effectiveness of gelatin solutions in humans. In particular there are no comparative studies which would allow one to conclude that gelatin solutions are just as effective as plasma or albumin.

Most authors are satisfied with stating that the preparations are effective [*1346*]; on closer examination one sees that most of the cases had only slight blood loss. Thus the following articles emphasize that infusion of 500 ml of gelatin solution was sufficient to eliminate "shock"; Haemaccel is the best documented of all gelatin preparations [*183, 212, 549, 679, 1027, 1028, 1259, 1803*], but here too there is lack of comparative studies with saline solution on one hand and plasma preparations on the other. In other studies large amounts of blood and vasopressors were administered at the same time as or shortly after gelatin. Thus it is impossible to make conclusive statements about the effectiveness of these preparations [*102, 1461, 1841*].

In particular there is lack of larger controlled and comparative statistics concerning the management of burns, where the effect of a plasma replacement substance is expressed clearly. FROESCHLIN [*479*] reports on 23 burn patients who were treated with Haemaccel; but the cases are not documented more precisely. The same applies to the 17 cases listed by BARDHAN et al [*102*]. The 6% Indian gelatin was effective for 4—6 hours in 10 patients. In older review articles [*1430*] there is some information concerning the clinical effectiveness of gelatin; however, these are preparations which are different from those available today in several respects (concentration, no modification). Objective documentation is usually lacking here as well.

Some further studies deal with Haemaccel but do not present any new facts [*19, 98, 877*].

HARRFELDT [*654*] describes 1 patient in whom blood pressure and pulse became measurable again after infusion of 500 ml OPG.

ARTZ [*79*] reports on his experience with 200 bottles of 3% MFG during the Korean War. 100 bottles were used in the division area, and the rest in hospitals behind the lines. ARTZ writes that MFG seems to have proved itself useful in this small series of wounded soldiers; he stresses, however, that the average evacuation time was only 3½ hours.

The article by FRAWLEY [*464*] reports on the same cases as ARTZ, but no more information can be gleaned here, since all patients received large amounts of blood following the gelatin treatment. There is no data concerning the further course.

### *w) Summary and Conclusions: Volume Replacement with Gelatin*

1. Gelatin solutions have been used since 1915 as plasma replacement substances. The most important of the preparations available today can be divided into 3 groups:

Oxypolygelatin (OPG, Gelifundol), modified fluid gelatin (MFG, Plasmagel, Physiogel) and gelatin crosslinked by means of urea bridges (Haemaccel).

2. Preparations used earlier were usually more highly concentrated than the ones used today; in the latter there is considerable variation of concentration, electrolyte content and MW from one preparation to another. Here too the results obtained with one solution can not be directly transferred to another. In the following, consideration is given to the characteristics of the preparations available today.

3. The physico-chemical properties of gelatin are generally less precisely known than those of dextran. The average molecular weights ($\overline{M}_w$ and $\overline{M}_n$) are lower; for gelatins approximately 70—90% of the molecules lying below the renal threshold.

4. The main portion of a gelatin solution is therefore excreted in the urine within a few hours. Nothing definite is known about plasma concentration and breakdown of gelatin which remains in the body, since specific methods of demonstration are lacking.

5. In normovolemic and hypovolemic individuals gelatin preparations cause an increase in diuresis; there is no definite evidence of irreversible kidney damage.

6. The histological changes in the kidney observed after gelatin infusions are very likely of a functional and temporary nature.

7. Gelatin preparations generally have no clinical antigenic effect. OPG may sometimes be antigenic in humans, but not MFG and Haemaccel.

8. Allergic side-effects are rare.

9. Gelatin preparations of the MFG type gel at 7—10° C.

10. Infusion of OPG, Haemaccel and MFG, in this order, have an increasing ability to increase the sedimentation rate.

11. Gelatins have no disaggregating effect; instead they cause cell aggregation in lower concentration and with lower MW than dextran.

12. There is no data concerning the influence of gelatin preparations on blood viscosity at shear rates which occur in the capillary beds in humans.

13. Under standard conditions gelatin preparations have no influence on the determination of blood groups.

14. Infusion of gelatin influences neither the resistance to infection nor the nonspecific resistance of the human organism; they have no carcinogenic effect.

15. The influence of gelatin solutions on blood coagulation probably corresponds to the dilution effect.

16. Specific pharmacological properties of gelatin solutions are unknown.

17. There are no studies concerning the influence on laboratory tests.

18. Storage of Physiogel for 4 and of Haemaccel for 3 years does not affect the stability of the preparation.

19. The volume effect of gelatin solutions in hypovolemic individuals does not quite correspond to the amount infused initially and then declines rapidly; the effect of Haemaccel and OPG is probably little better than that of MFG. The volume effect is approximately between the levels observed after infusion of equal amounts of electrolyte solution or plasma.

20. Gelatin solutions can cause a normalization of blood pressure in hypovolemic individuals. The ability of MFG and Haemaccel to improve cardiac output has not been fully investigated, and for OPG it has not been studied at all. The data available for MFG and Haemaccel show that the effect does not correspond to that of plasma. There is no data concerning a specific flow-improving effect of gelatin solutions.

21. Only few experimental results permit the assumption of a therapeutic effect comparable to that obtained with plasma in the treatment of severe shock conditions. These results were almost all obtained with older 5% or even more highly concentrated solutions of OPG. Only scattered studies using 3% MFG in a very few dogs show an effect comparable to

Table 11. *Advantages and disadvantages of dextran and gelatin preparations i clinical treatment of shock*

| | Gelatin | Dextran |
|---|---|---|
| Physico-chemical properties | insufficiently investigated | known |
| Water binding capacity | unknown in vivo | 20—25 ml/g in circulation |
| Breakdown in organism | not known exactly | complete |
| Renal function | no evidence of injurious effect | |
| Histology | no evidence of injurious effect | |
| Antigenicity | no evidence of clinical consequences | |
| Allergic reactions | less frequent than after plasma infusions | |
| Increase in sedimentation rate | + to +++ | dextran 40: lowering effect dextran 70: (+) |
| Aggregating effect | + | — |
| Disaggregating effect | — | dextran 40: ++ dextran 70: — |
| Lowering of raised blood viscosity | insufficiently investigated | dextran 40: yes dextran 70: slight |
| Gel point | MFG at 7—10° C | −0.6° C |
| Blood group determination | no influence | no influence |
| Defence against infection | no influence | no influence |
| Carcinogenicity | — | — |
| Influence on blood coagulation | according to dilution | in clinical doses (up to 1.5 g/kg bw) without consequence |
| Antithrombotic effect | unknown | +++ |
| Influence on laboratory tests | not investigated | yes, in certain methods |
| Stability | little known | good for 10 years |
| Volume effect | poorer than plasma | dextran 40: initially very strong, shorter tha dextran 70 dextran 70: like plasma initially somewhat stronger |
| Influence on hemodynamics | little investigated | dextran 70: approximately like plasma |
| Therapeutic effect | little investigated | dextran 70: approximately like plasma |
| Therapeutic effectiveness in treatment of burns | little known | dextran 70: initially like plasma |

that obtained with plasma. These experiments are not shock studies, but rather determination of the bleeding index. For the preparations available today there are no usable results of shock studies in dogs and other large animals, nor do the shock models used in rabbits allow conclusions with regard to the therapeutic effectiveness in hypovolemic patients.

22. The are no clear, verifiable data concerning the clinical utility of gelatin preparations in treatment of serious shock states. Compared with plasma and dextran there is very few data. It can be assumed on the basis of several articles that gelatin preparations have proved useful in the treatment of less severe shock situations. The experience of the Americans with 200 bottles of 3% MFG during the Korean War shows that satisfactory results can be obtained with gelatin preparations and with average evacuation times of 3½ hours under ideal conditions (total air superiority) if enough blood was available in the field hospitals. The preparation Haemaccel is the best documented of all the gelatin solutions. Here too, comparative data about its effectiveness is lacking, especially with regard to management of burns. There is only scarce data regarding the clinical use of Physiogel (documented are 150 patients, almost all of whom also received massive blood transfusions). There are no studies concerning the treatment of burns with this preparation.

23. *Table 11* compares the most important advantages and disadvantages of dextran 70 and the gelatin preparations available today.

## 3. Polyvinyl pyrrolidone (PVP)

### *a) Definition*

Unlike dextran and gelatin, polyvinyl pyrrolidone (PVP) is not a product of a substance which occurs biologically, but is a completely *synthetic* [*1677*] *polymer of vinyl pyrrolidone (Fig. 17).*

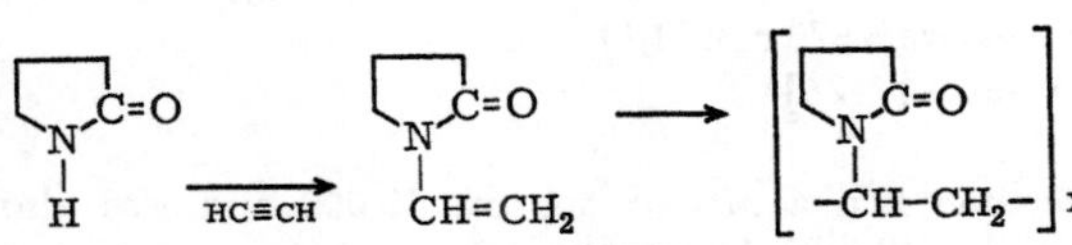


Fig. 17. Polymerization of vinyl pyrrolidone (center) to PVP (right). The pyrrolidone formula is at the left

Since this substance can not be broken down at all in the body, it is practically no longer used today.

Large amounts of PVP were used during World War II by the German army. This experience was the basis of a thorough study of a few fundamental problems involved in the use of synthetic colloids as plasma expanders. For this reason a short survey based on the literature follows. It deals with some of the interesting questions with regard to this problem, although from the practical standpoint they are only historically important. Nevertheless there are still sizable supplies of PVP in several developing countries and this replacement substance is still used clinically to a moderate extent. We ourselves have had no practical experience with PVP in Switzerland.

Some European countries still manufacture PVP, but it is primarily intended for export. In the USA, PVP may be used only upon vital indication if absolutely no other colloids are available. One patient may never receive a total of more than 1000 ml. This stipulation has to be printed on each bottle, and for this reason PVP was never placed on the market.

In 1939 the only volume replacement substances available in Germany were preserved whole blood and crystalloid solutions. Therefore extensive studies were made with *polyvinyl alcohol,* but this substance was dropped because it caused secondary anemia. Then HECHT and WEESE [*684*] tested polyvinyl pyrrolidone. At first it was named *Hämodyn,* but later is was brought onto the market under the name *Periston.*

## *b) The Various Preparations*

*Periston* (Bayer, Leverkusen).

| Conc. | NaCl | KCl | g/100 ml<br>$CaCl_2$ | $MgCl_2$ | $NaHCO_3$ |
|---|---|---|---|---|---|
| 4% | 0.7 | 0.042 | 0.005 | 0.0005 | 0.025 |

$\overline{M}_w$=25,000 (30,000, [*551*]) $\overline{M}_n$=15,000

Molecular weight distribution:
peak fraction=189,000 (see also [*1288*]), cf. Table 12 $\frac{\overline{M}_w}{\overline{M}_n}$ =2.0

colloid-osmotic pressure=670 mm $H_2O$
pH =approx. 6 (acc. [*1176*])
$\eta_{rel}$ =2

Before 1952 Periston had a $\overline{M}_w$ of approx. 50,000 and was also commercially available as Kollidon (BASF, Ludwigshafen).

*6% Periston N* (Bayer, Leverkusen) has a $\overline{M}_w$ of 12,000 ($\eta_{rel}$=1.6).

Table 12 provides a survey of the most important preparations.

## *c) Metabolism*

WILLENEGGER [*1523*] assumed that 95% of PVP with an average MW of 25,000 is excreted in the urine and that only fractions with an average MW of 140,000 can not be eliminated.

Table 12. *Physico-chemical data of the most important PVP preparations discussed in the literature*

| *Generic name*<br>Trade name | Concen-<br>tration | $\overline{M_w}$ | Molecular weight distribution<br>10% Low mol. fr. | <br>top fraction 10% | Electrolyte content<br>in g/100 ml | Manufacturer |
|---|---|---|---|---|---|---|
| Periston | 4% | 25,000 | 4100 [*551*] | 189,000 [*551*] | NaCl 0.70<br>KCl 0.042<br>$CaCl_2$ 0.05<br>$MgCl_2$ 0.0005<br>$NaHCO_3$ 0.025 | Bayer, Leverkusen |
| Periston-N<br>Neo Compensan | 6% | ~ 12,000 | — | — | NaCl 0.55<br>KCl 0.042<br>$CaCl_2$ 0.05<br>$MgCl_2$ 0.0005<br>$NaHCO_3$ 0.023 | Bayer, Leverkusen<br>Heilmittelwerke, Vienna |
| Periston (before 1952)<br>(Hämodyn, Kollidon) | 4% | 50,000 | — | — | — | Bayer, Leverkusen<br>BASF, Ludwigshafen |
| Plasgen | 3.5% | 50,000 [*551*] | 9600 [*551*] | 127,000 [*551*] | NaCl 0.9<br>KCl 0.042<br>$MgCl_2$ 0.0005<br>$CaCl_2$ 0.025 | Kyorin Pharmaceutical Co.,<br>Tokyo |
| Plasgen-L | 6% | 17,000 | — | — | NaCl 0.55<br>KCl 0.042<br>$CaCl_2$ 0.025<br>$MgCl_2$ 0.0005<br>$NaHCO_3$ 0.023 | Kyorin Pharmaceutical Co.,<br>Tokyo |

Table 12 (continued)

| *Generic name* Trade name | Concen- tration | $\overline{M}_w$ | Molecular weight distribution 10% Low mol. fr. | top fraction 10% | Electrolyte content Additions | Manufacturer |
|---|---|---|---|---|---|---|
| Isoplasma | 4% | — | — | — | $Na^+$ 144 mval/l<br>$K^+$ 6.7 mval/l<br>$Cl^-$ 150.6 mval/l | Vifor, Geneva |
| Subtosan | 3.5% | 50,000 | — | — | — | Specia, Paris |
| Parenteral P | 3.5% | 40,000 | — | — | $Na^+$ 140 mval/l<br>$K^+$ 6 mval/l<br>$Ca^{++}$ 4 mval/l<br>$Mg^{++}$ 3 mval/l<br>$Cl^-$ 120 mval/l<br>$Acetate^-$ 33 mval/l | Serag-Wiessner Naila/Munich |
| Compensan | 4% | 30,000 | — | — | — | Heilmittelwerke, Vienna |
| Kollosteril | 3.5% | 30,000 | — | — | $Na^+$ 137 mval/l<br>$Mg^{++}$ 2.5 mval/l<br>$K^+$ 4 mval/l<br>$Ca^{++}$ 3.3 mval/l<br>$Cl^-$ 110 mval/l<br>$Acetate^-$ 36.8 mval/l<br>Rutin 0.2 g/l | Dr. Fresenius, Bad Homburg |
| Elo Compen | 4% | 24,500 | — | — | Rutin 0.25 g/l | Leopold, Graz |

In an excellent article, RAVIN, SELIGMAN and FINE [*1161*] used PVP tagged with $^{131}I$ to show without question that molecules with a MW of less than 40,000 can be found in the tissues.

On the basis of studies by HECHT and SCHOLTAN [*685*] one must count on the organism retaining about 20% of the new PVP preparation with an average MW of 25,000.

*What happens to the Periston which is not excreted in the urine?*

There is no basis for believing that this foreign colloid is broken down by the organism [*1161, 1381*]. In animals and humans, primarily the RES, as well as other tissues, store the PVP not eliminated in the urine and may retain it for several years [*45, 48, 49, 50, 51, 103, 104, 203, 686, 757, 785, 972, 1025, 1161, 1250, 1289, 1464*].

Swelling of the tubular epithelium was often observed to be an expression of an acute storage phenomenon in the kidneys. It must be remembered, however, that similar symptoms occur in the kidneys after the use of other colloids and glucose solutions as well [*107, 280, 468, 903, 1450, 1451, 1453, 1560*].

Some believe that this deposit phenomenon is only temporary and without any functional importance [*903*]. On the other hand many authors regard the deposit of PVP as irreversible [*468, 757, 785, 1161, 1289*]. According to HÜSSELMANN [*757*] such deposits occur even with clinical dosages.

Great difficulties in interpretation of these reports arise because the changes are often only found months after infusion. Therefore it is important at what moment the histological investigation is made [*490, 903*].

Various authors have maintained that no functional impairment of the RES occurs because of the PVP deposit. Even so, other researchers [*1386, 1497*] observe a reduction in phagocytotic activity after the use of a PVP preparation having a $\overline{M}_w$ of approx. 40,000.

Considerable attention was raised when animal experiments showed that Periston had carcinogenic properties [*755, 930*]. HUEPER himself however could not duplicate his experiments later [*756*], and there is no evidence that PVP has ever caused a carcinoma in humans [*902*].

Since PVP can combine with numerous substances, the term "serum and cell cleanser" was coined [*1287, 1290, 1291, 1292, 1293*]; later a special form of PVP, *Periston "N"* was introduced for clinical use [*153*]. The average MW of this 6% Periston is 12,600. Convincing proof of a specific antitoxic property of this preparation can not be found and for this reason this therapy is now seldom used.

## *d) Volume Effect*

RAVIN and co-workers [*1161*] used PVP tagged with $^{131}I$ to measure the length of time PVP remains in the circulation. They found that it is proportionate to the molecular size. Fractions of 25,000 and less leave the circulation immediately and thus cause practically no volume effect.

HECHT and SCHOLTAN [*685*] found 18% of the infused PVP in the urine before the infusion was ended. 3 hours after the infusion was terminated, 48.3% was found in the urine. The objection to the studies of KORTH and HEINLEIN [*837*] is that volume replacement was only made 15 hours after the dogs were bled, i. e. after considerable spontaneous refilling had already taken place.

We will not discuss in detail here the numerous other articles about this topic and about therapeutic results, in view of the non-usage of this agent today. No clinician likes to assume the responsibility for a preparation which is not broken down in the human organism, and in view of our present knowledge of the role played by the RES in shock pathogenesis, it is felt unwise to subject it to any additional burden. For technical reasons it is almost impossible to produce preparations with such pure fractions that no PVP would remain in the organism. Even if one could, the volume effect would be approximately that of a pure electrolyte solution. Thus since PVP has no advantages compared with dextran and gelatin, there seems no reason to use the preparation. Regarding PVP and platelet adhesiveness see [*1801*]. This effect is however without clinical significance [*1745*].

### *e) Summary: Polyvinyl Pyrrolidone*

The synthetic polymer, polyvinyl pyrrolidone (PVP), is not broken down in the organism, and the body stores for an unlimited time the amount not excreted in urine. If a colloid is to be used as a volume replacement substance, it must contain fractions whose molecular weights are above the renal threshold. Thus most clinicians no longer use PVP preparations, as they have the disadvantage of permanent storage and have no advantages over dextran and gelatin.

## 4. Starch (Hydroxyethyl Starch)

### *a) Definition*

Hydroxyethyl starch was introduced in 1957 by WIEDERSHEIM [*1511*] as a plasma replacement substance. *Fig. 18* shows its structural formula. Unmodified starch is unsuitable for plasma replacement since it is immediately broken down by serum amylase. For this reason various modifications have been tested for some time [*1283*]. Of these, hydroxyethyl starch has proved to be the best. (In the following, HO-ethyl starch always stands for a 6% hydroxyethyl starch in 0.9% saline solution, unless stated otherwise.)

This plasma expander was tried for the following reasons [*389*]: According to current animal experiments, the therapeutic effectiveness of starch is said to be approximately that of dextran 75. Starch is an inexpensive, easily obtainable raw material for the manufacture of which, unlike dextran, no license is needed. The advocates of starch consider its main advantages to be that HO-ethyl starch is neither toxic nor antigenic and causes no disturbance of blood coagulation.

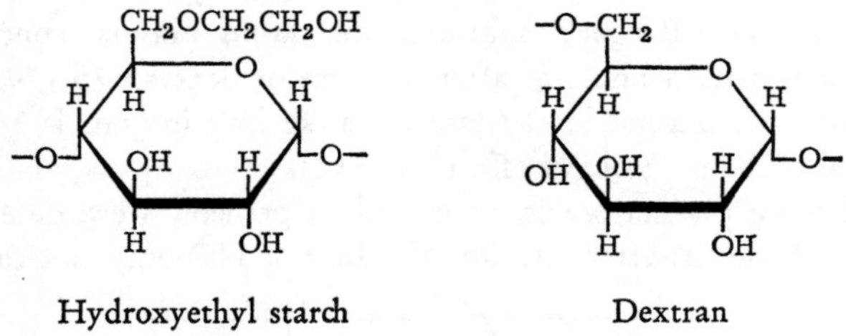


Fig. 18. Comparisons of the formulas for starch and dextran. The HO-ethyl starch molecule has much branching; that of dextran is linear. The linkages in HO-ethyl starch are mainly α-1—4, in dextran α-1—6 (acc. RUSSELL [*1232*])

SCHOCH [*1283*] provides a survey of the physico-chemical properties of the substance used to date. On the basis of $|\eta|$ (approx. 0,27) determinations, it is assumed that the preparation available must have properties similar to those of dextran 75 (see also [*357*]). Recent investigations [*269*] allow the assumption that $\overline{M}_w$ is about 400,000 and $\overline{M}_n$ is far below 100,000, i. e. it is a highly polydisperse solution (cf. [*1631, 1631 a, 1688*]).

## *b) Manufacture*

Only "waxy starches", the genetic variants which occur in rice and grain, are used; they have highly branched molecules. The amylopectin fraction of starch is suspended in water and mixed with dilute hydrochloric acid until the desired degree of hydrolysis is reached. This is done in such a way that the end product has the same viscosity as dextran 75. The neutralized material is mixed with dilute sodium hydroxide and is treated with ethylene oxide until 90% of the glucose units are substituted. The preparation is manufactured by MacGaw Laboratories, Inc., Glendale, Calif. On the label is printed: "For animal experiments only!"

HO-ethyl starch is not available commercially; the first clinical experiments were made at Johns Hopkins University.

## *c) Metabolism*

According to THOMPSON et al. [*1432*] HO-ethyl starch is very resistant to α-amylase and is broken down like dextran. No acute toxic effect could be determined with the use of up to 3 g/kg bw in 10 rats ([*1433*], see also [*1511*]). On the other hand, administration of 25 ml/kg bw daily for

4 weeks caused loss of weight in rabbits and because of this there is some suspicion of *toxic properties* [*1199*].

## *d) Plasma Concentration*

After removal of 30 ml of blood/kg bw and replacement of the same amount of a starch-Ringer's solution, the same plasma concentrations resulted in dogs after 4 hours as after infusion of dextran 75 [*1431, 1432*]. After 24 hours the plasma level (dose 25 ml/kg bw) in gods is 38.2 ± 1.4% [*1483*] (cf. also under "Volume effect", p. 144).

The following plasma levels, expressed in percent, were determined in 2 volunteers (A and B) after infusion of 1 liter of HO-ethyl starch [*101*]:

| | A | B |
|---|---|---|
| 10 min | 100 | 100 |
| 1 hr | 90 | 87 |
| 4 hrs | 82 | 67 |
| 10 hrs | 64 | 77 (?) |
| 24 hrs | 63 | 50 |

## *e) Renal Function*

Studies of
creatinin clearance,
PAH clearance,
maximum tubular reabsorption of glucose,
maximum tubular secretion of PAH
and further measurements of renal function revealed no differences compared to clinical dextran in dogs [*1433*].

After infusion of 25 ml/kg bw, 31.5 ± 1.4% is excreted in the urine in 24 hours [*1483*].

Silk [*1340*] has shown that HO-ethyl starch and dextran 75 both increase renal flow; the effect of dextran 75 is greater.

After exchange transfusions with HO-ethyl starch, 6% dextran 75 and physiological saline solution in 39 dogs, Murphy [*1066*] measured renal flow, resistance, pressure and hematocrit in the renal vessels, as well as excretion of urine. The Hct levels fluctuated between 5—30%. The effect of HO-ethyl starch was comparable to that of dextran; since HO-ethyl starch does not reduce diuresis, a specific vasodilator effect may be suspected.

24 hours after infusion, 12% and 20% of the infused HO-ethyl starch was found in the urine of the two volunteers. Plasma electrolyte changes were not observed [*101*].

### *f) Histological Investigations*

After infusion of 7.8—60 g of HO-ethyl starch/kg bw in dogs, the only morphological changes were swelling and vacuolization of the proximal tubuli, which, however, cause no functional disturbance. 6 days after the last infusion these phenomena had disappeared [*1483*].

### *g) Influence on Blood Coagulation*

In dog experiments of THOMPSON there were no significant differences between dextran and starch in regard to their prolongation of bleeding times, except that starch did not specifically depress fibrinogen concentration [*1433*]. However after infusion of 10—20 ml of HO-ethyl starch in dogs, CHENG et al. [*274*] observed a sharp drop in fibrinogen [*1681*]. In the experiments of GARZON [*493, 1681*] deep skin incisions were made as far as the fascia; for this reason the same objections must be raised as for a similar study in the dextran chapter. The prolonged bleeding times and the increased blood loss observed in that study did not appear to us to be directly related to clinical conditions (cf. also [*535 a*]).

LEWIS et al. [*885*] have measured bleeding time, platelet count and coagulation factors in dogs after marked hemodilution (Hct 20% of initial level!) with HO-ethyl starch, dextran 40 and 75. With the large doses used, all three substances produced a prolonged bleeding time, reduction of platelet adhesiveness and a fibrinoplastic effect. There was a significant difference with regard to plasma protein concentrations, where dextran 40 caused it to rise more quickly than HO-ethyl starch (see also [*1416*]). The differences in the levels, compared with dextran 75, were statistically insignificant.

In the two volunteers studied by BALLINGER, there was a drop in fibrinogen concentration, and bleeding and coagulation time increased [*101*].

### *h) Immunological Studies*

Preliminary studies by MAURER [*977*] revealed no signs of antigenic properties for HO-ethyl starch in rabbits and humans.

BRICKMAN et al. [*210*] have made in vitro immunological studies with leucocytes of 7 volunteers after infusion of 3 liters of HO-ethyl starch. On the basis of their results they assume that HO-ethyl starch has little antigenic properties; but they stress that the conclusions may only be drawn when experience is based on much larger figures.

### *i) Influence on Sedimentation Rate*

A 6% HO-ethyl starch solution acts like dextran 75; more highly concentrated starch increases the sedimentation rate.

When erythrocytes are washed, the admixture of HO-ethyl starch and dextran 40 or 75 produced minimal increments in erythrocyte binding of fibrinogen, $\alpha$- and $\gamma$-globulins. Electrophoresis of the plasma-polysaccharide mixture incubated with erythrocytes revealed a small but significant decrement in fibrinogen concentration and increment in $\alpha$, and $\alpha_2$ globulin concentration on addition of starch and dextran fractions [*1436*].

### *k) Pharmacological Properties*

Russell et al. [*1232*] compared the antithrombotic effect of HO-ethyl starch to that of dextran 40 and 75. The dextrans showed a significant protective effect, but no definite conclusions could be drawn concerning HO-ethyl starch.

HO-ethyl starch caused much less alteration in the platelet thrombus threshold than dextran [*147*].

### *l) Volume Effect*

Measured with the bleeding index in dogs, no difference could be determined between HO-ethyl starch, dextran 75 and blood ([*1432*], cf. also [*1416*]). In addition, blood volume increase, respiratory rate, pulse, blood pressure, pulse amplitude, hematocrit and hemoglobin changes in hemorrhagic shock are comparable to the levels found after infusion of the same amount of dextran 75 [*1433*].

There was likewise no important difference between these two colloids with regard to pH, $TCO_2$ and $pCO_2$ (see also [*1434, 1435*]). Takaori [*1414*] however, found a significant acidosis in hemodilution studies using HO-ethyl starch, but not with dextran.

### *m) Therapeutic Results*

**Animal Studies.** In irreversible hemorrhagic shock models in dogs, HO-ethyl starch proved to be slightly superior to dextran 75, but the differences were statistically insignificant [*100, 1345*].

In an original, new shock model with dogs, Vineyard et al. [*1470*] carefully compared 5 various replacement solutions. The amount to be infused was determined on the basis of arterial blood pressure and venous pressure. In the group which received HO-ethyl starch, a significantly greater number of animals survived compared with the group that received dextran 75. However in order to keep the animals alive, much greater amounts of HO-ethyl starch were required than of dextran, causing the Hct to drop more sharply. Compared with dextran 40 there were no significant differences with regard to survival. The effect of plasma and Ringer's solution was similar to that of HO-ethyl starch. It seems important to us in this model that all animals were retransfused with 200 ml of shed erythrocytes along with the test solution. The significance of this procedure is unclear, but the suspicion remains that the animals which received HO-ethyl starch or Ringer's solution profited from this procedure (see above with regard to Hct drop!).

DEFALCO [*345*] observed the following mortality rates in hemorrhagic shock in dogs:

| | |
|---|---|
| 0.9% NaCl solution plus blood (1:1) | 30% |
| blood | 40% |
| HO-ethyl starch plus blood (1 : 1) | 60% |

In preliminary studies with pigs, HO-ethyl starch has proved inferior to blood ([*478*], cf. also [*357*]).

In their model with dogs, DILLON et al. [*352*] obtained no survivors with a 7% HO-ethyl starch-Ringer's solution.

**Human studies.** BALLINGER [*101*] reports on the first results with 15 patients who were admitted in hypovolemic shock. Compatibility of HO-ethyl starch infusions was, without exception, good. There was immediate rise in blood pressure, and the success of the therapy was comparable to the effect of dextran 75. A later report [*389*] reveals that up to now 60 patients, 49 of whom were in hemorrhagic shock, were each treated successfully with 500—1500 ml of HO-ethyl starch; further data is available from LEE [*1730 a*], and [*1817 b*].

### *n) Summary: HO-ethyl Starch*

1. At present in the USA a 6% solution of hydroxyethyl starch in 0.9% saline is being tested extensively. This is not yet commercially available. On the basis of the scanty findings to date it may be assumed that this starch solution brings about therapeutic results comparable to those of dextran 75 in dogs and in humans. With certain preparations, however, *toxic properties* were observed.

2. Little has yet been published about the physico-chemical properties of this substance. It is sometimes assumed on the basis of viscosity determinations that the molecular weight is similar to that of dextran 75. However this assumption is not justified, since HO-ethyl starch has a different molecular structure. Various findings seem to indicate that this preparation contains very high molecular weight fractions and is highly polydisperse.

3. As yet there are no important advantages over dextran, since the antigenicity of dextran no longer plays a part in the preparations used today.

4. HO-ethyl starch and dextran 75 appear to behave similarly with regard to the influence on blood coagulation.

5. Nothing definite can be said yet concerning the antithrombotic properties.

6. With regard to the influence on erythrocyte aggregation and flow improvement, there is likewise no data available yet.

7. Without a doubt it will take several years to clear up all of the problems which are encountered when a new plasma substitute is introduced. In the case of dextran it became evident that some questions crop up, are understood and solved only after years of worldwide use. The advantage of an expander with a starch base would certainly be the relatively inexpensive raw material which is available everywhere and in sufficiently large supply.

### 5. Alginon

A plasma replacement solution containing 3.36% alginon is sold in Switzerland as Plasmaflex (Laboratoires Vifor S. A., Geneva). The manufacturer states that alginon (sodium salt of polymannuronic acid) with an average MW of 20,000 is obtained by partial hydrolysis of sodium alginate, a polysaccharide derivative extracted from marine algae. "Further: infusion of alginon does not cause dilution of hemoglobin in the blood since release of hemoglobin is promoted"! The rest of the data in the prospectus is also difficult to understand. 50% of the amount infused is already excreted 1 hour after infusion. There is reference to 5 Japanese articles from 1945 to 1957; we ourselves have found only 1 article by Takayama [*1418*] in the European literature. Because of the scanty data one can not recommend use of this preparation as a plasma expander (cf. also [*683, 1064*] and Hartmann, in [*355*]).

### 6. Levan

In 1963 Schechter [*1251, 1252*] published a preliminary report about the possible use of Levan as a plasma substitute. There are no results about the clinical use of this fructose polymer ($\overline{M}_n = 28{,}000$, $\overline{M}_w = 115{,}000$). See also [*1677*].

# D. Volume Replacement with Colloid-free Solutions

## I. Electrolyte Solutions

### 1. General Remarks

The idea of using colloid-free fluids for treating volume loss is attractive because of its simplicity. Since the solutions used for this purpose contain nothing but substances already found in the body, it is not necessary to discuss toxicity, metabolism, histological and immunological studies, allergic reactions, etc.

As early as 1879 KRONECKER and SANDER showed that dogs with great loss of blood could be kept alive with saline infusions (quoted in [*848*], cf. also [*352 a, 1717*]); in 1886 LANDERER made successful saline infusions in humans (quoted in [*848*]). At the same time, however, much was said against the use of saline solutions in hemorrhagic shock. COHNHEIM and LICHTHEIM [*1877*] found a high degree of edema in the stomach wall after infusion of electrolyte solutions [*1717*] (quoted in [*1514*]).

SCHEGA [*1253, 1254, 1255, 1256*] has thoroughly studied the problem of edema formation after infusion of electrolyte solutions in hypovolemic animals. He assumes that electrolyte solutions leave the vascular system in the stomach and intestinal tract at the same rate with which they are infused. Edema occurs also after use of PVP, but not after infusions of 6% dextran (see also [*1296*]). It appears that edema occurs very readily in traumatized tissue. Recently a sequestration of protein-rich fluid was found in the intestinal tract of rats and dogs after abdominal trauma, both in the wall and in the lumen [*458, 528 a*].

The data on this topic, however, varies quite considerably. Several authors warn of the danger of edema formation [*43, 216, 463, 1703*]. Others however have observed no unfavorable effects following rapid infusion of electrolyte solutions in normovolemic individuals under anesthesia [*83*]. Also after serious tissue trauma, such as burns [*1054*], no brain or lung edema nor heart insufficiency was observed following infusion of very large amounts of electrolyte solutions in animals and humans [*21, 462, 846, 1214*], see also [*1851*]. The state of renal function probably plays an important part here.

CRAWFORD and LUDEMANN [*310*] have infused 1—3 liters of 0.9% or 0.5 liters of 5% NaCl solution in healthy individuals without changes in renal blood flow occurring. These authors further point out that humans, compared with dogs, are able to excrete a sodium excess only slowly and therefore are prone to lung edema (cf. [*491*]); in dogs too the occurrence of pulmonary edema depends considerably on the state of renal function [*659*].

HOLM [*722*] assumes that the hypoalbuminemia which occurs after the infusion of electrolyte solutions can be partially explained by a retardation of albumin return into the intravascular space.

In most of the experimental studies mentioned in the previous chapters one can see that electrolyte infusions which correspond to the lost volume have a certain therapeutic effect. In many of these articles, the effect of the carrier solution was checked with a group of animals treated with 0.9% saline solution. In spite of temporary improvement [*1257*] as can be seen in many publications, the results of treatment with replacement equal to the volume lost is relatively poor compared with plasma and good colloids

[*42, 244, 352, 405, 542, 578, 684, 769, 780, 809, 925, 957, 1048, 1071, 1115, 1117, 1155, 1214, 1494*].

On the other hand COLEMAN et al. [*290*] recently showed that even the infusion of pure water in irreversible shock in dogs produces a protective effect, and that a 0.45% NaCl solution impairs hemolysis and is no less effective than 0.9% saline solution. TABOR [*1413*], however, found no effect with the administration of water in mice.

It was known at an early date that water and sodium ions [*410*] are important in the treatment of all hypovolemic shock conditions [*835, 1213, 1413*].

S. M. ROSENTHAL and R. C. MILLICAN [*1214*], two pioneers in this field, compiled their own experience and the results of the literature (287 references); they concluded that therapy of hemorrhagic shock with electrolyte solution can be successful only if several times the amount lost are infused early enough. For this reason, only investigations which follow this principle are mentioned below.

## 2. Volume Effect

*In dogs* after blood loss of a small percent of the bw, the blood volume can be maintained by infusion of 0.9% saline solution in an amount 2.5× that of the blood lost [*378*].

In normovolemic *volunteers* practically no increase in blood volume can be found 2 hours after an i. v. infusion of 1 liter of physiological saline solution [*151, 505*].

After infusion of 500 ml of lactated Ringer's solution we have found only a somewhat more rapid rise in blood volume in slightly hypovolemic, fully hydrated volunteers compared with control individuals ([*601, 604*], see Fig. 6; cf. also [*14, 376, 1106*]).

In recent years the articles of SHIRES and his associates as well as those of others have repeatedly advocated the use of large amounts of Ringer's lactate for treating hemorrhagic shock (survey in [*1332*], see also [*352 a*]). These authors have developed a method for simultaneous measurement of erythrocyte volume and plasma volume as well as interstitial fluid [*1328, 1329*]. After blood losses of 10% of the BV in dogs, the reduction of the extracellular space (ECS) corresponds to the amount of blood removed [*1332*]; after bleeding of 25% of the BV, however, a reduction of the ECS from 18—26% was determined (measured with $^{35}SO_4$ and other methods [*1331*]). This is attributed to a non-measurable redistribution of ECS fluid [*1329*]. When dogs in irreversible shock models received lactated Ringer's solution amounting to 5% of the bw in addition to the blood removed, there was no reduction of the ECS, but there was with blood alone or with blood plus 1% of the bw in plasma ([*1330*], cf. also [*984 a, 1707*]).

Almost identical results were observed in humans [*311*], but here the blood losses averaged only 1131 ml. Another article recommends giving the patient a balanced electrolyte solution in the dosage, "blood lost plus 10 ml/kg bw" [*786*].

Recent studies by MOORE [*1044*] lead one to believe that the observations of SHIRES were made with extremely dehydrated individuals. MOORE infused 6 patients who had been hypovolemic for 4 hours with normal saline solution amounting to 3.5 times the amount of blood which was lost within 4 hours (blood losses between 10.5 and 14.3% of the bw). The infusion was completed in 4 hours. With this therapy the plasma volume is temporarily normalized because about 1/4 of the electrolyte solution infused remains in the vascular system. Infusion of fluid per os has a similar effect.

*During the hypovolemic phase and after infusion the changes of the ECS are exactly as expected. No inexplicable deficits were observed.* The influx of albumin is not impaired by the infusion of saline solution; it is about 4 g/hr. At the end of the experimental period the albumin concentrations in the treated individuals were greater than in the control individuals. The globulins, however, were highly diluted during the infusion. On the other hand, hyperglobulinemia occurred in the control individuals who received neither fluid nor nourishment (cf. also p. 7). From these experiments MOORE concludes that *replacement therapy of this type* (electrolyte solution infused = 3.5 times amount of blood lost) *must be repeated after about 6 hours if no colloid-containing solutions have been given in the meantime.* In the experimental studies of SERKES and LANG [*1321*] as well, the results of SHIRES could be repeated neither in hemorrhagic shock nor in tourniquet shock; this means that here too the reduction of the ECS corresponded to the amount of blood lost, and no unexplainable deficits occurred (see also [*723*]). This has now been confirmed in several recent papers [*1591, 1611 a, 1691 b, 1783, 1792, 1805, 1813, 1844*].

The associates of MOYER [*352*] assume that extracellular fluid is "bound" to the ground substance in severe shock; however no definite evidence can be produced for this theory.

## 3. Therapeutic Results

### *a) Isotonic Solutions*

FRANK et al. [*463*] and NASTUCK and BEATTY [*1073*] observed no effect after additional infusion of glucose or electrolyte solutions during the late stages of hemorrhagic shock in dogs. Also working with dogs WOLFMAN et al. [*1548*] was able to reduce the mortality from 80% to 20% by infusing lactated Ringer's solution in a dosage of 25% of the ECS in addition to blood (see also [*1214, 1513*]).

In the irreversible shock model described on p. 148, SHIRES observed a survival rate of 20% with transfusion of blood only, and 30% after blood plus small amounts of plasma. After infusion of blood plus large amounts of Ringer's lactated solution, 70% of the animals survived.

With early treatment consisting of large amounts (up to 50% of the bw!) of electrolyte solutions without colloids, the following authors observed good results in animal experiments in the treatment of acute hypovolemia and hemorrhagic shock conditions: [*21, 22, 108 b, 202 a, 462, 535 a, 1083, 1117, 1182, 1229 a, 1229 b, 1229 c, 1245, 1413, 1470, 1611 a, 1838*].

Reviews can be found in EICHHOLTZ [*394*] and ROSENTHAL [*1214*]. In endotoxin shock large amount of electrolyte solutions do not seem to be favorable [*1796*].

None of these articles, however, provides evidence that therapy with electrolyte solutions alone produces better results than treatment with blood, albumin, and modern dextran preparations in doses which cause an identical volume effect and take into account the normal requirements of water and electrolyte (invisible loss, assisted respiration, etc.).

In certain situations electrolyte solutions seem to produce a better effect than plasma or artificial colloids; these are experimental situations which do not correspond to clinical conditions [*462, 1413*]. In other studies colloids with strong side-effects were used [*21, 22, 1117*], or a combination of shock and dehydration was investigated [*202 a*]. Also there are cases where the animals received massive overtransfusions [*1229 c*]. Some authors do not attempt to show any superiority of electrolyte solutions over colloids, but do show that early infusion of large amounts of electrolyte solution in slight to moderately severe shock can bring about amazingly good results [*1182*]; with regard to this there are no corresponding control experiments with good colloids [*1083, 1182, 1245*].

The possibility of treating hemorrhagic shock with large amounts of lactated Ringer's solution was recently studied thoroughly, particularly by DILLON et al. [*351, 352, 352 a*], associates of MOYER. In these studies all questions in this regard are discussed thoroughly and important conclusions are drawn; thus they warrant closer inspection.

All of the experiments of this group have taken place at various times during the last 17 years [*352*]. In the experiments over 100 dogs were used in a modified Wiggers technique, where all untreated control animals succumb and 50% of those which receive shed blood survive. In such a situation improving or worsening of survival chances due to the infusion solution tested can be observed very well.

The following types of therapy were tested (number of animals/mortality):

1. *Controls*, no treatment (6/6).

2. Retransfusion of shed *blood* (24/12).

3. Like 2, plus the same amount of *RL-8* (12/3). RL-8 is a lactated Ringer's solution, the pH of which is adjusted to 8.2—8.5 by the addition of 0.1 n NaOH.

4. Like 2, plus 3 times the amount of 5% *glucose solution* (7/6).

5. Like 2 plus the same amount of 10% *mannitol solution* (6/6).

6. Retransfusion of *half* of the shed blood plus *RL-8 according to formula* (8/1).

The formula is: volume of shed blood + [(volume of shed blood in ml) × (0.035 × Hct of the shed blood)].

*Example:* A dog in this group with a Hct of 40, from which 1 liter of blood was taken, receives 500 m of blood + [1000 + (1000 × 0.035 × 40) ml of lactated Ringer's solution] = 500 ml of blood + 2400 ml of lactated Ringer's solution.

The amount of Ringer's solution thus corresponds to the amount of blood removed in the following multiples:

with Hct 50: 2.75×,
with Hct 40: 2.4×,
with Hct 30: 2×.

7. *Retransfusion of half of the blood removed + RL-8 in a volume equal to that of the blood removed* (14/8).

8. Retransfusion of *half* of the blood removed plus *6% dextran* (MW?) in *0.9% NaCl solution with an amount equal to the amount of blood removed* (i. e. the dogs received massive overtransfusion!) (13/7).

9. Retransfusion of *half* of the blood removed plus *6% dextran* (MW?) in *10% fructose with an amount equal to the amount of blood removed* (see 8!) (8/6).

10. *RL-8 according to formula* (20/10).

11. *RL-6 according to formula* (7/6). RL-6 is a commercially available Ringer's solution (Na = 130, Cl = 109, Lactate = 28, K = 4, Ca = 3 mval/l) with a pH of 6.5.

12. *6% dextran* (MW?) in 0.9% saline solution in an amount equal to the amount of blood removed (9/7).

13. *7% Hydroxyethyl starch* in Ringer's solution in same dosage as 12 (9/9).

The statistical evaluation reveals the following:

*Blood retransfusion (2) results in:*

i. significantly lower mortality compared with 1, 4, 5, 11, 13,
ii. comparable mortality compared with 3, 7, 8, 9, 10, 12,
iii. higher mortality than 6.

The "formula" provided is based on experiments with dogs and huma which showed that the plasma volume increase after massive infusion water and salt was

$$0.077 \times H_2O \text{ load} + 1.152 \times \text{val Na load.} \qquad [35$$

In another article by the same author [351] another "formula" is give (amount of erythrocytes)×4+amount of plasma removed (in ml).

Although the authors theoretically place very strict requirements on t shock protocol for testing various types of therapy, they overlook t following important points in their experiments:

1. The weight of the experimental animals varies between 12—28 l
2. The number of experimental animals in each group varies betwe 6 and 24.
3. A comparison of the figures of untreated (6) animals and those tra fused with shed blood (24) shows that these controls were not carried simultaneously with all other types of therapy.
4. Several external experimental conditions changed during the cou of 17 years, as can be ascertained in the section, "methods".
5. It is assumed that all dogs have a BV of 8%, although this was measured.
6. The animals in the dextran group were all overtransfused, since rapid infusion of 6% dextran 70 or 80 initially causes a much larger bl volume, even if the volume replacement is equal.

Since the authors evaluate their data even further when statistically significant differences resulted, and draw their conclusions, the follow points must be emphasized: detailed data concerning the dextran prepa tions used is lacking; they were probably (17 years ago!) old preparati with high peak fractions. The authors believe that one may do with infusion of colloids in shock therapy since it is known that there are pec who have no plasma albumin and whose blood volume is normal in s of that. However such individuals have other proteins with colloid osm properties; there are no studies about the influence of this anomaly in sh The data given is in part contradictory; as in the text it is stated starch was used in Ringer's solution, but in the summary there is men of starch in NaCl.

Thus several points in these articles remain open, but the followin clear: The survival figures in this hemorrhagic shock model are the s whether the shed blood is retransfused or whether 2—3 times as n Ringer's lactate is given; this is true although the animals in the electro group have a hematocrit level of 15%, hemoglobin level of approx. 6 g and a hypoproteinemia of 50%. DILLON assumes that the BV in electrolyte groups was not normalized, but he provides no usable meas ments. The experiments also show the superiority of electrolyte solut over glucose and other crystalloid solutions.

In this respect the results of RUSH [*1229 c*] and TAKAORI [*1417*] are interesting; they reported that strong hemodilution with large amounts of electrolyte solutions, unlike colloids, does not cause long-term survivals (cf. also [*1415, 1416*]).

There are no statistically evaluated articles concerning the management of patients in *severe* hemorrhagic shock with the use of large amounts of balanced electrolyte solution [*1779, 1788*]; this method is at present being tested by the Americans in the Vietnam War (see [*616*]). In humans smaller blood losses can be treated successfully with infusion of 2—3 times as much electrolyte solution [*1229 b, 1836*]; other than price, however, there appear to be no advantages with this method (cf. [*1044 a*]).

There are statistically evaluated articles concerning the managment of burns with large amounts of electrolyte solutions. On the basis of the studies by MARKLEY [*952*], MOYER [*1054*] and WILSON [*1533*], one can assume that such electrolyte therapy produces results comparable to those of plasma in the initial treatment of burn shock in adults, but not in children; there has not yet been proof of superiority over the customary types of therapy with colloid and electrolyte solutions (see also [*617*]).

### *b) Hypertonic Solutions*

BROOKS et al. [*216*] used a hemorrhagic shock model of 90 minutes duration (BP 40 mm Hg) in dogs. They compared the effect of an infusion of 2.74% sodium bicarbonate (332 mval/l) or 1.8% NaCl solution *during* the hypotensive phase with the effect of 10% glucose and isotonic saline solution. In this model untreated control animals and recipients of hypertonic glucose or physiological saline solutions usually did not survive; on the other hand, animals which were infused with solutions having double osmolarity compared with plasma recovered. On the basis of these experiments the authors recommend increasing the plasma osmolality during treatment of hemorrhagic shock states by means of infusion of hypertonic solutions; this also enlarges the extracellular space and eliminates disturbances in the acid-base balance. The case history of a patient treated in this manner is given as an illustration. The experiments of BROOKS, however, are not incontestable, because

1. the infusion therapy is a prophylactic treatment here,
2. the number of experimental animals is not the same in the various groups,
3. some of the animals were treated with antibiotics,
4. there are no controls with colloids.

In letters to the editor of *Lancet* these experiments were criticized for other reasons: Controls with double the amount of isotonic saline solution are lacking [*727*], the BV effect of the various infusion solutions is not known

[*988*]. J. B. WALKER [*1475*] comments that she already described the favorable effect of high percent saline solutions in shock patients as early as 1936. The answer of BROOKS [*217*] to these letters is not able to dissipate the justified doubt about the value of his work (see also [*386*]).

BERGENTZ and BRIEF [*136*] have likewise shown the importance of osmolality; in their experimental procedure they compared physiological (0.3 molar) and hypertonic (0.6 molar) saline solutions and Tris buffer = Tham (0.6 molar). Correction of acidosis with Tham produced no advantages over 0.6 m saline solution in agreement with the results of BROOKS (see also [*1513, 1603*]). It is interesting that in these experiments as well, the sharp drop in Hct in the groups treated with hypertonic solutions did not influence the chances of survival.

In hemorrhagic shock in dogs, BÜCHERL [*230*] observed no effect of hypertonic solutions. However REINERT [*1173*] observed an increase in survival rate in a small series of rats after infusion of 1.8% NaCl solution. MESSMER [*1007*] has shown that the infusion of hypertonic sugar or electrolyte solutions causes a sharp increase in flow in the splanchnic region. In severe hemorrhagic shock in rats, hypertonic solutions together with retransfusions of blood brought about a significant increase in survival time and the number of survivors compared with blood retransfusion plus isotonic solutions; the chemical structure of the dissolved substance apparently was unimportant (see also [*1603*]). Like BERGENTZ [*136*], MESSMER [*1007*] assumes that the protective effect of hypertonic solutions depends on the increase of osmolality and not on the presence of Na ions (see also [*108 a, 162 a, 1753*]).

BRAND [*202 a*] used an electrolyte-glucose mixture with an osmolality of 360 mosm. Before the beginning of the experiment however his animals were severely dehydrated; because of this it is not surprising that infusion of blood or colloid alone has poorer results than infusion of the slightly hypertonic solution.

## II. Non-electrolyte Solutions

It is certain that isotonic glucose solutions provide a slight protective effect in the treatment of hypovolemic shock conditions of all kinds; even so, no one doubts any longer that *solutions containing sodium* always produce better results (cf. control experiments in the previous chapters and [*1214*]).

The value of giving hypertonic non-electrolyte solutions in *addition* to blood replacement is not yet clear and the results are contradictory (cf. [*352, 1007*]). There are no corresponding studies in humans [*1753*].

## III. Summary and Conclusions: Volume Replacement with Colloid-free Solutions

1. Death occurs in most cases after several hours despite temporary improvement if a blood loss which permits no spontaneous improvement is replaced with the same amount of electrolyte solution.

2. Animal and human studies show that blood volume barely can be maintained for a few hours after replacement of the blood lost with 2—3 times as much isotonic electrolyte solution. A relatively larger portion of the electrolyte solution infused remains in the vascular system in hypovolemia than in normovolemia.

3. Some authors assume that an unproportionally large reduction of the interstitial space (IS) occurs in hypovolemic shock. It is not clear where this fluid goes; perhaps it is bound to the ground substance. Other studies however in hypovolemic individuals showed no unproportionally large reduction of the IS.

4. In animal experiments, early replacement of lost blood with *large* amounts of electrolyte solutions without colloids in hemorrhagic shock produces results as good as those obtained with blood, plasma derivatives or artificial colloids. There is no proof that this type of therapy is superior; there are no results of careful comparative studies in humans.

5. There are reasons to believe that blood transfusion plus additional transfusion of Ringer's solution with a pH of 8 in a dose 2—3 times as large as the amount of blood lost in hemorrhagic shock in dogs can produce better results than blood replacement alone; but there are no convincing human studies with regard to this.

6. There seems to be no danger of edema formation with infusion of large amounts of electrolyte solutions when cardiac and renal functions are intact; however there are no precise data about this risk in shock patients who have cardiac or renal damage.

7. Additional use of hypertonic solutions (regardless of the substance dissolved) along with blood transfusion has a favorable hemodynamic effect; nothing is known about the therapeutic value in humans, and in animal experiments the results are contradictory.

8. Maintaining normal plasma osmolality is more important than correcting metabolic acidosis in order to increase the chances of survival in animal experiments.

9. In the treatment of all hypovolemic shock conditions, solutions containing electrolytes are much more effective than glucose solutions. For this reason it is stressed that all colloidal substances should *always* be infused *in media containing electrolytes* in treatment of shock (no salt-free albumin or dextran in 5% glucose should be used!).

PART THREE

# Discussion

There is no doubt that complete restoration of the circulating blood volume as early as possible is the most important therapy in larger blood loss and all forms of hypovolemic shock. While this *principle* is not con tested, views about various details differ, e. g. about the most favorabl *route of application* for volume replacement.

## A. Oral Therapy

The simplest method for volume replacement is certainly *oral ad ministration of hypotonic saline solution.* Isotonic saline solutions woul be desirable, but they can usually not be swallowed by the patients du to the unappetizing taste. The p. o. therapy, however, is suitable *only fo the treatment of smaller volume losses* (up to 30% of the BV at most) o *as an additional measure* when i. v. replacement is incomplete. It seem appropriate to support the spontaneous refilling of the vascular system b such a procedure. After multiple injuries patients are often incapable o taking fluid orally (unconsciousness!) and therapy of this kind shoul only be started if one is certain that there is *no injury to the gastrointestin tract* and that therapy can be started immediately after the volume loss. *risk* does exist in that patients who may receive such treatment often have tendency to vomit and thus are subjected to the danger of aspiration. Fro the standpoint of the anesthesiologist as well, this procedure is undesirable there is to be *anesthesia and surgery* shortly after the treatment for shock.

The effectiveness of administering fluid orally is limited in that th absorption of water is retarded after trauma. This applies also to fluid which are administered by means of enema. Goldberg and Fine [*533* showed in 1945 that intestinal absorption of water and glucose in hemor rhagic shock in animals is soon greatly impaired, while absorption of physic logical saline solution is impaired only in later stages. Tinckler [*1443* recently showed that water reaching the jejunum directly by means of tube is absorbed after trauma, but fluid which is drunk by the patient is nc (inadequate intestinal motility). It is also known from burn experimen [*15*, *1212*] that early (before shock is established) oral administratio of hypotonic electrolyte solutions is able to maintain the plasma volume i less severe cases (burns of up to 20% of the body surface). Allgöwer [*35* used this method successfully at an earlier date. It seems to be *appropriate as first aid treatment when insufficient or no i. v. fluid infusion is possible* and when there are no contraindications. This type of therapy can be recommended especially in situations where the *volume loss* takes places *relatively slowly*, as in burns, war and catastrophe situations. One must realize however that volume replacement by this means only takes place slowly compared with i.v. administration in humans, and that the organism depends upon the mobilization of its own colloid reserves. *The administration of water and electrolytes is the most important factor in volume replacement therapy; for this reason there is no doubt that the oral administration of hypotonic electrolyte solutions, perhaps by means of a tube, is much better than no therapy at all* (cf. [*1836 a*]).

## B. Intra-arterial Infusion

Recommendations continually appear for *intra-arterial administration* of infusion solutions in severe hemorrhagic shock [*949, 1236, 1364, 1449, 1580*]. In 1955 this problem was thoroughly clarified by GURD [*624*]. He showed that the site of infusion is unimportant as long as sufficient volume can be supplied during a certain period of time (see also [*640*]). In these studies it can also be seen that too rapid infusion when normovolemia has almost been reached or overtransfusion worsens the prognosis. Furthermore intra-artierial infusions are seldom used clinically for shock therapy, since it is usually much more difficult and time-consuming to find a good approach to an artery than to one or more veins. On the other hand there is no objection to intra-arterial infusion if an artery has already been catheterized, perhaps intra- or postoperatively. One can assume that *i. a. infusion has a better effect* than i. v. infusion when the pressure in the aorta *in terminal stages* has already fallen so far that adequate *perfusion of the coronaris* is no longer possible. *In all other situations there is no good evidence which would support the superiority of i. a. over i. v. infusion, so long as there is the possibility of infusing an equal volume in the same period of time.*

Thus in clinical situations it is recommended that one inserts venous catheters percutaneously or by cut down at an early stage (i. e. perhaps even preoperatively) in patients threatened by shock so that infusions can be made quickly and in sufficient amounts should the need arise. The risk of a properly (aseptically) introduced venous catheter is surely less than the danger which faces a patient in severe shock when it is impossible to provide immediate and sufficient volume replacement.

## C. Hemoglobin, Oxygen Transport

Along with volume replacement, all measures should be taken in order to provide sufficient oxygen supply to the tissues (cf. [*1095*]). The factors which influence oxygen transport fall into three main categories [*119*]:

## I. The Gas Phase

Further division can be made; the column at the right lists the idea: conditions which are to be achieved in each subdivision

| | *Ideal conditions* |
|---|---|
| Inspired air | sufficient $pO_2$ |
| Airways | unobstructed, low resistance |
| Lungs | normal volume, capacity and compliance |
| Alveolar ventilation | sufficient for maintaining normal $pCO_2$; evenly distributed for geographical matching with capillary perfusion |

## II. The Blood Phase

| | *Ideal conditions* |
|---|---|
| Arterial $pO_2$ | sufficient for full utilization of the $O_2$-carryin; capacity of blood |

In the treatment of shocked patients and patients who are severely ill one should generally strive for the most ideal conditions possible pari passı with volume replacement (i. e. ventilation with oxygen!). This is illustratec by the following parameters which for the most part determine the blooc phase of oxygen supply and which are already influenced in a negative wa) by the primary blood loss.

| | |
|---|---|
| Oxygen content | dependent on Hb concentration and $pO_2$ |
| Cardiac output | lowered |
| Blood volume | lowered |
| Flow distribution | disturbed |
| Pulmonary circulation | lowered, because dependent upon the BV; als( relation to the alveolar ventilation is disturbe( |

Normal oxygen transport in the blood is further dependent on th( "milieu intérieur" which is provided by the *isoiony* (constant ion compositioı and number of ions), *isotonicity* (constant osmotic pressure) and *isohydr*} (constant hydrogen ion concentration); also *temperature* and the amount o: *buffers* present are important.

## III. The Tissue Phase

In this category belong the capillaries and the tissues which guarante( adequate oxygen supply by means of normal permeability and metabolism This phase is also disturbed in shock. In the ideal situation, i. e. where ther( are no changes in the vital organs, all factors can be normalized by earl)

replacement of the lost blood by means of an erythrocyte free solution; the $O_2$ content (dependent on the Hb concentration) is the only exception to this. It can be seen in Table 13 and Fig. 19 (from [*119*]) that the amount of circulating Hb is the limiting factor in treatment of shock with erythrocyte free solutions.

Table 13

| | | Respiration of | |
|---|---|---|---|
| | | room air art. $pO_2$ 100 mm Hg* | 100% $O_2$ art. $pO_2$ 650 mm Hg |
| 15 g Hb | Hb $O_2$ | 19.60 ml | 20.10 ml |
| | dissolved $O_2$ | 0.30 ml | 1.95 ml |
| | Total | 19.90 ml | 22.05 ml |
| 10 g Hb | Hb $O_2$ | 13.00 ml | 13.40 ml |
| | dissolved $O_2$ | 0.30 ml | 1.95 ml |
| | Total | 13.30 ml | 15.35 ml |
| 5 g Hb | Hb $O_2$ | 6.50 ml | 6.70 ml |
| | dissolved $O_2$ | 0.30 ml | 1.95 ml |
| | Total | 6.80 ml | 8.65 ml |

* A Hb saturation of 97% is assumed.
Normal Hb levels: Males 14.5—18.1 g-%
Females 12.5—16.7 g-%

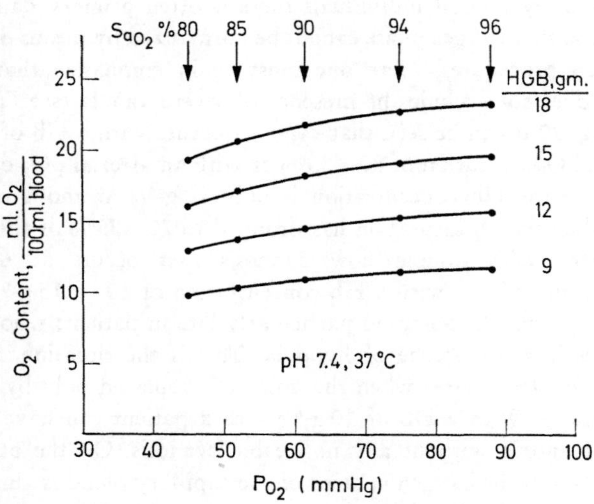


Fig. 19. The $O_2$ carrying capacity of blood depends on the Hb concentration and the arterial oxygen partial pressure. $Sa_{O_2}$=oxygen saturation of arterial blood; $P_{O_2}$=oxygen partial pressure. (From BENDIXEN et al. [*119*].)

*The dependency of $O_2$ transport in ml/min upon cardiac output (norm 5—6 l/min) and various Hb concentrations* can be seen in *Table 14* (fr( [*119*]):

Table 14

| cardiac output | Hemoglobin 15 g room air | 15 g 100% $O_2$ | 10 g room air | 10 g 100% $O_2$ | 5 g room air | 5 g 100% $O_2$ |
|---|---|---|---|---|---|---|
| 10 l | 1990 | 2205 | 1330 | 1535 | 680 | 865 |
| 5 l | 995 | 1103 | 665 | 768 | 340 | 433 |
| 2.5 l | 498 | 552 | 333 | 383 | 170 | 217 |

It can be seen from these data that a reduction of the Hb to 10 g- can be compensated by a relatively slight increase in the cardiac outp especially when the patient is ventilated with pure oxygen.

It is also clear that one may replace blood losses of up to approximat( 30% of the BV without danger in previously healthy young patients using erythrocyte-free solutions, if these solutions provide continual refilli of the blood volume and an increase in cardiac output. On the other ha one must recognize that the following factors limit the compensati capability of the circulation for hypoxia [*119*]:

Advanced age, coronary heart disease, cardiopulmonary diseases, obesi acidosis, hyperthyroid state and fever. Antiadrenergic agents, sedati\ narcotics and anesthetics also have a similar effect.

In seriously injured individuals there is often primary damage to lı function, so that the gas phase cannot be normalized by means of therapeı ventilation procedures. Here one must again emphasize that absence cyanosis does not exclude the presence of severe anoxia (see *Fig. 20*).

In Fig. 20 it can be seen that *cyanosis* occurs with a Hb of 15 g-% a an arterial $O_2$ saturation of 80—85% or with an arterial $pO_2$ of 45 mm I If however the Hb concentration is only 10 g-%, cyanosis only becor visible when the $O_2$ saturation has dropped to 70—75% or the $pO_2$ is o: 35 mm Hg. With double flow cyanosis first occurs at 60—70% saturation in patients with a Hb concentration of 10 or 15 g-%. Genera speaking, cyanosis is observed particularly late in patients who can incre flow rates in the presence of hypoxia. This is the situation, for examj after larger blood losses when the volume is replaced only by erythrocy free solutions. With a Hb of 10 g-% such a patient can have a danger degree of anoxia without any noticeable cyanosis. On the other hand, low flow states the oxygen content of the capillary blood is almost as low that of venous blood and cyanosis occurs early. If the oxygen absorption the tissues is high and the flow rate very low, cyanosis can occur althoı the arterial oxygen saturation is 100%.

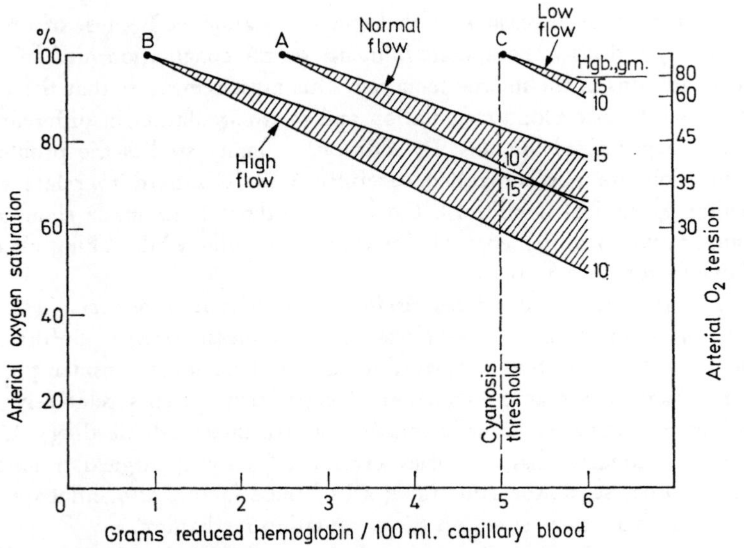


Fig. 20. Relation between arterial $O_2$ saturation, $O_2$ tension in mm Hg and reduced Hb content in capillary blood with Hb concentrations of 10 or 15 g/100 ml of blood

It is assumed that cyanosis occurs with a 5 g-% reduced Hb content in capillary blood (cyanosis threshold).

A: Relationships with normal blood flow, assuming that capillary blood consists of approx. $^2/_3$ venous and $^1/_3$ arterial blood and the a. v. difference of reduced Hb is 3.76 g-%.

B: Relationships with double cardiac output, assuming that the ratio in capillary blood is 1:1, arterial to venous, and that a. v. difference in reduced Hb is 1.9 g-%.

C: Represents a "low flow" state. Flow is reduced by $^1/_3$; it is assumed that the capillaries contain approximately 90% venous blood and only 10% arterial blood. The a. v. difference in reduced Hb is approximately 5.6 g-%. (From BENDIXEN et al. [*119*].)

# D. Shock Models

It is extremely difficult to base conclusions concerning therapy in humans on the results of experiments with hemorrhagic shock in animals [*1329*]. *The following factors influence mortality in experimental hemorrhagic shock:*

Species [*1585*], sex, age, season, time of day, room temperature [*1782*], humidity of the air, endemic diseases (worms, cysticerci), nutritional status and hydration conditions.

Even more important are premedication and *type of anesthesia.* With regard to this, RUSHMER [*1230*] states that results obtained with anesthetized animals may be applied only with the greatest caution to non-anesthetized animals and to humans (see also [*106, 1092, 1177, 1359, 1363, 1426, 1593, 1828, 1834*]). One must also consider the fact that most experiments are made (for technical reasons) with *heparinized* animals. Because of this th is already a decisiv therapeutic influence on the coagulation mechanism a the conditions in the microcirculation. One must remember that the varic colloids influence blood coagulation and microcirculation in different wa in non-heparinized humans. In addition, in many studies the problems respiration are not controlled carefully, and it is hard to relate expe mental to clinical conditions. Only few authors have made simultanec comparative measurements with various substitutes while taking all of t above factors into account.

*For the evaluation of the usefulness of plasma expanders in huma it is important to have careful controls and measurements.* Unfortunat there are however few comparative studies. One must consider that pu hemorrhagic shock as used in animal experiments occurs relatively rar in humans (butchers' injuries, massive gastro-intestinal bleeding). Usua there are extensive tissue injuries, crushing, fractures, surgical trauma, a disease processes at the same time; all of these factors also influence sho especially with their effect on the coagulation mechanism.

Although traumatic shock can only be standardized with great difficul in animal experiments the importance of volume effect is such that it is st valuable to study its therapeutic influence in animals despite the poi mentioned. In a well-standardized animal experiment, the importance of t volume factor alone can be evaluated. In modern laboratories such fact as room temperature and humidity can be standardized for the most pa veterinaries are able today to provide standardized animals which have be nourished well and which are free of disease. Careful planning can take ir consideration such factors as season, date, and state of hydration. If o then uses the same type of anesthesia, ventilation and anticoagulation in cases, such animal experiments can provide important information. Howev the careful transfer of these results to clinical conditions compared with t findings in humans is important.

A further problem which affects both experimental shock research a clinical shock treatment is the *consideration of the daily requirements of t organism with regard to water, electrolytes and calories.* Only fe researchers take into account that the often lengthy shock experime require parenteral administration of water and electrolytes; this is often t case if one is not simultaneously studying the effect of dehydration, e. g. is appropriate in experiments which are to resemble situations like those war. But in such cases one must consider the important differences betwe animals and humans with regard to the spontaneous refilling of the vascul system. In humans this occurs much more slowly than in the usual labor tory animals. It is often seen that after intensive shock treatment a patien normal daily requirements of water and electrolytes are ignored for t most part or are even completely forgotten. This often applies to patie with whom peroral nourishment is theoretically possible but who have been subjected to severe trauma and are able to eat only small amounts. Many difficulties in restoring normal renal function after severe blood losses are simply based on the fact that it was realized too late that the patient did not receive his normal water requirement for several hours, not to mention additional fluid losses which often occur in such patients because of tubes, fistulas, drains, tracheotomy, etc.

*For good shock management one must therefore prescribe sufficient amounts of water, electrolytes and calories to cover the normal daily requirement, existing deficits and other possible losses in addition to providing sufficient volume replacement.*

## E. Problems of Blood Volume Determination

Because of the great importance of the volume factor in the management of shock, mortality studies in animal experiments for evaluating the therapeutic effect of plasma substitutes in man should go hand in hand with exact methods for determination of blood volume. A large number of books, review articles and original papers in recent years are dedicated to questions of methodology of blood volume determination. Some of the more important publications in this field are listed at the end of the bibliography. From these publications one can conclude the following:

1. BV determinations in man with an error of ±5% are possible with the methods known today [*36, 328, 593, 1527*]. With ideal conditions, the error is about ±3%.

2. The measurement of the BV as the sum of the erythrocyte- and plasma volumes (EV+PV) by means of two independent tracer substances provides the most accurate results [*328, 1319*].

3. If only 1 tracer is used, erythrocyte marking gives more reliable results than plasma marking when there is disturbed capillary permeability [*1775*]. In hemorrhagic shock the capillary permeability for RIHSA is unchanged [*1319*].

4. The most common, most reliable and simplest tracers which can be used are $^{51}Cr$ for the erythrocytes and $R^{131}IHSA$ or $R^{125}IHSA$ for determination of the plasma volume. Evans blue dye (=T 1824) can also be used, but this method is much more complicated if it is to provide accurate results.

5. The use of a semi-automatic electronic measuring device like the Volemetron and a radioactive plasma tracer measured in centrifuged plasma produces results equal to the usual methods of measurement [*272, 273, 1832*], so long as the necessary correction factors for the Hct are taken into account ([*615*], original unpublished results). Otherwise the figures for BV are higher compared with the summation methods.

6. To assure complete mixing in all cases, removal of several blo samples is important after injection of the tracer if the hemodynam conditions are not stable and/or the capillary permeability for the trac is increased. In all other situations removal of a small amount of blo after 10 minutes is sufficient for plasma marking substances. Extrapolati to 0 time is no more accurate than using the average figures from 10- a 30-minute sample [*66*].

7. One should not use a tourniquet for taking blood samples aft complete mixing of the tracer [*328*]. A Hct measurement should be ma along with every BV determination in the same sample. The use of a plas catheter placed in a big vein for isotope injection and taking samples dc not disturb the result if proper flushing is carried out (own unpublish results).

8. It has been shown that reliable results can be obtained by plasn tagging alone using RIHSA even after hemorrhage (30% of the BV) a transfusions, by taking a single 5, 10 or 20-minute sample [*160, 1489, 171* (cf. [*66*]).

9. With stable hemodynamics the same results may be obtained by mea of marking albumin with $^{125}I$ or $^{131}I$ or gamma globulin with $^{131}I$ [*152* or erythrocytes with $^{59}Fe$ or $^{51}Cr$ [*1036, 1686 a, 1698*].

Thus it can be assumed that reliable results are provided by the metho used by us for BV determination after removal of 400—500 ml of bloc and infusion of various blood replacement substances. We always us $R^{131}IHSA$ as a marking substance, the Volemetron as the measuring devi with 10-minute blood tests. In the studies with infusion of homologo plasma we never used a tourniquet and with every BV determination v measured the radioactivity in whole blood as well as in plasma. Taking t Hct correction factors into account resulted in the same figures (see [*615*] the detailed description of these data forms the subject of a separa publication.

The validity of the results of our BV determinations is confirmed by t studies of numerous other authors, some of whom use other methods (s Tables 5, 6, 9, 10).

## F. Colloid Osmotic Pressure, Filtration, Interstitial Pressure

More than a hundred years ago [*1859*] Claude Bernard (quoted [*363*]) recognized the importance of colloids for maintaining a norm BV. The classic work of Starling [*1379*] at the turn of the centu laid the cornerstone for our ideas about oncotic pressure. In gener his views are still valid today; he realized that proteins are also able pass the capillary endothelia, but he assumed that the amount was negligibl

Today we know that normal capillaries are also permeable to greater or smaller amounts of proteins according to regional differences, but that at the same time comparable quantities reach the circulation by way of the lymphatic system [*1044*].

The transcapillary transfer of macromolecules (MW greater than 10,000) is a matter of either *pinocytosis or cytopemsis.* Pinocytosis is vesicular transport into or out of the cell, and cytopemsis is vesicular transport of macromolecules across a membrane between two extracellular phases [*1179*]. Among other explanations for these phenomena are the "pore theories", whereby pores of various sizes, the largest of which are probably to be found on the venous side of the capillary bed, permit the passage of molecules of varying size (see also [*1021*]). These theories are predominantly working hypotheses which still need confirmation in humans under normal and pathological conditions.

The physico-chemical relationships are somewhat better clarified. It is known that filtration in the capillaries is a function of blood pressure ($P_B$), tissue pressure ($P_T$), extravascular ($t_T$) and intravascular ($t_B$) colloid osmotic pressure [*715*]; the following formula is valid:

$$\text{Filtration} = k\,(t_B - t_T + P_T - P_B).$$

The *pressure in the interstitial tissue* has been studied intensively in recent years by Guyton [*627*]. He assumes that there is a negative pressure of approx. —6.4 mm Hg in the interstitium under normal conditions. This pressure becomes positive only when edema occurs. These results are confirmed in humans as well; Perren (1967, Lab. f. exp. Surgery, Davos-Platz, personal information) has found negative pressures of the same magnitude in the interstitium of the lower leg, but after surgery of lower leg fractures these pressures become positive. Guyton [*628*] further showed that the elasticity of interstitial fluid is very low with negative pressures but increases considerably when positive levels are reached; this is also confirmed by clinical experience with patients suffering from edema (finger pressure!). He assumes [*629*] that under normal conditions the interstitial fluid is bound almost 100% to the gelatinous matrix of the ground substance and only becomes mobile when the interstitial pressure becomes positive, i. e. rises above 1 atmosphere (compare also [*1771*]).

These findings may possibly be able partially to *explain the effectiveness of large amounts of balanced electrolyte solutions in the treatment of hemorrhagic shock.* In the opinion of Dillon [*352*] and of Shires [*1322*] it is completely unimportant to maintain colloid osmotic pressure in treatment of hemorrhagic shock, but we believe that there have still been far too few careful studies with humans to justify taking over this concept in the clinic. Transcapillary refilling and possibly refilling through the lymphatic system occurs much more rapidly in laboratory animals than it does in humans; thus it is conceivable that the good laboratory results can not l reproduced in their full scope. The favorable findings in humans reporte by SHIRES [*1322*] are not surprising when one considers what we ha stated above concerning the daily requirements of water and electrolyte *There has not yet been any evidence that infusion of extremely lar amounts of electrolyte solutions is more advantageous than replaceme therapy with colloids plus water and electrolytes for satisfying the actu requirements in clinical treatment of shock.* According to most clinicians o therapeutic efforts should be directed toward restoring normal conditions the "milieu intérieur" as quickly as possible [*1696*].

HOPKINSON [*1696*] has shown that during a short period of hypovolem without hypotension, the interstitial (IS) fluid pressure fell but was restor to normal by reinfusing the shed blood. After a period of hypotensive sho the interstitial fluid pressure remained low and was not restored to norm by replacement of the shed blood alone. The addition of 5% bw Ringe solution restored the IS fluid pressure to normal. The use of dextran 70 or instead of Ringer's lactate lowered the IS fluid pressure further. The surviv rate of dogs treated by blood replacement plus Ringer or dextran is t same, suggesting that increased tissue perfusion and $O_2$-consumption a more important than replacement of extracellular fluid losses in the trea ment of hypotensive shock.

WEESE [*1495*] assumes that in treatment with artificial colloids t organism uses the foreign colloids to stabilize the colloid osmotic pressur and stores its own *proteins in deposits;* thus urea nitrogen and non protei nitrogen are not increased and the blood amino acids are unchanged [*146*

We see a possible explanation for the effectiveness of large amounts electrolyte solutions in that the extravascular colloid osmotic pressure dro while the associated rapid massive influx of albumin does not cause t intravascular pressure to rise as quickly as is often assumed. It is al conceivable that the lymph circulation and thus the influx of water, electr lytes and proteins is increased by means of infusion of large amounts electrolyte solutions (cf. [*535 a*]).

# G. Comparison of the Various Possibilities which are Available for Replacement of Blood Loss

*Blood* is still the most important therapeutic substance for treatme of severe blood losses. Certainly however several restrictions are necessa with regard to the principle that blood should *always* be replaced wi blood. It is certain today that the total hepatitis frequency (non-icte plus icteric cases) after blood transfusions is much higher than was pre ously assumed; thus one should stipulate that blood should be given on when the oxygen supply of the organism unconditionally requires it [*1654*

*1654 h*]. On the basis of clinical experience and many animal experiments, one may permit the Hct to drop to approximately 30% (or the Hb to 10 g-%) after refilling of the vascular system in patients who have no cardio-pulmonary disease, if perfect pulmonary function is assured and the oxygen requirement is not much increased. This means that with men of "normal" build, blood losses up to about 1½ liters (i. e. about 30% of the BV) may be replaced with erythrocyte-free solutions if there is no preexisting anemia. The other important reason which suggests a modification of the rule cited above is the fact that a patient can not be retransfused with his own blood. The dangers of immunological complications are becoming more and more clear, and it has recently become known that such complications can sometimes also have functional consequences in the form of rapid plasma loss.

Because of the danger of hepatitis, no more nonpasteurized *plasma preparations* should be used today in treatment of shock. Thus only PPS or albumin can be considered. Since these are available only in limited supply and are exceedingly expensive, the use of artificial colloidal solutions is becoming more and more common. No final judgment can be made yet concerning the possibility of using *electrolyte solutions* alone. It is conceivable that in the future we may have to revise our ideas concerning the importance of colloid osmotic pressure; on the other hand there seems to be no reason why one should not maintain a normal oncotic pressure whenever this is possible.

In German-speaking countries only two of the *artificial colloidal solutions* are considered today: *dextran and gelatin.* In America, Canada, England and most of the Scandinavian countries only dextran preparations can be sold. *PVP* is practically no longer used because it can not be broken down at all by the organism. Only preliminary reports exist concerning *starch* and *levan;* no preparations made with these substances are available commercially. Finally *Alginon* can not be described as an effective plasma replacement substance. *Thus in the next chapter there is discussion as to whether or not there are good reasons for preferring preparations from one or the other of the dextran or gelatin groups.*

First the *disadvantages* must again be mentioned which all *artificial colloidal solutions* have compared with blood and plasma. They contain no enzymes, antibodies, nor coagulation factors. They have only a slight or no buffer capacity and can not take over the transport functions of the body proteins. However it must be emphasized that even the best plasma preparations such as PPS and albumin likewise contain few or no antibodies since the gamma globulin fraction has been separated. Pasteurization leads to further changes which cause these plasma preparations to be no longer identical with fresh blood with regard to enzyme content, coagulation factors, etc. [*1745 a*].

There is as yet no evidence that these more or less theoretical disadva tages would have a negative effect in initial shock therapy. Most importa would be the absence of coagulation factors, but this hardly is importa clinically, since the absent oxygen carrying capacity limits the administrati of artificial colloids anyway, and the organism in general possesses sufficie reserves for the compensation of hemodilution of this amount. Perfect r placement is not even possible with *autologous* fresh blood; here too an coagulants of some kind must be added, and any storage of blood in vit brings with it decisive changes in the coagulation process. Besides, individu plasma fractions such as gamma globulin or fibrinogen can be given tod in those cases where there is a deficit or a therapeutic effect can be expecte

## H. Dextran or Gelatin?

In 1957 GRÖNWALL [*575*] listed the *requirements* which an artifici colloid infusion solution should fulfill (see p. 49 f.). We confirmed that de tran 70 corresponds to these requirements for the most part, while gelat does not fulfill point 4 with regard to intravascular persistence. Nor do gelatin in any way fulfill the point dealing with the same problem in t requirements set up in 1963 by the American *National Research Coun* [*1074*]: "It should be retained to the extent of 50% of the infused volun for at least 6, and preferably for 12 hours".

We do not know whether this is the only reason why gelatin prepar tions are not permitted to be sold in the USA (see [*1500 a*] p. 40 and 30C it is possible that the absence of sufficient data concerning breakdown the human organism and therapeutic effectiveness also play a pa LUNDSGAARD [*925 b*] quotes a remark by PENNELL [*1122 a*] according which the gelatin preparations commercially available in Europe tod fulfill the American requirements as plasma substitutes. In a personal no (May 31, 1967) R. B. PENNELL, Boston, Chairman of Committee on Plasn and Plasma Substitutes, N.R.C., informed us: "The statement shou probably have been qualified by the phrase: (Physiogel is) acceptable f emergency stockpiling. We would accept your statement that dextran probably preferable to gelatin if dextran is freely available. Dextran ar human serum albumin are the only two agents for plasma volume expansic currently stockpiled in our country".

*Thus it remains a fact that gelatin preparations are not common in t USA.*

In 1944 SWINGLE [*1407*] wrote: "According to most investigato gelatin is not as effective as plasma, but more efficacious than saline Shortly afterwards WILLENEGGER [*1520*] wrote: "Gelatin has a poor effe similar to that of saline solutions", and "Gelatin solutions have been tak up again, whose inadequate effect has long been known ..." In spite of th gelatin solutions were again brought onto the market at the beginning of the 1960's in Germany and in Switzerland!

This step would seem justified if, in the meantime, the equal value of these new gelatin preparations, compared with plasma, had been adequately proved in hemorrhagic shock in *animal experiments*. We have compiled the findings reported in the literature with regard to this in the section on therapeutic results, p. 125 f. The result is that very few studies [*578, 1048, 1115*] in severe hemorrhagic shock show an equal value of 5% and even more highly concentrated solutions [*882 a*] of *OPG* and plasma; there is one study with 5 dogs concerning 3% *MFG* [*1117*]. In addition there are the studies with rabbits published by LUNDSGAARD [*925 b*] in 1967. No such data exists concerning *Haemaccel* (cf. [*432 b*]); the experiments of LUTZ [*937*] refer to a light shock model (1 hour hypotension). Studies about the therapeutic influence of expanders on hemorrhagic and other forms of shock should also be made in *irreversible* models, since only here can one determine possibly specific properties of the expander which are independent of the volume effect. Such studies exist for dextran (e. g. [*100, 426, 891, 996, 1103, 1345, 1547*]), but not for gelatin. We have already pointed out the doubtful usefulness of experiments which determine the bleeding index (see p. 126 f.).

A whole series of articles deals with other forms of shock and shows the inferiority of gelatin to plasma:

1. *Rifle bullet wounds* (SWINGLE [*1408*]).

2. *Tourniquet shock:* Contrary to GRODINS [*569*], SWINGLE found a single injection of 5% (!) gelatin in dogs ineffective and writes: "The gelatin was apparently not retained in the circulation but rapidly passed through the injured capillaries in the limb" (see also [*434*]). KLEINBERG [*828*] found gelatin to be about equal to or less effective than physiological saline solution; SERKES [*1317*] showed the superiority of plasma over physiological saline solution (see also [*636*]). Only SCOTT et al. [*1305*] showed a similar effect in dogs after infusion of 7% (!) gelatin solution compared with fresh plasma.

To us the most important articles seem to be those dealing with:

3. *Burn experiments*, where the inferiority of gelatin to plasma or other replacement substances is clear, as can be seen in several studies [*238, 527, 984, 1115, 1214*].

*It is obvious from all of this that there are no animal experiments which would have justified the therapeutic use of gelatin rather than dextran in hemorrhagic shock.*

It would therefore seem that careful hemodynamic *studies in humans* are needed to confirm the effectiveness of gelatin. As it was stated in Part One, such studies would have to show primarily that gelatin is capable of raising effectively cardiac output and increasing flow in the microcirculation of hypovolemic patients. The effect of Physiogel on cardiac output has been studied neither in animals nor in humans, and the only study with Haemaccel shows a particularly poor effect. For OPG as well there is only one such study. Verifiable data about the effect on microcirculation compared with plasma or albumin are not available for any of the three types of gelatin.

The observation of LUNDY [*927*] confirms the poor hemodynamic effect of gelatin; to maintain sufficient blood pressure he often had to use vasopressors when he used gelatin (MW 43,000, Upjohn) in place of 6% dextran.

The supporters of Physiogel [*925*] refer to the favorable experience with gelatin during the *Korean War*. Here no more than 200 bottles were used, 100 of them in the division area. Thus there can scarcely be a comparison with the 4000 bottles of dextran which were used in Korea. A quotation from ARTZ [*78*] states [*924*] that no difficulty with MFG because of the *high gel point* was recorded during the winter months in Korea. ARTZ himself emphasizes [*78*] however that there are no data on the question whether cold hindered the administration of gelatin. SCHMIDT [*1263*] states that the high gel point still represents a practical disadvantage in peaceful situations as well.

It is also argued that there is practically no difference in the *volume effect* of gelatin and dextran preparations after larger blood losses [*924*]. That this is not the case in humans can be seen in Table 9 (p. 121); besides, one must consider that the three articles mentioned which favor gelatin were written in 1951 and 1952. The gelatin preparations used at that time are not identical with those used today (usually it was more highly concentrated OPG).

As a *side-effect of the dextrans* the influence on blood coagulation is mentioned [*925, 925 a, 925 b*]; each time the inconclusive article by GARZON [*493*] is mentioned. In the section on dextran we have discussed this question thoroughly. It is generally accepted today that a substitution therapy using erythrocyte-free colloids is only desirable to a maximum volume of 1500 ml. The slight influence on blood coagulation (see also [*668*]) occurs in normal adults only with doses of over approx. 1500 ml/24 hours and it has been shown clinically that this influence is unimportant. For reasons of oxygen supply, larger amounts are infused without simultaneous infusion of blood only as an exception. It must be noted that higher doses of dextran 70 *can* be infused, especially when further blood loss occurs during the replacement therapy, because then there is also loss of dextran. In emergency situations where no other colloid is available, an increased bleeding tendency is less of a risk than untreated hypovolemia; for this reason, as an exception, the dose should be increased. Thus one can hardly speak of a particular narrowing of the therapeutic span of dextran [*673, 674, 925*] because of its influence on hemostasis, all the more since certain of these authors [*668,*

*674*] assume that widespread intravascular clotting processes often occur in shock, and for this reason they recommend giving heparin and fibrinolysin.

If so-called *bloodless surgery* (massive hemodilution) should acquire practical importance in the future, colloids which have no influence on blood coagulation, even in very high dosages, would naturally be desirable.

According to the results available at this time, strong hemodilution with dextran and starch is possible. Experience with gelatin till now (K. MESSMER, personal information, 1968 [*1008*]) has resulted in almost 100% mortality, while equally strong hemodilution with dextran 70 regularly results in survival. For his experiments MESSMER used Haemaccel or Physiogel; the autopsy of the gelatin animals always revealed massive accumulation of ceberospinal fluid in the subdural and ventricular space, and in some cases cerebral edema. In addition, K. MESSMER has just shown that Haemaccel is a very potent histamin liberator. [Abstracts 4th Congr. Europ. Soc. f. Exp. Surgery, April 1969, Davos; Europ. Surg. Res. 1 (1969)]. A very undesirable side effect of a plasma expander! Corresponding studies with OPG have not been published.

Strong hemodilution with dextran 70 is also possible in *humans;* this can be seen in an article by FITTS [*447 a*], who performed surgery on a member of the Jehovah's Witnesses because of a colon carcinoma. The anemic patient refused blood transfusion. Postoperatively his blood volume was maintained with dextran because of severe bleeding into the stomach, whereby the Hb decreased to 2.4 g-%. The patient was discharged in good general condition.

It is quite possible that the good results with dextran in hemodilution and shock studies can be attributed to the *antithrombotic effect,* in which case a suspected side-effect would actually be an advantage. It would be very difficult to find substances which would not affect the blood coagulation at all and at the same time have effective antithrombotic properties [*1654 f*].

It is further stated [*924, 925 a, 925 b*] that dextrans are associated "with questionable side-effects on *renal function*". As has been stated above (see p. 72 f.) careful studies provide no such evidence as long as the basic principles of water and electrolyte therapy are considered (which also applies to therapy with all other natural and artificial colloids). In this respect one must again emphasize that colloids for volume replacement should be given in electrolyte solutions and not in glucose solutions, and that the administration of mannitol, sorbit, or similar osmotic diuretics requires precise knowledge of the changes produced by them [*330*]. These changes are: temporary plasma volume increase; at first a drop and then continual rise in serum sodium; reduction of total body water; incomplete spontaneous refilling of the vascular system after blood loss and administration of mannitol.

In this context the use of low molecular weight dextran (dextran 40) is not a point for discussion since it is not considered to be an actual plasma replacement substance but rather a remedy. Since confusion always occurs, reference is again made to the following articles:

Couch [*304*] and Collins [*293*] have written critical review articles about low molecular weight dextran. Both unfortunately contain numerous mistakes, and the literature has not been summarized thoroughly. The questions raised have been discussed in this book in the respective chapters.

One also encounters the opinion [*666*] that PPS is equal to low molecular dextran with regard to the disaggregating effect, but reference to corresponding data is lacking. On the other hand, Groth [*586, 587*] has shown that albumin solutions with the same oncotic effect bring about results similar in many respects to those caused by dextran 40; but along with this he attributes specific properties to Rheomacrodex.

The supporters of *gelatin* [*668, 671, 673, 674, 924, 925, 925 a, 925 b, 1738, 1738 a*] maintain that it generally has the following advantages over dextran:

1. Gelatin is not supposed to be *antigenic*. This applies to MFG, but not to OPG. The dextran preparations used today are likewise non-antigenic in humans.

2. Gelatin preparations are said to have *no influence on the hemostatic mechanism*. This may apply to small doses, but for large infusions in hypovolemic individuals there is not enough evidence.

3. Gelatin is said to be *pharmacologically inert*. One must question whether this fact is really an advantage in all situations. Haemaccel is contraindicated in shock as a result of thrombo-embolism and fat-embolism. The pharmacological properties of dextran (antithrombotic effect) could very well be partially responsible for the good results in treatment of shock.

4. Even with the infusion of several liters, *no side-effects* are said to have been observed. It can be seen in the literature that side-effects also occur after infusion of gelatin. It is difficult to give precise data about the relative frequency of such reactions since gelatin preparations are used so much less frequently than dextran. It is definite that the frequency of side-effects is smaller for dextran than it is for blood preparations.

5. The amount of residual gelatin which is not excreted through the kidneys is said to be broken down into *amino acids by the body's own proteases*. However we know of no article which would support this view, e. g. by means of gelatin tagged with radioactive substances. Since all gelatin preparations are chemically influenced, it seems possible that they might not be broken down completely by the body's own proteases. In addition there is no data concerning the *rate of breakdown*. Such studies are certainly difficult to carry out since there are no specific methods for demonstrating

gelatin in the tissues, blood and urine. It has been shown that the portions of dextran which are not excreted are completely broken down in the organism.

6. Because of their low average molecular weight, gelatin preparations are *very quickly excreted through the kidneys* and have an *osmotic diuretic effect*. It is not by chance that the English and American authorities require that an expander should remain in the vascular tree as long as possible. It is argued that longer retention is not necessary in civilian conditions; but economic aspects are also closely bound to this (see below). Besides, there are no exact quantitative data concerning the extent of the *osmotic diuresis* which is said to be produced by gelatin preparations in humans in hemorrhagic shock. When it is clinically indicated, osmotic diuresis is generally brought about by means of substances with a much lower MW, such as mannitol or sorbit. Whether gelatin can cause the same degree of osmotic diuresis seems questionable. There is no clear proof of a favorable effect of osmotic diuresis in hemorrhagic shock in humans and we have already mentioned the dangers of using osmotic diuretic agents.

7. In vitro gelatin preparations are said to be *less viscous* than dextran. This fact has nothing to do with the influence on viscosity in vivo. This depends primarily upon to what level the Hct can be reduced. There are no adequate studies about the influence of gelatin preparations on pathologically raised viscosity in humans. Dextran 40 lowers increased blood viscosity.

8. There is said to be no danger of *impairment of urine flow*. After administration of dextran 70 and 40 in clinical dosage when basic principles of water and electrolyte balance have been heeded, there is also no impairment.

9. The *lower price* of gelatin is also emphasized, but the difference compared with that of dextran 70 is minimal. When one buys a colloid-containing solution, one primarily thinks of the volume or colloid osmotic effect and not of the amount of water; thus the objection arises that volume replacement therapy with gelatin preparations would be more expensive than with dextran 70. With rabbits it has been shown [*925*] that approximately twice as much Physiogel is required, compared with dextran 70, to obtain the same therapeutic effect. This has been confirmed in humans [*1811*]. The amount of human dried plasma, PPS or albumin necessary to produce a volume effect comparable to that of dextran 70 costs considerably more in most countries.

If considerably more gelatin than dextran 70 is required to obtain the same volume effect, then greater supplies must also be stockpiled; this presents *storage space problems* which are not to be underestimated, especially in military and civil defence spheres, and it would entail great expense. For the same reasons the *problem of transport* is more difficult and also results in financial consequences.

10. After storage for 4 years, no flake formation is said to occur in Physiogel, while flaking was observed in some bottles in the dextran reserves of the American army. This flaking was caused by great temperature fluctuations and/or defects in the glass containers and covers. It has been shown that dextran solutions can be kept for 10 years when stored correctly; dry dextran substance can be stored for an unlimited period. There are only few data concerning the storage capabilities of gelatin preparations other than Physiogel.

11. On the basis of 5 experiments in dogs LUNDSGAARD [*1719*] feels that Physiogel should be preferred to dextran for treating patients who were massively irradiated in an atomic war, since there is no influence on coagulation. However he has not shown that patients with a hemorrhagic diathesis could be improved or saved by Physiogel administration.

12. Referring to the work of ROTHSCHILD [*1793*] and RIEGER [*1707, 1787*] dextran is said to impair protein synthesis [*1738 a*]. However ROTHSCHILD stated 1961: "a toxic effect on albumin production has not been shown". On the basis of his animal experiments with long term administration of large amounts of high molecular weight dextran he assumes that dextran depresses albumin synthesis by a colloid osmotic mechanism. These experiments have no application to the clinical use of dextran but represent a proof for the fact that dextran is an effective colloid. This applies also to the papers of RIEGER [*1707, 1787*] who observed hypoalbuminemia after dextran and gelatin infusions. The 2 dog experiments [*1787*] are not conclusive.

Toxicological testing is absent (for Physiogel there is one article with results from 110 mice). The volume effect is too slight and does not last long enough (cf. [*613, 1811*]). There are insufficient hemodynamic studies. Along with these aspects and economic considerations, the following *disadvantages of MFG preparations and Haemaccel* must also be taken into account:

1. The *calcium content* of these solutions precludes the infusion of ACD blood immediately after a gelatin infusion through the same apparatus. Rapid infusion of larger amounts can be dangerous with an injured myocardium, especially in digitalized patients.

2. The *chloride content* in Haemaccel is too high (162.2 mval/l).

3. The *sodium content* of 120 mval/l in Plasmagel (in Physiogel?) is too low.

4. The gelatin preparations of the MFG type *gel at 7—10° C, which is a serious disadvantage in military medicine.*

5. *Physiogel* is *buffered* at a pH of 6.83 [*1382*].

The supporters of MFG as a colloid for shock prophylaxis and shock therapy [*668, 671*] have recently stated: "Efforts must be directed toward *developing an optimal gelatin preparation*" [*925, 925 a*]. Thus they are not satisfied with the present preparations, although it can not be contested that these preparations are usable as it is.

Our comparison of the two most important types of plasma substitutes can be closed by referring again to a distinguished worker in this field: "Dextran is probably preferable to gelatin if dextran is freely available. Dextran and human serum albumin are the only two agents for plasma volume expansion currently stockpiled in our country (USA)" (PENNELL, 1967, see p. 168).

# I. Practical Conclusions

1. Pasteurized plasma protein solutions (PPS), albumin and dextran 70 are the best plasma substitutes available today for catastrophy stockpiles. PPS and albumin can be manufactured only in limited quantity, and they are extremely expensive; thus it seems appropriate to stockpile larger quantities of dextran 70 for the needs of the army and civil defence. In times of peace these stores could certainly be used in the civilian sphere.

2. In daily practice and in the clinic, dextran 70 is the choice for a plasma expander to be used in volume losses up to approx. 1000—1500 ml in formerly healthy normal individuals. An effective antithrombotic prophylaxis is introduced at the same time by dextran 70. Where protein loss is prominent, use of PPS or albumin is recommended. When using erythrocyte-free solutions one must be sure that the Hct does not drop below 30% after volume replacement. (Do not overlook preexisting anemia!) In such cases and with larger blood losses, transfusion of whole blood is absolutely indicated. Along with volume replacement in the initial phase of shock treatment, the most important measure is the assurance of optimal respiratory function for full use of the available $O_2$ carrying capacity. The prophylaxis of hypovolemic conditions is important for the improvement of results in shock treatment. In situations where one can predict volume losses it is recommended to start volume replacement early, not waiting for the first signs of hypovolemia. Thus in all major surgery, volume replacement with dextran 70 infusion is started when narcosis is begun; infusion of blood is added when it is dictated by the oxygen requirements of the organism.

# J. Concluding Remarks

Our discussion shows that important aspects are still open for shock research in the field of blood replacement. Particularly needed are precise metabolic data on the question of the extent to which volume replacement is possible with erythrocyte-free solutions in humans. The entire problem of *oxygen supply, transport and consumption* at various Hct levels under shock conditions in humans has been little investigated or not at all. Further data is necessary concerning the importance and regulation of the *colloid osmotic pressure.* Closely allied with this are problems of *interstitial pressure;* with respect to this there are no reliable measurements under normal conditions and with various pathological conditions in humans. The possibility of volume replacement with large amounts of *balanced electrolyte solutions* must be studied precisely, and the advantages and disadvantages as well as the risks of this procedure must be clarified. Very little is known concerning the importance of *buffering* electrolyte solutions in humans. More evidence concerning the part played by individual plasma fractions in shock should be collected.

## K. Outlook

As long as the manufacture of plasma preparations depends upon blood donors, we are forced to use *artificial colloidal solutions.* On the basis o available results it seems unlikely that plasma substitutes equal to or bette than dextran can be manufactured on a gelatin or starch base. Should i become evident that the risk of hepatitis transfer is not present with deep frozen erythrocytes, one should investigate whether solutions of erythrocyte with artificial colloids can be used. Clarification of this possibility in th near future seems appropriate, since in many countries large amounts o erythrocytes are available in the manufacture of plasma; only a smal portion of these erythrocytes are used clinically. It is also conceivable that i the future artificial colloids can be developed or so modified that a certai oxygen transport and release capacity can be obtained. The discovery o such a substance would make it possible to manufacture an almost perfec blood replacement substance for initial treatment of shock. Unfortunatel there is as yet no basis for believing that this might soon be the case. Unt such a time we will continue searching for new ways to reduce the risks o blood transfusions, and we will have to restrict the administration of bloo to such cases where it is indicated as urgent.

## PART FOUR

# Summary

1. *Smaller blood losses* of 500—1000 ml are compensated for by the human organism by means of *mobilization of interstitial fluid and proteins* within 18—48 hours. A healthy individual solves this problem without difficulty, but even relatively small blood losses can be a heavy burden on the diseased organism; thus they should be replaced early.

2. Moderate blood losses can be compensated for by means of oral water and electrolyte administration but the volume refilling occurs slowly. If oral therapy is undesirable or impossible, administration of 4% pasteurized plasma protein (PPS), 5% albumin, or a 6% solution of dextran 70 (in 0.9% NaCl, $\overline{M}_w$ 70,000, Macrodex) with large volume loss as well causes a volume increase which corresponds to the amount administered and which continues until the circulating blood volume has been restored by the body's own mechanisms.

3. The use of fresh plasma, human dried plasma and stored pooled plasma can not be justified for the replacement of small and moderate blood losses because of the risk of hepatitis transfer. Besides, the volume effect provided by fresh plasma does not always correspond to the amount infused, for immunological reasons.

4. For the same reasons (especially hepatitis risk) blood transfusions should be prescribed only when the oxygen supply of the organism is in jeopardy because of lack of erythrocytes. On the basis of clinical experience and the findings of animal experiments, it can be assumed that the *replacement of 1000—1500 ml of blood (approx. 30% of the BV)* can be made *with erythrocyte-free solutions* in adults, if there is no preexisting anemia and when one can be assured that respiration is adequate. If the latter is disturbed, it should be improved by means of ventilation with 100% $O_2$, since increasing the erythrocyte volume above normal does not lead to an improvement of oxygen supply.

5. After restoration of the blood volume with erythrocyte-free solutions, the *Hct should not drop below* approx. 30% (the Hb not below 10 g-%).

6. *Blood transfusions* are absolutely indicated for treating *larger blood losses.*

7. The presently available *gelatin preparations* of the types, oxypolygelatin (Gelifundol, Biotest), modified fluid gelatin (Plasmagel, Braun or

Roger Bellon, Physiogel SRC) or Haemaccel (Hoechst) have not been clarified physico-chemically; they have also been relatively little investigated with regard to toxicology. The volume effect does not correspond to the amount infused, too little is known about their hemodynamic effect, and there is not enough experimental and clinical documentation of their therapeutic effectiveness. Most data support the opinion that gelatin preparations are inferior to equal amounts of plasma and dextran 70 in treatment of shock. The use of gelatins is therefore not economical. They can be used with lighter forms of shock, but dextran 70 is required under more difficult conditions.

8. There is more data concerning OPG and Haemaccel than MFG. *MFG* preparations have the disadvantage for military medicine that they *gel* at 7—10° C. *OPG* can have an *antigenic* effect in humans.

9. Gelatin preparations are not suitable for *military needs.* Since pasteurized plasma protein solutions and albumin preparations can only be manufactured in limited quantity and are very expensive, the creation of reserves of dextran 70 is recommended.

10. For *civilian conditions* as well, only the easy manufacture supports gelatin.

11. Compared with pasteurized plasma protein solution and albumin, dextran 70 has the advantage of a specific *antithrombotic effect.*

12. *Polyvinyl pyrrolidon* (PVP, Periston) should no longer be used today since it can not be broken down in the organism.

13. *Hydroxyethyl starch* is being tested at this time for its usefulness as a plasma replacement substance. We must wait for the results. In the light of experience up to this time it seems questionable whether this starting point can lead to preparations which are superior to dextran 70.

14. Results obtained by using large amounts (2—3 times the amount of blood lost) of *balanced electrolyte solutions* (e. g. with buffered lactated Ringer's solution) are as good as those obtained with blood and colloids for treating shock in animals. Until now these findings have not been sufficiently confirmed in humans.

15. *10% low molecular dextran* (dextran 40, Rheomacrodex) causes a marked increase in initial volume which, however, does not last as long as the increase caused by dextran 70. Dextran 40 has disaggregating properties, reduces increased blood viscosity and improves blood flow in the capillaries. There is as yet no proof of a better effect in initial clinical treatment of shock compared with dextran 70, pasteurized plasma protein solution and albumin.

Thus a 10% dextran 40 solution is a strong expander *yet not actually a plasma substitute.* Clear terminology with respect to this is particularly necessary as this example shows.

16. We recommend replacing smaller and moderately large blood losses with dextran 70, pasteurized plasma solution or albumin. We prefer dextran 70 for economic reasons and because of the additional antithrombotic effect; we reserve pasteurized plasma protein solutions and albumin for conditions which make protein replacement appear urgent. Blood is given additionally only with larger blood losses. It is most important to administer sufficient amounts of water and electrolyte to fill the daily requirements, existing deficits and additional pathological losses.

# Literature


1. Åberg, B., W. L. Bloom, and E. Hansson: Gastro-intestinal excretion of dextran-$C^{14}$. Acta physiol. scand. **52,** 188 (1961).
2. Abildgaard, U.: Acceleration of fibrin polymerization by dextran and ficoll. Interaction with calcium and plasma proteins. Scand. J. clin. Lab. Invest. **18,** 518 (1966).
3. Ablaza, S. G. G., G. T. Raber, G. Blanco, D. P. Morse, A. Adam, and H. T. Nichols: Intentional hemodilution. Arch. Surg. **87,** 32 (1963).
4. — — —, T. Shemanski, and H. T. Nichols: Intentional hemodilution. Arch. Surg. **91,** 893 (1965).
5. Adamkiewicz, V. W., and P. J. Sacra: Passive transfer of dextran anaphylactoid reaction in rats. Amer. J. Physiol. **205,** 357 (1963).
6. Adant, M.: Quelques effects de l'injection intraveineuse de dextran et de polyvinylpyrrolidone au chien normal ou hépatectomisé. Bull. Acad. roy. Méd. Belg. **19,** 264 (1954).
7. Adashek, E. P., and W. H. Adashek: The incidence of hepatitis in open heart surgery where massive blood transfusions are used. Bibl. haemat. fasc. **19,** 631 (1964).
8. Adelson, E., W. Crosby, and W. Roeder: Further studies of a hemostatic defect caused by intravenous dextran. J. lab. clin. Med. **45,** 441 (1955).
9. — Bleeding time prolongation after dextran infusion. Bibl. haemat. fasc. **7,** 275 (1958).
10. Adwan, K. O., and B. J. Wilson: The effect of treatment for chronic anemia on respiratory dynamics. Amer. Surg. **26,** 152 (1960).
11. Agersborg, H. P. K., jr., R. R. Overman, and C. M. Pomerat: Electrolytes and plasma expanders. Z. ges. exp. Med. **130,** 477 (1958).
12. Ahnefeld, F. W., u. M. Allgöwer: Der Schock — Entstehung, Verlauf und Therapie. Dtsch. med. Wschr. **87,** 425 (1962).
13. — Ergebnisse der Blutvolumenbestimmungen mit dem Volemetron. In: Horatz, K., u. R. Frey: Schock und Plasmaexpander, p. 114. Berlin-Göttingen-Heidelberg: Springer 1964.
14. —, M. Halmagyi u. K. Ueberla: Untersuchungen zur Bewertung kolloidaler Volumenersatzmittel. Anaesthesist **14,** 137 (1965).
15. — Die Verbrennungskrankheit — Entstehung, Diagnostik, Therapie. Darmstadt: Wehr und Wissen 1966.
16. Albert, S. N.: Blood volume. Springfield, Ill.: Thomas 1963.
17. —, J. Shibuya, C. S. Jain, and N. Minh: Conceptions and misconceptions of blood volume measurements. J. nat. med. Ass. **56,** 489 (1964).
18. —, S. C. Jain, J. Shibuya, and C. A. Albert: Mean corpuscular volume, osmolality, and viscosity of banked blood. Their significance in blood transfusions. Anesth. Analg. **44,** 338 (1965).
19. Alberti, A., e A. Sartore: Studio sull'impiego clinico di un nuovo sostituto plasmatico nel trattamento del „cranioleso". Minerva med. **31,** 120 (1965).
20. Alexander, R. S.: The systemic circulation. Ann. Rev. Physiol. **25,** 213 (1963).

21. ALEXANDER, K., u. H. G. HORST: Vergleichende Untersuchungen über die Wirkung von physiologischer Kochsalzlösung und Periston beim hämorrhagischen Schock der Katze. Arch. int. Pharmacodyn. **143**, 514 (1963).
22. ALLEN, F. M.: Theory and therapy of shock; varied fluid injections. Amer. J. Surg. **62**, 80 (1943).
23. ALLEN, J. C.: Effects of dextran, albumin and polyvinylpyrrolidone on the lipids in experimental nephrosis. Clin. Res. **7**, 278 (1959).
24. —, J. H. BAXTER, and H. C. GOODMAN: Effects of dextran, polyvinylpyrrolidone and gamma globulin on the hyperlipidemia of experimental nephrosis. J. clin. Invest. **40**, 499 (1961).
25. ALLEN, J. G., D. M. ENERSON, E. S. G. BARRON, and C. SYKES: Pooled plasma with little or no risk of homologous serum jaundice. J. Amer. med. Ass. **154**, 103 (1954).
26. —, D. DAWSON, W. A. SAYMAN, E. M. HYMPHREYS, R. S. BENHAM, and J. HAVENS: Blood transfusions and serum hepatitis: Use of monochloroacetate as an antibacterial agent in plasma. Ann. Surg. **150**, 455 (1959).
27. —, and W. A. SAYMAN: Serum hepatitis from transfusion of blood: epidemiologic study. J. Amer. med. Ass. **180**, 1079 (1962).
28. — Post-transfusion hepatitis. Calif. Med. **104**, 293 (1966).
29. — The advantages of the single transfusion. Ann. Surg. **164**, 475 (1966).
30. ALLEN, P. Z., and E. A. KABAT: Immunochemical studies on dextrans. J. Amer. chem. Soc. **78**, 1890 (1956).
31. ALLEN, T. H., R. A. WALZER, K. GREGERSEN, and M. I. GREGERSEN: Blood volume, bleeding volume, and tolerance to hemorrhage in the splenectomized dog. Amer. J. Physiol. **196**, 176 (1959).
32. ALLGÖWER, M.: Zur Frage der Zitrat-Toxizität bei Transfusionen mit Zitratblut. Helv. chir. Acta **14**, 483 (1947 a).
33. — Über die Wirkung von Heparin, polyanetholsulfosaurem Natrium (Liquoid Roche) und tribasischem Natriumcitrat auf menschliche Leukozyten in vitro. Schweiz. med. Wschr. **77**, 131 (1947 b).
34. —, u. W. REIF: Zur Frage der Zitrat-Toxizität mit Zitratblut. Helv. chir. Acta **16**, 75 (1949).
35. —, u. J. SIEGRIST: Verbrennungen. Berlin-Göttingen-Heidelberg: Springer 1957.
36. —, u. E. STUDER: Methodik und Ergebnisse einer Schnellbestimmung des Blutvolumens mit Iod$^{131}$ in der Klinik. Arch. klin. Chir. **301**, 123 (1962).
37. —, u. U. F. GRUBER: Current status of plasma expanders. Rev. int. Serv. Santé Armés **37**, 751 (1964).
38. — — Die Rolle von Leber und Darm im Schock. Schweiz. med. Wschr. **95**, 1087 (1965).
39. — — Noch einmal: Verbrennung und Rheomacrodex. Bemerkungen zur Arbeit von G. BIRKE u. S. O. LILJEDAHL. Schweiz. med. Wschr. **96**, 1692 (1966).
40. — Schock. In: H. HELLNER, R. NISSEN u. K. VOSSSCHULTE: Lehrbuch der Chirurgie, 5. verb. Auflage, p. 85. Stuttgart: Thieme 1967.
41. —, u. U. F. GRUBER: Schockpathogenese und ihre Differentialdiagnose. Chirurg **38**, 97 (1967).
41a. — Bemerkungen zum Problem der Plasmaersatzstoffe in der Wehr- und Katastrophenmedizin. Anaesthesist **16**, 12 (1967).
41b. —, u. C. BURRI: Schockindex. Dtsch. med. Wschr. **92**, 1947 (1967).
42. ALLISON, J. B., W. H. COLE, W. W. WALCOTT, S. GELFAN, W. S. ROOT, and M. I. GREGERSEN: Objective evaluation of transfusion therapy in hemorrhagic shock. Amer. J. Physiol. **156**, 191 (1949).

43. Almgård, L. E., S. O. Liljedahl, and B. Nylén: Electric burns of the abdomen. Acta chir. scand. **130,** 550 (1965).
44. Alstadter, R.: Blutersatzmittel. Ärztl. Sammelbl. **49,** 31 (1960).
45. Altemeier, W. A., L. Schiff, E. A. Gall, J. Gisueffi, D. Hamilton, D. Freiman, and H. Braunstein: Long term studies on the effect of polyvinylpyrrolidone retention in human patients. Surg. Forum **4,** 724 (1954).
46. Amberson, W. R.: Blood substitutes. Biol. Rev. **12,** 48 (1937).
47. American Defense Medical Purchase Description: Dextran injection, 6%, 500 cc. Nr. 5, Sept. 24, 1965. Commanding Officer, U.S. Navy Supply Depot (Code 1051), 5801 Tabor Ave., Philadelphia, Pa., 1965.
48. Ammon, R., u. W. Müller: Der Einfluß hoher Periston-Gaben auf den Kaninchenorganismus unter besonderer Berücksichtigung der Speicherorgane. Dtsch. med. Wschr. **15,** 465 (1949).
49. —, u. G. Braunschmidt: Das Schicksal von Periston im Organismus. Biochem. Z. **319,** 370 (1949).
50. —, u. E. Depner: Ausscheidung und Verhalten verschiedener Polyvinylpyrrolidontypen im Organismus. Z. ges. exp. Med. **128,** 607 (1957).
51. —, u. G. Mohn: Der fluoreszenzmikroskopische Nachweis des Polyvinylpyrrolidons. Acta histochem. **6,** 66 (1958).
52. — Das Vorkommen von Dextranase in menschlichem Gewebe. Enzymologia **25,** fasc. 4, 245 (1963).
53. Amspacher, W. H., and A. R. Curreri: Use of dextran in control of shock resulting from war wounds. Arch. Surg. **66,** 730 (1953).
53a. Andersen, M. A., J. R. Border, and C. V. Mouritzen: Acidosis, catecholamines and cardiovascular dynamics. Ann. Surg. **166,** 344 (1967).
54. Andersen, S. B.: Blood volume in elderly anemic patients following blood transfusions. Lancet **I,** 717 (1960).
55. —, and T. G. Gabuzda: Simultaneous determination of plasma volume with T-1824 and $^{131}$I-labelled autologous and homologous paraprotein. Clin. Sci. **26,** 41 (1964).
56. Anderson, M. C., R. E. Geurkink, and D. N. Sims: Use of low molecular weight dextran to prolong bowel viability in strangulation obstruction. J. Amer. med. Ass. **192,** 564 (1965).
57. Anderson, R. A., E. Hardenbergh, and J. T. Fulmer: Effect of low molecular weight dextran on freezing injury in the mouse foot. Fed. Proc. **23,** 2 P.I. (1964).
58. — — Frostbite treatment in the mouse with low molecular weight dextran. J. surg. Res. **5,** 256 (1965).
59. Andreucci, S.: La tipizzazione del sangue e l'uso di un nuovo plasmaexpander: l'Emagel. Minerva anest. **29,** 342 (1963).
60. Angelo, G. J., D', L. M. Ameriso, and J. B. Tredway: Survival after mesenteric arterial occlusion by treatment with low molecular weight dextran. Circulation **27,** 662 (1963).
60a. Ankeney, J. L., L. H. Coffin, and A. S. Littell: Experimental evidence that vasoconstriction in hemorrhagic shock does not result in anaerobic metabolism. Ann. Surg. **166,** 365 (1967).
61. —, D. S. Renner, F. L. Leverett, and E. M. Beheler: Hemodynamic changes associated with hemodilution priming of a rotating disk oxygenator. Ann. thorac. Surg. **1,** 142 (1965).
61a. Appel, W., V. Wirmer u. S. Ebenezer: Beeinflussung klinisch-chemischer Untersuchungen durch Dextran. Anaesthesist **17,** 95 (1968).

61b. Appel, W., u. V. Wirmer: Quantitative Mikrobestimmung von Dextran in Körperflüssigkeiten. Z. klin. Chem. u. klin. Biochem. 6, 452 (1968).
62. Arborelius, M.: Arteriella cirkulationsrubbningar och gangrän i nedre extremiteterna. Svensk. Läk. Tidn. 60, 4 (1963).
63. Arbulu, A., and A. P. Thal: The hemodynamic effects of alpha- and beta-andrenergic blockade. Surgery 60, 60 (1966).
64. Ardry, M. R., et O. Risbec: Les gélatines modifiées utilisées comme substituts du plasma humain. Détermination quantitative. Incidences sur l'exploration des protéines sériques. Ann. pharm. franç. 12, 428 (1954).
65. Areskog, N. H., G. Arturson, G. Grotte, and G. Wallenius: Studies on heart lymph. Arch. Dis. Childh. 39, 182 (1964).
66. Armstrong, D. J., and D. C. Finlayson: The effect of spinal anesthesia on blood volume in man. Canad. anaesth. Soc. 14, 399 (1967).
67. Armstrong, J. B., J. A. Downey, M. H. Ferguson, and H. R. Williams: A comparison of dextran, polyvinylpyrrolidone, and isotonic saline infusion in the human. Canad. J. Biochem. 32, 636 (1954).
68. Armstrong, J. R., and I. Cohn: Effect of low molecular weight dextran on experimentally induced tumor implantation of the peritoneum. Surg. Forum 17, 100 (1966).
69. Arn, H.: Über Plasmatransfusionsreaktionen. Blut 4, 137 (1958).
70. Arndt-Hanser, A.: Serologische Untersuchungen nach Dextraninfusionen. Bibl. haemat. fasc. 5, 181 (1956).
71. Aronsson, T., G. Arturson, and G. Wallenius: Determinations of serum protein in the presence of dextran. Scand J. clin. Lab. Invest. 18, 458 (1966).
72. Arturson, G.: Pathophysiological aspects of the burn syndrome. Acta chir. scand. suppl. 274 (1961).
73. —, K. Granath, L. Thorén, and G. Wallenius: The renal excretion of low molecular weight dextran. Acta chir. scand. 127, 543 (1964).
74. —, and G. Wallenius: The intravascular persistence of dextran of different molecular sizes in normal humans. Scand. J. clin. Lab. Invest. 16, 76 (1964 a).
75. — — The renal clearance of dextran of different molecular sizes in normal humans. Scand. J. clin. Lab. Invest. 16, 81 (1964 b).
76. — Capillary permeability in experimental rapid freezing with rapid and slow rewarming. Acta chir. scand. 131, 402 (1966 a).
77. — Dextran: Plasma volume expanders—clinical experience with low molecular weight preparations. Med. postgrad. 4, 28 (1966 b).
78. Artz, C. P., J. M. Howard, Y. Sako, A. W. Bronwell, and T. Prentice: Clinical experiences in the early management of the most severly injured battle casualties. Ann. Surg. 141, 285 (1955).
79. — —, and J. P. Frawley: Chemical observations on the use of dextran and modified fluid gelatin in combat casualties. Surgery 37, 612 (1955).
80. —, and T. Fitts: Replacement therapy in shock. J. Trauma 2, 358 (1962).
81. — Volume replacement in shock. Surg. Gynec. Obstet. 122, 112 (1966).
82. Ashwin, J. G., and L. B. Jaques: The effect of phosphorus$^{32}$, reserpine and stypturon on thrombus formation in rats. Thromb. Diath. haemorrh. 5, 543 (1961).
83. Askrog, V.: The cardiovascular response of normal anaesthetized man to rapid infusion of saline. Brit. J. Anaesth. 38, 455 (1966).
84. Atik, M., and R. Gutierrez-Saenz: Production of acute nephrosis by incompatible (heterologous) blood transfusion and the protective effect of low molecular weight dextran. Surg. Forum 12, 48 (1961).

85. ATIK, M., B. MANALE, and J. E. PEARSON JR.: Some hemodynamic aspects of transfusion reaction with special reference to acute renal failure. Surg. Forum **13**, 383 (1962).
86. — — — Prevention of acute renal failure. Hemodynamic observations of transfusion reactions. J. Amer. med. Ass. **183**, 455 (1963).
87. — Prevention of acute renal failure. Amer. J. Surg. **108**, 384 (1964).
88. — Acute renal failure, a preventable complication. J. Trauma **6**, 701 (1966).
88a. — Dextran 40 and Dextran 70. Arch. Surg. **94**, 664 (1967).
89. AUB, J. C.: Studies in experimental traumatic shock: I. The basal metabolism. Amer. J. Physiol. **54**, 388 (1920).
89a. Australian Drug Evaluation Committee: Notes on current drugs: Low molecular weight dextran and oliguria/anuria. Med. J. Austr. i, 648 (1966).
90. BACH, H. G., u. H. GRAEFF: Klinische Daten zur Wirksamkeit des niedermolekularen Dextrans. Geburtsh. Frauenheilk. **24**, 506 (1964).
91. BAKER, C. H., and J. W. REMINGTON: Fluid shifts after hemorrhage. Amer. J. Physiol. **201**, 910 (1961).
92. — Fibrinogen-$I^{131}$, T-1824, and red-cell $Cr^{51}$ spaces following hemorrhage. Amer. J. Physiol. **205**, 527 (1963).
93. BAKER, R. J., W. C. SHOEMAKER, F. SUZUKI, R. J. FREEARK, and E. L. STROHL: Low molecular weight dextran therapy in surgical shock. Part 1: Control group and shock patients resuscitated prior to low molecular weight dextran therapy. Arch. Surg. **89**, 373 (1964 a).
94. —, W. C. SHOEMAKER, F. SUZUKI, R. J. FREEARK, E. L. STROHL, and J. CAREY: Low molecular weight dextran therapy in surgical shock. Part 2: Patients in shock treated with low molecular weight dextran. Arch. Surg. **89**, 379 (1964 b).
95. —, J. N. ST. VILLE, F. SUZUKI, and W. C. SHOEMAKER: Evaluation of red cell equilibration in hemorrhagic shock. Arch. Surg. **90**, 538 (1965).
96. —, and W. C. SHOEMAKER: Changing concepts in treatment of hypovolemic shock. Med. Clin. N. Amer. **51**, 83 (1967).
97. BALATRESI, P., e M. RISTORI: Correlazione tra emotrasfusioni massive ed alterazione di alcuni meccanismi della coagulazione in chirurgia toracica. Acta anaesth. (Padova) **16**, 753 (1965).
98. BALDASSARRE, M.: Un plasma-expander a basso peso molecolare: L'Emagel (indagini clinico-sperimentali). Acta anaesth. (Padova) **16**, 817 (1965).
99. BALESTRA, L., e G. C. MERETO: Alcuni aspetti dell'emocoagulazione doppo trattamento con Emagel: test di tolleranza all'eparina in vitro e fibrinolisi. Minerva anest. **31**, 418 (1965).
100. BALLINGER, W. F., II, T. F. SOLANKE, and W. L. THOMPSON: The effect of hydroxyethyl starch upon survival of dogs subjected to hemorrhagic shock. Surg. Gynec. Obstet. **122**, 33 (1966).
101. —, G. F. MURRAY, and E. E. MORSE: Preliminary report on the use of hydroxyethyl starch solution in man. J. surg. Res. **6**, 180 (1966).
102. BARDHAN, P. N., B. COYAJI, and M. RAM: Treatment of shock with gelatin as plasma expander. Indian J. med. Res. **51**, 871 (1963).
103. BARFUSS, F., u. O. EICHLER: Periston bei wiederholter Darreichung. Arch. exp. Path. Pharmakol. **206**, 346 (1949).
104. BARGMANN, W.: Über Milzveränderungen nach Zufuhr des Blutflüssigkeitsersatzes Periston. Virchows Arch. **314**, 162 (1947).
105. BARK, J.: Das Verhalten verschiedener Labortests zur Beurteilung der Verträglichkeit eines Plasmaexpanders. In: K. HORATZ u. R. FREY: Schock und Plasmaexpander, p. 106. Berlin-Göttingen-Heidelberg: Springer 1964.

106. Barlow, G., and D. H. Knott: Hemodynamic alterations after 30 minutes of pentobarbital sodium anesthesia in dogs. Amer. J. Physiol. **207,** 764 (1964).

107. Barner, F. R.: Über Eisen- und Periston-(Kollidon-)Speicherung. Z. ges. inn. Med. **23,** 1074 (1952).

108. Baue, A. E., G. Hermann, and R. S. Shaw: Study of bank blood toxicity. Surg. Gynec. Obstet. **113,** 40 (1961).

108 a. —, E. T. Tragus, and W. M. Parkins: Effects of increased osmolality and correction of acidosis on blood flow and oxygen consumption in hemorrhagic shock. J. surg. Res. **7,** 349 (1967).

108 b. — —, S. K. Wolfson, A. L. Cary, and W. M. Parkins: Hemodynamic and metabolic effects of Ringer's lactate solution in hemorrhagic shock. Ann. Surg. **166,** 29 (1967).

109. Baumgartl, F., H. Zintgen u. F. Zureda: Untersuchungen über Blutersatzmittel. Arch. klin. Chir. **285,** 353 (1957).

110. — Die Prüfung von Blutersatzmitteln und die physiologische Regeneration Dtsch. med. Wschr. **83,** 2045 (1958).

111. Bayliss, W. M.: Methods of raising a low arterial pressure. Proc. roy. Soc. B. **89,** 381 (1916)

112. Beck, W.: Schock- und Kollapsbekämpfung mit Dextran, einem neuen Blutflüssigkeitsersatzmittel. Med. Welt 753, 1951.

113. Bedarida, G., P. L. Cipolli, B. Magrassi, S. Marigo, e R. Turpini: Studio sperimentale e clinico sopra un plasmaexpander nella terapia di sostituzione della massa circolante. Minerva anest. **29,** 328 (1963).

114. Beecher, H. K., F. A. Simeone, C. H. Burnett, S. L. Shapiro, E. R. Sullivan, and T. B. Mallory: The internal state of the severly wounded man on entry to the most forward hospital. Surgery **22,** 672 (1947).

115. — Surgery in World War II. Vol I: The physiologic effects of wounds. Office of the Surgeon General, Dpt. of the Army, Washington, D. C. 1952.

116. Beerhalter, H., J. Hölzle u. G. Harbauer: Der Einfluß neuartiger Dextrankombinationspräparate auf Kreislauf, Atmung, Urinausscheidung und Elektrolyte. Arch. klin. Chir. **316,** 620 (1966).

117. Behrends, W., u. N. Steinhardt: Virushepatitis nach Bluttransfusionen. Dtsch. med. Wschr. **86,** 207 (1961).

118. Bell, L. G.: Plasma expanders in the armed services of the United States. U.S. armed Forces med. J. **5,** 1331 (1954).

119. Bendixen, H. H., L. D. Egbert, J. Hedley-Whyte, M. B. Laver, and H. Pontoppidan: Respiratory care. St. Louis: Mosby 1965.

120. Bennett, P. N., D. P. Dhall, F. N. McKenzie, and N. A. Matheson: Effects of dextran infusion on the adhesiveness of human blood-platelets. Lancet **II,** 1001 (1966).

121. Bentall, H. H., B. Smith, M. Al Omeri, D. G. Melrose, and S. Allwork: Blood-loss after cardiopulmonary bypass. Lancet II, 277 (1964).

122. Bergan, J. J., O. H. Trippel, H. A. Kaupp, and J. C. Kukral: Low viscous dextran in treatment of severe limb ischemia. J. Amer. med. Ass. **188,** 451 (1964).

123. —, O. H. Trippel, H. A. Kaupp, J. C. Kukral, and W. F. Nowlin: Low molecular weight dextran in treatment of severe ischemia. Arch. Surg. **91,** 338 (1965).

123 a. BERGAN, J. J., E. TEIXEIRA, P. DORIS, J. ARBIT, and I. MORAES: Augmentation of blood flow during venous occlusion. Surgery **62**, 366 (1967).

124. BERGENTZ, S.-E., O. EIKEN, and I. M. NILSSON: The effect of dextran of various molecular weight on the coagulation in dogs. Thromb. Diath. haemorrh. **6**, 15 (1961).

125. —, L.-E. GELIN, C.-M. RUDENSTAM, and B. ZEDERFELDT: Indications for the use of low viscous dextran in surgery. Acta chir. scand. **122**, 343 (1961).

126. —, and I. M. NILSSON: Effect of trauma on coagulation and fibrinolysis in dogs. Acta chir. scand.. **122**, 21 (1961).

127. —, L.-E. GELIN, C.-M. RUDENSTAM, and B. ZEDERFELDT: The viscosity of whole blood in trauma. Acta chir. scand. **126**, 289 (1963).

128. —, O. EIKEN, and L.-E. GELIN: Rheomacrodex in vascular surgery. J. cardiovasc. Surg. **4**, 388 (1963).

129. —, L.-E. GELIN, and C.-M. RUDENSTAM: Microcirculation in tumors. Acta chir. scand. **125**, 443 (1963).

130. — — —, and B. ZEDDERFELDT: Alterations of the viscosity (shear rate:shear stress ratio) of whole blood in trauma. Bibl. anat. **4**, 676 (1964).

131. — — — — Experiences of treatment with low viscous dextran in surgery. Bibl. anat. **4**, 520 (1964).

132. —, C.-M. FAJERS, L.-E. GELIN, and C.-M. RUDENSTAM: Intravascular aggregation of long duration and its consequences. Bibl. anat. **7**, 207 (1965).

133. —, L.-E. GELIN, S.-E. LINDELL, and C.-M. RUDENSTAM: The effect of trauma on equilibration of $Cr^{51}$ tagged red cells. Bibl. anat. **7**, 242 (1965).

134. —, och U. F. GRUBER: Central ventrycksmättning vid cirkulations insufficiens. Nord. Med. **74**, 868 (1965).

135. —, L.-E. GELIN, I. ISAKSSON, B. JOHANSSON, and S. OLSSON: A report on a burn catastrophy. Acta chir. scand. **129**, 257 (1965).

136. —, and D. K. BRIEF: The effect of pH and osmolality on the production of canine hemorrhagic shock. Surgery **58**, 412 (1965).

137. —, Å. FRITJOFSSON, and S. OLSSON: The effect of Rheomacrodex and albumin on kidney function in the early post-operative period. Scand. J. clin. lab. Invest. **17**, suppl. 86, 128 (1965).

138. —, T. FALKHEDEN, and S. OLSSON: Diuresis and urinary viscosity in dehydrated patients: Influence of dextran 40 000 with and without mannitol. Ann. Surg. **161**, 582 (1965).

139. — Pathophysiologie der Mikrozirkulation. In: O. H. JUST u. H. LUTZ: Genese und Therapie des hämorrhagischen Schocks, p. 68. Stuttgart: Thieme 1966.

140. —, and D. DANON: Alterations in red cells of traumatized rabbits. II. Preferential sequestration of old cells. Acta chir. scand. **132**, 26 (1966).

141. BERGER, R. L., T. P. BOYD, and P. S. MARCUS: A pattern of blood-volume response to open heart surgery. New Engl. J. Med. **271**, 59 (1964).

141a. BERGGREN, A., and K. GRANATH: Dextran 40. Lancet II, 802 (1966).

142. BERGMANN, H.: Zur Frage der posttransfusionellen Hyperbilirubinämie. Wien. klin. Wschr. **76**, 207 (1964).

143. BERGSTRÖM, J., H. BUCHT, J. EK, B. JOSEPHSON, and L. WERKÖ: The effect of intravenous infusion of large quantities of dextran solution on kidney function in man. Scand. J. clin. Lab. Invest. **11**, 82 (1959).

144. BERK, J. L., J. F. HAGEN, W. H. BEYER, and R. NIAZMAND: The effects of epinephrine on arteriovenous shunts in the pathogenesis of shock. Surg. Gynec. Obstet. **124**, 347 (1967).

145. BERLIN, N. I.: Determination of red blood cell life span. J. Amer. med. Ass. **188**, 375 (1964).

146. BERMAN, H. J.: Platelet agglutinability as a factor in hemostasis. Bibl. anat. **4,** 736 (1964).
147. —, N. E. NIESSEN, and G. P. FULTON: Hemostatic responses in hamsters 24 hours after infusion with hydroxyethyl starch: A preliminary report. In: Third Conference on Artificial Colloidal Agents, p. 99. Nat. Acad. Sci., Nat. Res. Counc., Washington, D. C. 1965.
148. BERNE, C. J.: Diagnosis of compensated hypovolemic shock. Amer. J. Surg. **103,** 412 (1962).
149. BERNSTEIN, E. F.: Methods of measurement of red blood cell aggregation. In: Conference on evaluation of low molecular weight dextran, p. 53. Nat. Acad. Sci., Washington, D. C. 1963.
150. BERSON, S. A., and R. S. YALOW: The use of $K^{42}$ or $P^{32}$ labeled erythrocytes and $I^{131}$ tagged human serum albumin in simultaneous blood volume determinations. J. clin. Invest. **31,** 572 (1952).
151. BERTRAND, J. J., T. V. FEICHTMEIR, N. KOLOMEYER, J. O. BEATTY, P. L. MURPHY, W. D. WALDSCHMIDT, and E. B. MCLEAN: Clinical investigations with a heat-treated plasma protein fraction—Plasmanate. Vox Sang. **4,** 385 (1959).
152. BESSELING, J. L., A. B. BULL, J. M. E. DUPLESSIS, and I. M. MASON: The rapid warming of blood for massive transfusion by radiofrequency induction. Sth Afr. med. J. **39,** 137 (1965).
153. BEUCHELT, H.: Zur Wirkung von Periston-N. In: Medizin und Chemie „Bayer" Leverkusen, Bd. 5, p. 235. Weinheim/Bergstraße: Verlag Chemie 1956.
154. BEUTL, K., A. ROGGEN, and H. NITSCHMANN: Physiogel; chemische und physikochemische Charakterisierung. Helv. chir. Acta **33,** 343 (1966).
155. BICHSEL-WERDER, E., u. A. HÄSSIG: Über die Beeinflussung der Serumbaktericidie durch kolloidale Plasmaersatzlösungen. Path. Microbiol. **28,** 713 (1965).
156. — Über die Bedeutung der Blutbaktericidie bei der Konservierung von Vollblut und Erythrocytensedimenten. Schweiz. med. Wschr. **96,** 1583 (1966).
157. BIENENSTOCK, J., and E. L. T. HARDING: Low molecular weight dextran (Rheomacrodex) in ischaemic ulceration of the skin. Lancet **I,** 524 (1964).
158. BIGAZZI, P. L.: Stato attuale della terapia mediante sostituti del plasma. Minerva anest. **29,** 319 (1963).
159. BIGELOW, W. G.: The microcirculation. Canad. J. Surg. **7,** 237 (1964).
159a. BILLMEYER, F. W., JR.: Measuring the weight of giant molecules. Chemistry **39,** 8 (1966).
160. BIRKE, G., S. O. LILJEDAHL, L. O. PLANTIN, and Å. RIEGER: Blood volume and plasma protein. I. Changes in blood volume and plasma proteins after bleeding in the splenectomized dog. Acta chir. scand. **132,** 477 (1966).
161. — — Nierenschädigungen bei ausgedehnten Verbrennungen mit Berücksichtigung der Behandlung mit Rheomacrodex. Schweiz. med. Wschr. **96,** 525 (1966).
161a. — — Noch einmal: Verbrennung und Rheomacrodex. Schweiz. med. Wschr. **97,** 823 (1967).
162. BIRKELAND, S.: The question of the reliability of blood volume determinations in severe pathological states where the circulation is unstable, possibly with manifest clinical shock. Acta chir. scand. suppl. **357,** 136 (1966).
162a. BLACK-SCHAFFER, G., E. P. GALL, R. T. SHIMIZU, and H. S. ESPARZA: The pathogenesis of the intestinal lesion of deep hypothermia and a proposed relationship to that of irreversible shock, including a note on a mechanism for the normal turnover of intestinal epithelium. Surgery **61,** 904 (1967).

163. Blackburn, E. K.: Indications for blood transfusion. Practitioner **195, 174** (1965).
164. Blalock, A.: Shock, further studies with particular reference to effects of hemorrhage. Arch. Surg. **29,** 837 (1934).
165. Bliss, J. Q., and P. B. Stewart: The selective response of skin to autologous and non-autologous plasma in non-sensitized subjects. Canad. med. Ass. J. **76,** 847 (1957).
166. — —, and J. L. Fuller: The selective cutaneous response to autologous and non-autologous plasma in dogs. Brit. J. exp. Path. **39,** 30 (1958).
167. —, D. G. Johns, and A. S. V. Burgen: Transfusion reactions due to plasma incompatibility in dogs. Circulat. Res. **7,** 79 (1959).
168. —, and J. D. Walker: Histamine release by homologous plasma in the dog. Canad. J. Biochem. **37,** 326 (1959).
169. Bloch, J. H., C. H. Pierce, W. G. Manax, G. W. Lyons, and R. C. Lillehei: Experimental cardiogenic shock. Arch. Surg. **91,** 77 (1965).
170. — — —, and R. C. Lillehei: Treatment of experimental cardiogenic shock. Surgery **58,** 197 (1965).
171. — —, and R. C. Lillehei: Reduction of external cardiac work in the treatment of cardiogenic shock. Circulation **32,** suppl. **2,** 52 (1965).
172. —, R. H. Dietzman, C. H. Pierce, and R. C. Lillehei: Theories of the production of shock. Brit. J. Anaesth. **38,** 234 (1966).
173. Blocker, T. G.: Physiology and treatment of shock. Texas St. J. Med. **51,** 620 (1955).
174. Blombäck, B., S. Gardell, B. Löfström, and E. Zetterqvist: Effekt av operationstrauma och infusion av olika dextranfraktioner på blödnings- och koagulationsfaktorer. Nord. Med. **69,** 155 (1963).
175. Bloom, W. L. Intravenous injection of dextran for the expansion of plasma volume. Amer. J. Med. **11,** 238 (1951 a).
176. — Present status of plasma volume expanders in the treatment of shock. Arch. Surg. **63,** 739 (1951 b).
177. — Plasma volume expansion of clinical trials of dextran fractions of defined molecular weight in normovolemic patients. Bibl. haemat. **7,** 277 (1958).
178. —, D. S. Harmer, M. F. Bryant, and S. S. Brewer: Coating of vascular surfaces and cells. A new concept in prevention of intravascular thrombosis. Circulation **26,** 690 (1962).
179. —, N. O. Fowler, J. A. Ward, and R. H. Franch: Hemodilution and changes in hemostasis induced by dextran: An experiment in dogs with and without plasma volume expansion. J. surg. Res. **3,** 152 (1963).
180. —, D. S. Harmer, M. F. Bryant, and S. S. Brewer: Coating of vascular surfaces and cells—A new concept on the prevention of intravascular thrombosis. Proc. Soc. exp. Biol. **115,** 384 (1964).
181. Bludau, W., u. L. Lendle: Plasmagel als Plasmaersatzflüssigkeit. Med. Pharm. Mitt. **32,** 1705 (1958).
182. Bock, K. D.: Schock, Pathogenese und Therapie. Berlin-Göttingen-Heidelberg: Springer 1962.
183. Böhmert, F., u. I. München: Schockbekämpfung mit einem neuartigen Plasmaexpander. Chirurg **34,** 228 (1963).
184. Bohmansson, G., H. Rosenqvist, G. Thorsén, and O. Wilander: Clinical experiences with dextran as a plasma substitute. Acta chir. scand. **94,** 149 (1946).
185. Bollman, J. L., R. C. Knutson, and J. S. Lundy: Volemic substances for replacement of blood. Arch. Surg. **63,** 718 (1951).

186. Bonchek, L. I., and N. S. Braunwald: Modification of thrombus formation on prosthetic heart valves by the administration of low molecular weight dextran. Ann. Surg. **165**, 200 (1967).

187. Borden, C. W., and W. H. Hall: Fatal transfusion reactions from massive bacterial contamination of blood. New Engl. J. Med. **245**, 760 (1951).

188. Border, J. R., E. Gallo, and W. G. Schenk: Alterations in cardiovascular and pulmonary physiology in the severly stressed patient: A rational plan for the management of hypotension. J. Trauma **6**, 176 (1966).

189. Borgström, S., L.-E. Gelin, and B. Zederfeldt: The formation of vein thrombi following tissue injury. Acta chir. scand. suppl. **247** (1959).

190. Borow, M., L. Aquilizan, A. Krausz, and A. Stefanides: The use of central venous pressure as an accurate guide for body fluid replacement. Surg. Gynec. Obstet. **120**, 545 (1965).

191. Boschenstein, F. K., J. A. Reilly, M. D. Yahr, and J. W. Correll: Effect of low molecular weight dextran on cortical blood flow. Arch. Neurol. **14**, 288 (1966).

192. Bouma, S.: Over het onstaan van acute nierinsufficientie door operaties aan de aorta abdominalis distaal van de nierarterien. Diss. Amsterdam 1963.

192a. Bounous, G., N. G. Sutherland, A. H. McArdle, and F. N. Gurd: The prophylactic use of an "elemental" diet in experimental hemorrhagic shock and intestinal ischemia. Ann. Surg. **166**, 312 (1967).

193. Bouvier, C. A., O. Koralnik et J. Gruendlinger: Troubles aigue de l'hémostase au cours de états de choc. Schweiz. med. Wschr. **94**, 1377 (1964).

194. Bowman, H.: Clinical evaluation of dextran as a plasma volume expander. J. Amer. med. Ass. **153**, 24 (1953).

195. Boyan, C. P., and W. S. Howland: Blood temperature: A critical factor in massive transfusion. Anesthesiology **22**, 559 (1961).

196. — — Problems related to massive blood replacement. Anesth. Analg. **41**, 497 (1962).

197. — — Cardiac arrest and temperature of bank blood. J. Amer. med. Ass. **183**, 58 (1963).

198. — Cold or warmed blood for massive transfusion? Ann. Surg. **160**, 282 (1964).

199. —, P. S. Underwood, and W. S. Howland: The effects of operation, anesthesia and plasma expanders on blood viscosity. Anesthesiology **27**, 279 (1966).

199a. — Treatment of hemorrhagic shock: Changing concepts. Clin. Med. 33 (1967).

200. Boyd, A. M., F. Fletcher, and A. H. Ratcliffe: Supportive therapy. An improved type of dextran. Lancet II, 59 (1953).

201. Boyd, T. F., and E. Joseph: Low molecular weight dextran in place of blood transfusion in thoracic surgery. Clin. Res. **11**, 392 (1963).

202. Braasch, D., u. G. Gössling: Erythrrozytendeformierung und Quellung durch Plasmafaktoren nach schweren Verbrennungen. Pflügers Arch. ges. Physiol. **289**, 1 (1966).

202a. Brand, E. D., T. K. Suh, and M. C. Avery: Reversal of postoligemic shock in the cat by hypervenobaric massive fluid therapy. Amer. J. Physiol. **211**, 1232 (1966).

203. Brass, K.: Morphologische Befunde bei Mensch und Kaninchen nach wiederholter Periston-(Kollidon-)Zufuhr. Frankfurt. Z. Path. **63**, 95 (1952).

204. Braude, A. I., J. F. Sanford, J. E. Bartlett, and O. T. Mallery: Effects and clinical significance of bacterial contaminants in transfused blood. J. lab. clin. Med. **39**, 902 (1952).

205. —, D. Williams, J. Siemienski, and R. Murphy: Shock-like state due to transfusion of blood contaminated with gram-negative bacilli; successful treatment with antibiotics and arterenol. Arch. intern. Med. **92**, 75 (1953).

206. — Transfussion reactions from contaminated blood; their recognition and treatment. New Engl. J. Med. **258**, 1289 (1958).

207. Breckenridge, I. M., and W. F. Walker: Blood-loss in open-heart surgery with low-molecular-weight dextran. Lancet **I**, 1190 (1963).

208. Brewer, D. B.: Renal clearances of dextrans of varying molecular weights. Proc. roy. Soc. Med. **44**, 561 (1951).

209. Brewer, S. S.: The sthenoplastic effect of dextran on platelets — the mechanism for prevention of thromboembolism. Xth Congr. int. Soc. Hematology, Abstr. K 13, Stockholm 1964.

210. Brickman, R. D., G. F. Murray, W. L. Thompson, and W. F. Ballinger: The antigenicity of hydroxyethyl starch in humans. J. Amer. med. Ass. **198**, 1277 (1966).

211. Bridenbaugh, L. D., and D. C. Moore: Local infiltration or peripheral nerve block anesthesia for surgery on the patient in shock. Clin. Anesth. **2**, 79 (1965).

212. Brinkmann, E. R., u. A. Kellersmann: Der Schock und seine Behandlung mit dem Plasmaexpander Haemaccel. Med. Klin. **58**, 1074 (1963).

213. British Pharmacopoeia: Dextran 150 injection—Dextran 110 injection—Dextran 40 injection. Addendum **1966**, 28 (1966).

214. Brock Neely, W.: Dextran: Structure and synthesis. In: M. L. Wolfrom, and R. S. Tipson: Adv. Carbohydr. Chem. vol. **15**, p. 341. New York: Academic Press 1960.

215. Broghammer, H., u. W. Fritsche: Blutgasanalytische Untersuchungen von Plastikbeutelkonservenblut bei Verwendung von ACD- und IAG-Stabilisator. Klin. Wschr. **44**, 519 (1966).

215a. Brohult, J., and J. Gillquist: The effect of low molecular dextran in posttraumatic anemia. Acta chir. scand. **133**, 91 (1967).

216. Brooks, D. K., W. G. Williams, R. W. Manley, and P. Whiteman: Osmolar and electrolyte changes in haemorrhagic shock. Hypertonic solutions in the prevention of tissue damage. Lancet **I**, 521 (1963).

217. —, and W. G. Williams: Osmolar and electrolyte changes in haemorrhagic shock. Lancet **I**, 891 (1963).

218. Bronwell, A., C. P. Artz, and Y. Sako: Evaluation of blood loss from a standardized wound after dextran. Surg. Forum **5**, 809 (1955).

219. Brues, A. M., W. E. Cohn, S. S. Kety, I. T. Nathanson, A. L. Nutt, D. M. Tibbettis, P. C. Zamecnik, and J. C. Aub: The toxic factors in experimental traumatic shock. II. Studies on electrolyte and water balance in shock. J. clin. Invest. **24**, 835 (1945).

220. Brunschwig, A., N. Corbin, and C. Johnston: Intravenous gelatin. Ann. Surg. **118**, 1058 (1943).

221. Bryant, M. F., W. L. Bloom, and S. S. Brewer: Use of dextran in preventing thrombosis of small arteries following surgical trauma. J. med. Ass. Georgia **50**, 580 (1961).

222. —, S. S. Brewer, and W. L. Bloom: Use of dextran in preventing thrombosis of small arteries. Clin. Res. **10**, 49 (1962).

223. BRYANT, M. F., W. L. BLOOM, and S. S. BREWER: Experimental study of the antithrombotic properties of dextrans of low molecular weigth. Amer. Surg. 29, 256 (1963).
224. — A new method of preventing postoperative thrombosis in small arteries. Sth med. J. 57, 391 (1964).
225. —, W. L. BLOOM, and S. S. BREWER: Study of the anti-thrombotic properties of dextrans of large molecular weight. J. cardiovasc. Surg. 5, 48 (1964).
226. — — — Use of dextran in thrombophlebitis, experimental and clinical studies. Amer. Surg. 32, 12 (1966).
227. BUCHBORN, E.: Schock und Kollaps. In: G. v. BERGMANN, W. FREY u. H. SCHWIEGK: Handbuch der inneren Medizin, 4. Aufl., p. 952. Berlin: Springer 1960.
228. — Stoffwechselveränderungen im Schock und ihre Bedeutung für die Schockbehandlung. Internist 3, 522 (1962).
229. BÜCHERL, E. S.: Die moderne Differentialtherapie des Schocks. Regensb. Jb. Ärztl. Fortbild. 12, 7 (1964).
230. — Neue Gesichtspunkte zur Pathogenese und Therapie verschiedener Schockformen. Berlin. Med. 15, 695 (1964).
231. BUCKWALTER, J. A., J. L. FERGUSON, R. J. JOHNSON, and R. T. SOPER: Blood volume measurements with a new instrument. Arch. Surg. 86, 874 (1963).
232. BULL, J. P., C. R. RICKETTS, J. R. SQUIRE, W. D'A. MAYCOCK, S. J. L. SPOONER, P. L. MOLLISON, and J. C. S. PATERSON: Dextran as a plasma substitute. Lancet I, 134 (1949).
233. — Historical landmarks in the study and treatment of blood loss. Brit. J. clin. Pract. 10, 743 (1956).
234. — Transfusion fluids. Ann. roy. Coll. Surg. Engl. 33, 175 (1963).
235. — Circulatory responses to blood loss and injury. Progr. Surg. 4, 35 (1964).
236. BUNKER, J. P.: Citric acid intoxication. Anesth. Analg. 36, 82 (1957).
237. BURRI, C., D. DE GASPARO, U. F. GRUBER u. M. ALLGÖWER: Die Wirkung verschiedener Plasmaersatzstoffe im hämorrhagischen und Verbrennungsschock. Helv. chir. Acta 31, 150 (1964).
238. —, u. M. ALLGÖWER: Die Wirksamkeit zweier Plasmaexpander im experimentellen Verbrennungsschock. Schweiz. med. Wschr. 94, 816 (1964).
239. — — Zur Funktion des reticuloendothelialen Systems (RES) nach Plasmaexpandern. Helv. chir. Acta 31, 533 (1964).
240. — — Der therapeutische Effekt verschiedener Plasmaexpander im experimentellen hämorrhagischen Schock. Chirurg 36, 1 (1965).
241. —, W. MÜLLER u. M. ALLGÖWER: Untersuchungen über Venendruck bei Blutverlust und Übertransfusion. Arch. klin. Chir. 316, 655 (1966).
242. —, u. P. MATTER: Die Beeinflussung der Durchblutung im Rundstiellappen durch niedermolekulares Dextran (NMD). Z. ges. exp. Med. 140, 170 (1966).
242a. —, u. M. ALLGÖWER: Klinische Erfahrungen mit der Messung des zentralen Venendruckes. Schweiz. med. Wschr. 97, 1414 (1967).
243. BUSHART, W., u. P. RITTMEYER: EEG-Untersuchungen im Schock. Münch. med. Wschr. 24, 1296 (1966).
244. BUTTLE, G. A. H., A. KEKWIG, and A. SCHWEITZER: Blood substitutes in treatment of acute haemorrhage. Lancet II, 507 (1940).
245. BUTTON, L. N., J. G. GIBSON II, and C. W. WALTER: Simultaneous determination of the volume of red cells and plasma for survival studies of stored blood. Transfusion 5, 143 (1965).

246. BUXTON, R. W.: Clinical and metabolic changes following trauma. J. m Ass. Georgia 53, 3 (1964).
247. BYGDEMAN, S.: Vascular reactivity in cats during induced changes in the a basa balance of the blood. Acta physiol. scand. suppl. 222 (1963).
248. —, och R. ELIASSON: Dextran — ett medel för profylax och behandling trombos. Svensk. Läk. Tidn. 63, 2743 (1966 a).
249. — — Effect of dextran in vitro on the adenosine diphosphate induc adhesiveness of human blood platelets. Thromb. Diath. haemorrh. 15, 4 (1966 b).
250. — —, and B. GULLBRING: Effect of dextran infusion on the adenosine phosphate induced adhesiveness and the spreading capacity of hum blood platelets. Thromb. Diath. haemorrh. 15, 451 (1966 c).
251. — —, and S. R. JOHNSON: Relationship between postoperative changes adenosinediphosphate induced platelet adhesiveness and venous thro bosis. Lancet I, 1301 (1966).
252. BYRNE, J. J.: Symposium on shock: Introduction. Amer. J. Surg. 110, 2 (1965).
253. — Current concepts—shock. New Engl. J. Med. 275, 543/659 (196
254. CAILAR, J. DU, G. PALEIRAC et B. ROQUEFENIL: Influence du dextran à l poids moléculaire (environ 40 000) sur les mécanismes de l'hémosta Ann. Anest. 6, 3 (1965).
255. CAMPBELL, D. H., J. B. KOEPFLI, L. PAULING, N. ABRAHAMSON, W. DAND KER, G. A. FEIGEN, F. LANNI and A. LE ROSEN: The preparation a properties of a modified gelatin (oxypolygelatin) as an oncotic substit for serum albumin. Texas Rep. Biol. Med. 9, 235 (1951).
256. CAPORALE, A., e C. CASTELLO: Trattamento del traumatizzato grave e tera pre- e post-operatoria con un nuovo sostituto del plasma. Minerva an 29, 408 (1963).
257. CARBONE, J. V., F. W. FURTH, R. SCOTT, and W. H. CROSBY: A hemosta defect associated with dextran infusion. Proc. Soc. exp. Biol. 85, 101 (1954
258. CAREY, J. S., F. SUZUKI, R. A. MLADICK, R. J. BAKER, and W. C. SHOEMAK Hemodynamic effects of low viscosity dextran in surgical shock. Su Forum 15, 22 (1964).
259. —, N. W. WOODWARD, P. A. MOHR, F. SUZUKI, R. S. BROWN, R. J. BAK and W. C. SHOEMAKER: Circulatory response to low viscosity dextran clinical shock. Surg. Gynec. Obstet. 121, 563 (1965 a).
260. —, R. S. BROWN, N. W. WOODWARD, Y. TAO, and W. C. SHOEMAKER: Cc parison of hemodynamic responses to whole blood and plasma expand in clinical traumatic shock. Surg. Gynec. Obstet. 121, 1059 (1965 b).
261. —, N. W. WOODWARD, R. BROWN, P. MOHR, P. SEWARD, and W. C. SHOEM KER: Hemodynamic responses to whole blood and blood substitutes clinical shock. Surg. Forum 16, 31 (1965 c).
261a. —, R. S. BROWN, P. A. MOHR, D. O. MONSON, S. T. YAO, and W. C. SH MAKER: Cardiovascular function in shock. Responses to volume load and isoproterenol infusion. Circulation 25, 327 (1967).
262. CARGILL, W. H., and H. D. BRUNNER: Metabolism of $C^{14}$ labeled dextran the mouse. J. Pharmacol. exp. Ther. 103, 339 (1951).
263. CARRIER, O., B. H. DOUGLAS, and J. W. CROWELL: Two factors affecting circulating red cell mass J. surg. Res. 4, 136 (1964).
264. CARTMILL, T. B., R. K. RICKS, H. E. GARRETT, J. A. WILLIAMS, and M. E. BAKEY: Blood volume measurements in cardiovascular surgical patie Surg. Gynec. Obstet. 121, 1269 (1965).

265. CASBERG, M. A., T. G. BLOCKER, W. C. LEVIN, and E. F. DUNTON: Pasteurized human plasma. Amer. J. Surg. **97**, 597 (1959)
266. CASTANEDA, A. R., E. BERNSTEIN, F. BANGSTADT, and R. L. VARCO: The effect of polyvinylpyrrolidone, mannitol, dextrose and of various dextrans on red blood cell charge. Bibl. anat. **7**, 262 (1965).
267. CAVAZZA, F., e G. CATANZARITI: Ricerche clinico-sperimentali su un nuovo sostituto del plasma. Minerva anest. **29**, 402 (1963).
268. CECCO, L. DE, e F. LUCISANO: Possibilità di impiego di un nuovo sostituto plasmatico in ostetricia e ginecologia. Minerva anest. **29**, 421 (1963).
269. CERNY, L. C., C. A. DANIELS, and R. C. GRAHAM: Physicochemical properties of hydroxyethyl starch. In: Third Conference on Artificial Colloidal Agents, p. 20. Nat. Acad. Sci., Washington, D. C., 1965.
270. CHADDUCK, W. M., W. G. CRUTCHFIELD, and M. ROBERTS: Use of dextran for prevention of thrombosis in arterial segments obstructed with gradual occlusion clamps. Surg. Gynec. Obstet. **121**, 491 (1965).
271. CHALMERS, T. C., R. S. KOFF, and G. F. GRADY: A note on fatality in serum hepatitis. Gastroenterology **48**, 22 (1965).
272. CHAPLIN, H., JR., and P. L. MOLLISON: Correction for plasma trapped in the red cell column of the hematocrit. Blood **7**, 1227 (1952).
273. — —, and H. VETTER: The body-venous hematocrit ratio: Its constancy over a wide hematocrit range. J. clin. Invest. **32**, 1309 (1953).
274. CHENG, E., B. LERNER, S. LICHTENSTEIN, K. E. KARLSON, and A. A. GARZON: Effect of hydroxyethyl starch on hemostasis. Surg. Forum **17**, 48 (1966).
275. CHIEN, S.: Quantitative evaluation of the circulatory adjustments of splenectomized dogs to hemorrhage. Amer. J. Physiol. **193**, 605 (1958).
276. —, and S. BILLIG: Effect of hemorrhage on cardiac output of sympathectomized dogs. Amer. J. Physiol. **201**, 475 (1961).
277. — Role of sympathetic nervous system in surviving acute hemorrhage. Amer. J. Physiol. **206**, 21 (1964).
278. CHRISTOPHERSON, E. B., A. G. MAY, J. A. DE WEESE, and C. G. ROB: Hemodynamic alterations in arteries with critical stenosis during acute hemorrhage. Surg. Gynec. Obstet. **121**, 832 (1965).
279. — — — — The hemodynamic effect of low molecular weight dextran in arteries with critical stenosis during acute hemorrhage. Surgery **60**, 402 (1966).
280. CLARK, J. H., M. V. SHELANSKI, D. MORSE, W. CHERRY, and C. MORSE: Effects of intravenous polyvinylpyrrolidone-solutions on the circulatory system. J. Philadelphia Gen. Hosp. **2**, 35 (1951).
281. CLARKE, R.: Recent advances in haemorrhage and shock. Brit. med. J. **II**, 721 (1957).
282. —, M. R. FISHER, E. TOPLEY, and J. W. L. DAVIES: Extent and time of bloodloss after civilian injury. Lancet **II**, 381 (1961).
283. CLAUSS, R. H., H. CHOLLET, S. J. GIANNINI, and A. HENDERSON: A simple method for the pretransfusion removal of potassium from stored whole blood. Surg. Forum **7**, 23 (1956).
284. COATES, J. B.: Surgery in World War II. Vol. II: General surgery. Office of the Surgeon General, Dept. of the Army, Washington, D. C., 1955.
285. —, and E. M. MCFETRIDGE: Blood program in World War II. Office of the Surgeon General, Dept. of the Army, Washington, D. C., 1964.

286. COHEN, S. N., and W. J. DOUGHERTY: Hepatitis among recipients of bloc from narcotic addicts; special report presented at Xth Conf. of Epidem Intellig. Serv., Commun. Dis. Center, U. S. Publ. Hlth. Serv., Atlanta, 1963
287. COHN, H. E., and W. F. BALLINGER: Experimental shock. In: W. F. BALLII GER: Research methods in surgery, p. 197. Boston: Little/Brown 1964.
288. COHN, J. N., and M. H. LURIA: Studies in clinical shock and hypotension. Amer. med. Ass. 190, 891 (1964).
289. — — Systemic and regional hemodynamic effects of low molecular weigl dextran in man. Clin. Res. 13, 59 (1965).
289a. — —, R. C. DADDARIO, and F. E. TRISTANI: Studies in clinical shock an hypotension. Circulation 35, 316 (1967).
289b. — Central venous pressure as a guide to volume expansion. Ann. intern. Me 66, 1283 (1967).
290. COLEMAN, F., J. W. CROWELL, E. E. SMITH, and R. M. WILSON: A hypoton solution for emergency blood substitution. Surgery 60, 392 (1966).
291. COLLINS, W. L., and L. W. FABIAN: Halothane anestesia during hypovolemi hypotension. In: L. R. ORKIN: Management of the patient in shock. Cli Anesth. 2, 119 (1965). Oxford: Blackwell.
292. COLLINS, G. M., and J. LUDBROOK: The intrinsic effect of low molecul weight dextran on resistance to blood flow in man. Surg. Gynec. Obste 123, 774 (1966).
293. — — The rheologic properties of low molecular weight dextran: fact c fancy? Amer. Heart J. 72, 741 (1966).
294. Committee on Plasma and Plasma Substitutes: The incidence, mortality an prevention of post-transfusion hepatitis. Nat. Acad. Sci., Nat. Res. Counc Washington, D. C., 1965.
295. CONWAY, J.: Cardiovascular response to sustained hypervolemia in the ur anesthetized dog. Circulation 28, 706 (1963).
296. — Hemodynamic consequences of induced changes in blood volume. Ci culat. Res. 18, 190 (1966).
297. COONSE, G. K., P. S. FOISIC, H. F. ROBERTSON, and O. E. AUFRANC: Traumati and haemorrhagic shock; experimental and clinical study. New Engl. Med. 212, 647 (1935).
298. COPE, O., and S. B. LITWIN: Contribution of the lymphatic systems to th replenishment of the plasma volume following a hemorrhage. Ann. Sur 156, 655 (1962).
299. CORÀ, D., S. DEBIASI, A. MAGGIA, and S. CORTESI: The circulating bloo volume as a factor regulating salt excretion in man. Clin. Sci. 22, 23 (1962).
300. CORLEY, R. D., and N. R. JOSEPH: Red cell charge as affected by low viscosit dextran. Proc. soc. exp. Biol. 122, 1171 (1966).
301. CORMIER, J. M., et J. SULZER: Utilisation clinique d'un dextran de faible poid moléculaire. Presse méd. 72, 3429 (1964).
302. COTTIER, H.: Vergleichende histologische Untersuchungen über die Wirkun wiederholter intravenöser Injektionen größerer Mengen von isogener Blutplasma und Physiogel bei Mäusen. Helv. chir. Acta 33, 376 (1966).
303. COTTIER, P., A. BASEVI u. H. J. SCHAFROTH: Die Wirkung eines Gelatine expanders Physiogel auf die Nierenfunktion. Helv. chir. Acta 33, 38 (1966).
304. COUCH, N. P.: The clinical status of low molecular weight dextran. Clin Pharmacol. Ther. 6, 656 (1965).

305. COURNAND, A., R. L. RILEY, S. E. BRADLEY, E. S. BREED, R. P. NOBLE, H. D. LAUSON, M. I. GREGERSEN, and D. W. RICHARDS: Studies of the circulation in clinical shock. Surgery 13, 964 (1943).

306. —, R. P. NOBLE, E. S. BREED, H. D. LAUSON, E. DE F. BALDWIN, G. B. PINCHOT, and D. W. RICHARDS: Chemical, clinical and immunological studies on the products of human plasma fractionation. VIII. Clinical use of concentrated human serum albumin in shock, and comparison with whole blood and with rapid saline infusion. J. clin. Invest. 23, 491 (1944).

307. COX, E. F., C. T. FLOTTE, and R. W. BUXTON: Dextran in the treatment of thrombophlebitis. Circulation 28, 706 (1963).

308. — — — Dextran in the treatment of thrombophlebitis. Surgery 57, 225 (1965).

308a. CRAIG, L. C.: Fractionation and characterization by dialysis. In: P. ALEXANDER, and R. J. BLOCK: A laboratory manual of analytical methods of protein chemistry, vol. I, p. 103. London: Pergamon Press 1960.

309. CRAIG, W., H. K. GRAY, and J. S. LUNDY: Present status of plasma volume expanders in the treatment of shock: Clinical results in surgery. Arch. Surg. 63, 742 (1951).

310. CRAWFORD, B., and H. LUDEMANN: The renal response to intravenous injection of sodium chloride solutions in man. J. clin. Invest. 30, 1456 (1951).

311. CRENSHAW, C. A., P. C. CANIZARO, G. T. SHIRES, and A. ALLSMAN: Changes in extracellular fluid during acute hemorrhagic shock in man. Surg. Forum 13, 6 (1962).

312. CREUTZFELDT, W., H.-J. SEVERIDT, H. SCHMITT, E. GALLASCH, H. J. ARNDT, H. BRACHMANN, G. SCHMIDT, u. U. TSCHAEPE: Untersuchungen über Häufigkeit und Verlauf der ikterischen und anikterischen Transfusionshepatitis. Dtsch. med. Wschr. 91, 1813 (1966).

313. — —, H. BRACHMANN, G. SCHMIDT u. U. TSCHAEPE: Untersuchungen zur Prophylaxe der Transfusionshepatitis durch Gamma-Globulin. Dtsch. med. Wschr. 91, 1905 (1966).

314. CRITZ, J. B., and A. W. MERRICK: Serum electrolyte and hematocrit changes in young rabbits following hemorrhage. Amer. J. Physiol. 196, 173 (1959).

315. CRONBERG, S., S. BELFRAGE, and I. M. NILSSON: Fibrinogen-transmitted hepatitis. Lancet I, 967 (1963).

316. —, B. ROBERTSON, I. M. NILSSON, and J.-E. NILÉHN: Suppressive effect of dextran on platelet adhesiveness. Thromb. Diath. haemorrh. 16, 384 (1966).

317. CROOK, J. A., JR., and E. L. BRACKNEY: Blood volume changes associated with surgery. Amer. Surg. 30, 706 (1964).

318. CROSBY, W. H.: Misuse of blood transfusion. Blood 13, 1198 (1958).

319. — Trends in blood transfusion. Ann. N. Y. Acad. Sci. 115, 399 (1964).

320. CROWELL, J. W., S. H. BOUNDS, and W. W. JOHNSON: Effect of varying the hematocrit ratio on the susceptibility to hemorrhagic shock. Amer. J. Physiol. 192, 171 (1958).

321. —, R. G. FORD, and V. M. LEWIS: Oxygen transport in hemorrhagic shock as a function of the hematocrit ratio. Amer. J. Physiol. 196, 1033 (1959).

322. —, and E. E. SMITH: Oxygen deficit and irreversible hemorrhagic shock. Amer. J. Physiol. 206, 313 (1964).

323. CSEH, G., and I. K. SZABO: Significance of the chemical structure of polysaccharides in the activation of lipoprotein lipase. Acta physiol. Acad. Sci. hung. 25, 117 (1964).

324. CUELLO, L., K. BHANGANADA, J. D. MACK, and C. W. LILLEHEI: Hemodiluti in extracorporeal circulation. In: Conference on Evaluation of Lc Molecular Weight Dextran, p. 114. Nat. Acad. Sci., Washington, D. ( 1963. (Note: The full name of the first author reads correctly L. MAINARDI, cf. MAINARDI 1964, nr. 945. The above heading probably is d to a mistake.)

325. CYRUS, A. E., JR., A. S. CLOSE, L. L. FOSTER, D. H. BROWN, and E. H. ELLISO Effect of low molecular weight dextran on infarction after experimen occlusion of the middle cerebral artery. Surgery **52**, 25 (1962).

326. CZOK, G., K. TRAENKNER, G. SIEBERT, W. KIECKEBUSCH u. K. LANG: Bioch mische, physiologische und morphologische Untersuchungen über „Mo fizierte, flüssige Gelatine (MFG)", ein Blutersatzmittel. Klin. Wschr. 511 (1959).

327. DAGHER, F. J., and F. D. MOORE: Equilibrium behavior of tagged erythr cytes in experimental "irreversible shock". J. surg. Res. **4**, 554 (1964).

328. —, J. H. LYONS, D. C. FINLAYSON, J. SHAMAI, and F. D. MOORE: Blo volume measurement: A critical study. Prediction of normal values: Co trolled measurement of sequential changes: Choice of a bedside metho Adv. Surg. **1**, 69 (1965). Chicago: Yearbook Med. Publ.

329. — —, J. LISTER, and F. D. MOORE: Hemorrhage in normal man. The effe of angiotensin. J. surg. Res. **6**, 66 (1966).

330. — —, M. R. BALL, and F. D. MOORE: Hemorrhage in normal man. II. Effe of mannitol on plasma volume and body water dynamics following acu blood loss. Ann. Surg. **163**, 505 (1966).

331. DAHLGREN, S.: Njurförändringar efter infusion med lågvisköst dextra Nord. Med. **70**, 1258 (1963).

332. DANIEL, W. J., S. D. MOHAMED, and N. A. MATHESON: Treatment mesenteric embolism with dextran 40. Lancet **I**, 567 (1966).

333. DANOWSKI, T. S., J. R. ELKINGTON, and A. W. WINKLER: Movements of bo water in response to acute blood loss. Amer. J. Physiol. **147**, 306 (1946).

334. DARGAN, E. L., W. METCALF, E. J. HEHRE, and A. OHIN: Clinical evaluati of a new dextran plasma expander. J. Amer. med. Ass. **179**, 203 (1962).

335. DAVIDSOHN, I., and K. STERN: Blood transfusion reactions: Their causes a identification. Med. Clin. N. Amer. **44**, 281 (1960)

336. DAVIES, J. W. L., and E. TOPLEY: A critical evaluation of red cell and plas volume techniques in patients with civilian injuries. J. clin. Path. **12**, 2 (1959).

337. —, C. R. RICKETTS, and B. N. WILLIAMS: Plasma volume expansion by rap infusion of a low molecular weight dextran. Brit. J. Pharmacol. **21**, 2 (1963).

338. — Methods of assessment of blood loss in the shocked and injured patie Brit. J. Anaesth. **38**, 250 (1966).

339. DAVIS, R. A.: Shock and allied forms of failure of the circulation. New Yor Grune & Stratton 1949.

340. —, L. E. SYPHERS, A. J. LESSER, S. M. GARSTKA, and R. E. ROTHE: Intractal post-operative shock. Western J. Surg. **69**, 1 (1961).

341. — Blood volume dynamics. Springfield, Ill.: Thomas 1962.

341a. DAVIS, J. H., J. W. BENSON, M. WOLFE, B. NELSON, and W. E. ABBOTT: T effect of capillary permeability on the maintenance of plasma volu following the administration of dextran and albumin. Surg. Forum **5**, 4 (1954).

342. DAVIS, R. B., and M. J. PALMER: Thrombocytopenia and release of platelet amines induced by thrombin and bacterial lipopolysaccharide. Brit. J. exp. Path. **46**, 554 (1965).

343. DEAVERS, S., E. L. SMITH, and R. A. HUGGINS: Rate of disappearance from the circulation of multiple injections of T-1824 and $I^{131}$ tagged albumin. Cardiovasc. Res. Center Bull. **2**, 43 (1963).

344. —, R. A. HUGGINS, and E. L. SMITH: Influence of autologous and homologous blood exchange on the bleeding volume of dogs. Amer. J. Physiol. **210**, 146 (1966).

345. DEFALCO, A. J.: The use of hydroxyethyl starch in the treatment of acute hemorrhagic shock in dogs. In: Third Conference on Artificial Colloidal Agents, p. 104. Nat. Acad. Sci., Washington, D. C., 1965.

346. DERN, R. J., R. P. GWINN, and J. J. WIORKOWSKI: Studies on the preservation of human blood. I. Variability in erythrocyte storage characteristics among healthy donors. J. lab. clin. Med. **67**, 955 (1966).

347. DEUTSCH, E.: Die Antikoagulantien in der Therapie der peripheren arteriellen Durchblutungsstörungen. Wien. klin. Wschr. **76**, 151 (1964).

348. — Indikationen und Gefahren der Antikoagulantienbehandlung. Wien. med. Wschr. **115**, 595 (1965).

349. DEVITT, J. E., F. N. BROWN, and W. G. BEATTIE: Fatal bleeding ulcer. Ann. Surg. **164**, 840 (1966).

350. DHALL, D. P., D. R. HARPER, F. N. MCKENZIE, and N. A. MATHESON: Aggregation of human platelets by dextran. Nature (London) **210**, 745 (1966).

350a. DIETZMAN, R. H., G. W. LYONS, J. H. BLOCH, and R. C. LILLEHEI: Relation of cardiac work to survival in cardiogenic shock in dogs. J. Amer. med. Ass. **199**, 825 (1967).

350b. —, J. H. BLOCH, J. A. FEEMSTER, Y. IDEZUKI, and R. C. LILLEHEI: Mechanisms in the production of shock. Surgery **62**, 645 (1967).

351. DILLON, J., L. J. LYNCH JR., R. MEYERS, and H. R. BUTCHER: The treatment of hemorrhagic shock. Surg. Gynec. Obstet. **122**, 967 (1966).

352. — — — —, and C. A. MOYER: A bioassay of treatment of hemorrhagic shock. I. The role of blood, Ringer's solution with lactate, and macromolecules (dextran and hydroxyethyl starch) in the treatment of hemorrhagic shock in the anesthetized dog. Arch. Surg. **93**, 537 (1966).

352a. — Importance of sodium-containing crystalloid solutions in hemorrhagic shock. Med. Ann. D. C. **35**, 473 (1966).

353. DINTENFASS, L.: Thixotropy of blood and proneness to thrombus formation. Circulat. Res. **11**, 233 (1962).

354. — A preliminary outline of the blood high viscosity syndromes. Arch. intern. Med. **118**, 427 (1966).

355. Division of Medical Sciences: Artificial Colloids for Intravenous Use. Nat. Acad. Sci., Washington, D. C., 1962.

356. Division of Medical Sciences: Second Conference on Artificial Colloidal Agents. Nat. Acad. Sci., Washington, D. C., 1963.

357. Division of Medical Sciences: Third Conference on Artificial Colloidal Agents. Nat. Acad. Sci., Washington, D. C., 1965.

358. DOBERNECK, R. C., M. P. REISER, and E. YUNIS: Acute renal failure after hemolytic transfusion reaction. Surg. Gynec. Obstet. **119**, 1069 (1964).

359. —, and B. ZIMMERMANN: Early mechanisms of homeostasis after hemorrhage in man. J. surg. Res. **4**, 36 (1964).

360. Donovan, J. C., C. J. Lund, and L. Whalen: Simultaneous determinations o blood volumes using Evans blue and sodium radiochromate. Surg. Gynec Obstet. **119**, 1031 (1964).
361. Dow, J. W., J. F. Dickson III, N. A. Hamer, and H. L. Gadboys: Anaphylactoid shock due to homologous blood exchange in the dog. J. thor Surg. **39**, 449 (1960).
362. Drake, C. T., and F. J. Lewis: The plasma volume expanding effect of lov molecular weight dextran in the hypothermic dog. Surg. Forum **12**, 18 (1961).
363. Drucker, W. R., W. D. Holden, B. Kingsbury, N. Hofmann, and L. Graham: Metabolic aspects of hemorrhagic shock. Metabolic studies on th need for erythrocytes in the treatment of hypovolemia due to hemorrhage J. Trauma **2**, 567 (1962).
364. Drury, A. N: The treatment of wound shock. Medical Research Council Committee on Traumatic Shock and on Blood Transfusion. London H. M. Stationery Office 1940.
365. Dubiel-Tomaszewski, W., W. R. Stern, and D. P. Hall: The use of lov molecular weight dextran (Rheomacrodex) as an anticoagulant in lef atrial to femoral artery by-pass. J. thorac. cardiovasc. Surg. **50**, 221 (1965)
366. Dubois-Ferrière, H.: La maladie post-opératoire et le shock traumatique Genève: Imprimerie du „Journal de Genève" 1945.
367. Duff, J. H., H. M. Scott, D. I. Peretz, G. W. Mulligan, and L. D MacLean: The diagnosis and treatment of shock in man based on hemodynamic and metabolic measurements. J. Trauma **6**, 145 (1966).
368. Dugdale, M., J. D. Nofzinger, and F. Murphey: Some effects of low molecular weight dextran on coagulation. Thromb. Diath. haemorrh. **11**, 11 (1966).
369. Duke, M., V. D. Herbert, and W. H. Abelmann: Hemodynamic effects o blood transfusion in chronic anemia. New Engl. J. Med. **271**, 975 (1964).
370. Dumont, A., et A. Goffaux: Détermination du groupe sanguin après perfusion intraveineuse de „dextran". Acta chir. belg. **50**, 215 (1951).
371. Duesberg, R., u. H. Spitzbarth: Klinik und Therapie der Kollapszustände Stuttgart: Schattauer 1963.
372. Dybkjaer, E., and F. Kissmeyer-Nielsen: Undersøgelser over indvirkninger af Rheomacrodex pa plasma in vitro. Ugeskr. Laeg. **125**, 715 (1963).
373. —, E. Berg, and F. Kissmeyer-Nielsen: Coagulation studies in extracorporea circulation. Acta chir. scand. **128**, 350 (1964).
374. —, and P. Elkjaer: The use of heated blood in massive blood replacement Acta anesth. scand. **8**, 271 (1964).
375. Eberlein, J., u. H. Dobberstein: Kreislaufmessungen an Blutspendern bei rascher Infusion eines neuen Plasmaexpanders. Arzneimittelforsch. **12**, 494 (1962).
376. Ebert, R. , E. A. Stead jr., and J. G. Gibson: Response of normal subjects to acute blood loss. Arch. intern. Med. **68**, 578 (1941).
377. Ebert, R. V.: Clinical characteristics of American dextran. Bibl. haemat. fasc 7, 270 (1958).
378. Eckert, C., T. E. Weichselbaum, R. Sights, and V. Miller: Study of the effect of the administration of dextran and physiologic saline solution on the colloidal osmotic pressure of the plasma in splenectomized dogs following hemorrhage. Surg. Forum **4**, 731 (1954).
379. Eckstein, M., and J. Lindner: The histochemistry of the plasma substitution especially with dextran. Ann. histochim. suppl. **2**, 163 (1962).

380. Editorial: A transfusion accident. Lancet II, 1204 (1953).
381. Editorial: Alleged fatal blood transfusion. Brit. med. J. II, 1277 (1953).
382. Editorial: Reactions to dextran. Med. J. Austr. 40, 926 (1953).
383. Editorial: Metabolism of the plasma expanders dextran and polyvinylpyrrolidone. Nutr. Rev. 11, 281 (1953).
384. Editorial: Plasma volume expanders and blood typing. J. Amer. med. Ass. 154, 1398 (1954).
385. Editorial: Infected blood transfusion. Brit. med. J. II, 334 (1958).
386. Editorial: Hypertonic sodium for "irreversible" oligaemic shock. Lancet I, 539 (1963).
387. Editorial: More on shock. New Physician, A-24, 1965.
388. Editorial: Drugs and placental barrier. Brit. med. J.II, 219 (1966).
389. Editorial: Potential plasma substitute—as effective as dextran. J. Amer. med. Ass. 197, 30 (1966).
390. EDMUNDS, L. H., JR., J. FOLKMAN, A. B. SNODGRESS, and R. B. BROWN: Prevention of brain damage during profound hypothermia and circulatory arrest. Ann. Surg. 157, 637 (1963).
391. EGER, W.: Der Einfluß von Plasmaexpandern auf die unspezifische Resistenz des Organismus. Med. exp. 8, 176 (1963).
392. —, u. E. SCHULZ: Experimentelle Untersuchungen über den Einfluß von Chlorpromazin auf das Dextranödem der Leber. Anaesthesist 14, 332 (1965).
393. EHRLY, A. M.: Wirkung von niedermolekularem Dextran auf Erythrozytenaggregate beim Sludgephänomen. Med. Klin. 61, 989 (1966).
394. EICHHOLTZ, F., u. Y. HAGIHARA: Nebenwirkungen der kolloidalen Blutersatzmittel. Hippokrates 32, 248 (1961).
395. EICHLER, J., and G. STEPHAN: Verhalten der Blutgerinnungsfaktoren nach Infusion von Plasmaexpandern. Anaesthesist 13, 102 (1964).
395a. —, G. STEPHAN: Vergleichende Untersuchungen nach Infusion von Plasmaexpandern. Münch. med. Wschr. 109, 1420 (1967).
396. EICHLER, O., I. APPEL u. F. SEBENING: Versuche über Dextran-Infusionen und ihre physiologischen Folgeerscheinungen. Klin. Wschr. 32, 127 (1954).
397. EIGLER, F. W., u. K. BONHOEFFER: Die Viskosität verschiedener Blutersatzmittel und ihrer Mischungen mit heparinisiertem Rinderblut bei Temperaturen von 8, 21 und 38° C. Thoraxchirurgie 10, 254 (1963).
398. EIKEN, O.: Thrombotic occlusion of experimental grafts as a function of the regional blood flow. Acta chir. scand. 121, 410 (1961).
399. EINHEBER, A., and D. CARTER: Failure of ten per cent low molecular weight dextran as a blood substitute after oligemic shock in primates. J. Trauma 6, 630 (1966).
400. EISEMAN, B., and P. BOSOMWORTH: Vasodilator agents in management of wound shock. Nat. Acad. Sci., Washington, D. C. 1963 a.
401. — — Evaluation of low molecular weight dextran in shock: Pharmacology and pertinent rheology. Nat. Acad. Sci., Washington, D. C., 1963 b.
402. EISINGER, R. P.: Failure of expanded plasma volume to induce exaggerated natruresis in hypertensive man. Amer. J. med. Sci. 249, 216 (1965).
403. EKELUND, L.-G.: Determination of blood volume. Scand. J. clin. Lab. Invest. 17, suppl. 86, 53 (1965).
404. EKDAHL, P.-H., and B. ZEDERFELDT: In vitro studies on the conjugation of cholic acid in human liver homogenates. I. Effect of Rheomacrodex on the liver conjugation of cholic acid. Acta chir. scand. 126, 326 (1963).

405. ELDER, J. D., W. M. PARKINS, and H. M. VARS: Observations on modifi fluid gelatin as a plasma volume expander. Bibl. haemat. fasc. **7**, 2 (1958).

406. ELIAS, G. L., F. N. GURD, L. G. HAMPSON, and A. S. V. BURGEN: Comparis of effectiveness of autologous and non-autologous plasma in oligem shock in dogs. Circulat. Res. **11**, 857 (1962).

407. ELIASSON, R., and U. SAMELIUS-BROBERG: The effect of various dextran fra tions on the suspension stability of the blood after intravenous injecti in cats. Acta physiol. scand. **58**, 211 (1963).

408. —, och U. F. GRUBER: Rheomacrodex inverkan på njurfunktionen. Opus med. suppl. **2**, 83 (1965).

409. — The antithrombotic properties of dextran. Med. postgrad. **4**, 18 (1966).

410. ELKINGTON, J. R., A. W. WINKLER, and T. S. DANOWSKI: The importance volume and tonicity of body fluids in salt depletion shock. J. clin. Inve **26**, 1002 (1947).

411. EMERSON, C. P., and R. V. EBERT: A study of shock in battle casualties. An Surg. **122**, 745 (1945).

412. ENERSON, D. M.: Cellular swelling: I. Hypothermia, graded hypoxia, and t osmotic effects of low molecular weight dextran on isolated tissues. An Surg. **163**, 169 (1966).

413. —, and H. M BERMAN: Cellular swelling: II. Effects of hypotonicity, lo molecular weight dextran addition and pH changes on oxygen consum tion of isolated tissues. Ann. Surg. **163**, 537 (1966).

414. —, and J. MEROLA: Cellular swelling: III. Effects of hypothermia and add tion of low molecular weight dextran on oxygen consumption an electrolyte composition of isolated tissues. Ann. Surg. **165**, 244 (1967).

415. ENGEL, F. L.: The significance of the metabolic changes during shock. An N.Y. Acad. Sci. **55**, 381 (1952).

416. ENGESET, J., A. L. STALKER, and N. A. MATHESON: Effects of dextran 40 c erythrocyte aggregation. Lancet **I**, 1124 (1966).

416a. — — — Turbidimetric measurement of red cell aggregation and effects dextran 40. Congr. brit. Microcirc. Soc., Aberdeen, 1967.

417. ERNST, C. B., W. J. FRY, R. O. KRAFT, and M. S. DE WEESE: The role of lo molecular weight dextran in the management of venous thrombosis. Sur Gynec. Obstet. **119**, 1243 (1964).

418. EUFINGER, H.: Die Behandlung des Schocks in der Chirurgie. Med. Wel 781, 1963.

419. — Schock und Plasmaexpander. In: K. HORATZ u. R. FREY: Schock un Plasmaexpander, p. 84. Berlin-Göttingen-Heidelberg: Springer 1964.

420. — Die Volumensubstitution beim Schock in der Chirurgie. Chir. Prax **9**, 193 (1965).

421. EVANS, A. J.: Management of shock in burns. Anglo-Germ. med. Rev. **2**, 17 (1963).

422. — The treatment of burns. In: D. N. MATTHEW: Recent advances in th surgery of trauma, p. 76. London: Churchill 1963.

423. EVANS, E. I., M. J. HOOVER, G. W. JAMES, and T. ALM: Studies on traumat shock. I. Blood volume changes in traumatic shock. Ann. Surg. **119**, 6 (1944).

424. EVANS, T. H., W. L. HAWKINS, and H. HIBBERT: Studies on reactions relatin to carbohydrates and polysaccharides. LXIV. Antigenicity of dextra produced by Leuconostoc mesenteroides. J. exp. Med. **74**, 511 (1941).

425. Evans, W. A., and D. Wong: Renal changes following the administration of low molecular weight dextran. Austr. J. Surg. 69 (1966).
426. Evans, W. E., and J. C. Darin: The additive effects of low molecular weight dextran in the treatment of endotoxin shock with hyperbaric oxygen. J. Trauma **5**, 213 (1965).
426a. Evonuk, E.: Hemodynamic and metabolic responses of infused low molecular weight dextran. Amer. J. Physiol. **212**, 514 (1967).
427. Ewald, R. A., and W. H. Crosby: Reported experiences with dextran in communist countries. Transfusion **3**, 376 (1963).
428. —, A. A. Young, and W. H. Crosby: Particle formation in dextran solutions. Mil. Med. **129**, 952 (1964).
429. —, J. W. Eichelberger jr., J. W. Yong, H. J. Weiss, and W. H. Crosby: The effect of dextran on platelet factor 3 activity: In vitro and in vivo studies. Transfusion **5**, 109 (1965).
430. Fadhli, H. A., D. P. Fine, and M. K. Maizji: Intra-arterial dextran in experimental surgery. J. Amer. med. Ass. **196**, 177 (1966).
430a. — — — Intra-arterial infusion of dextran. J. thorac. cardiovasc. Surg. **53**, 496 (1967).
431. Fåhraeus, R.: The movement of water in surviving tissue at different temperatures. A contribution to the pathogenesis of shock. Acta Soc. med. upsalien. **61**, 107 (1956).
432. Falholt, W.: The dye injection method for circulatory studies. Scand. J. clin. Lab. Invest. **10**, suppl. 35 (1957).
432a. Falk, V., B. Forkman, and K. E. Arfors: The permeability of the placenta to dextrans. Acta obstet. gynec. scand. **46**, 414 (1967).
432b. Farbwerke Hoechst AG, Abt. Behring-Präparate: Haemaccel, physiologischer Plasmaexpander der Behringwerke. Anaesth. prax. **2**, 72 (1967).
433. Fayot, G., et P. Huguenard: Impressions cliniques après 350 perfusions veineuses de dextran. Anesth. Analg. Réanim. **12**, 517 (1955).
434. Fekl, W., u. H. Bickel: Zu: Experimentelle Untersuchungen mit kolloidalen Volumenersatzlösungen. Anaesth. Resusc. **13**, 240 (1966). Berlin-Göttingen-Heidelberg: Springer 1966.
435. Fernbach, D. J.: Hazards of unneccessary blood transfusions. Anesth. Analg. **40**, 667 (1961).
436. Feurstein, V., u. H. Schroll: Die klinische Bedeutung des Kaliumanstieges im Konservenblut. Wien. klin. Wschr. **76**, 206 (1964).
437. — Grundlagen und Ergebnisse der Venendruckmessung zur Prüfung des zirkulierenden Blutvolumens. Anaesth. Resusc. **7**. Berlin-Göttingen-Heidelberg: Springer 1965.
438. Fine, J.: The bacterial factor in traumatic shock. Springfield, Ill.: Thomas 1954.
439. — Irreversible shock. New Engl. J. Med. **268**, 107 (1963 a).
440. — Shock and electrolyte disturbances: Etiology and classification of shock. Amer. J. Cardiol. **12**, 587 (1963 b).
441. — Panel discussion V. Amer. J. Cardiol. **12**, 628 (1963 c).
442. — Current status of the problem of traumatic shock. Surg. Gynec. Obstet. **120**, 537 (1965 a).
443. — Oligemia in surgical shock. Lancet **II**, 440 (1965 b).
444. Finlayson, D. C., F. J. Dagher, and L. D. Vandam: Diurnal variation in blood volume of man. J. surg. Res. **4**, 286 (1964).
445. Fischer, M., u. H. Wimmer: Aktivierung des fibrinolytischen Systems durch niedermolekulares Dextran. Bibl. haemat. fasc. **23**, 1278 (1965).

445a. Fischer, M., K. Lechner und F. Pesendorfer: Erfahrungen mit Rheo macrodex bei der Behandlung arterieller Durchblutungsstörungen. Med Welt 17, 712 (1966).

445b. — Ein Plasma-Expander auf Gelatine-Basis und sein Effekt auf Blutgerin nung, Fibrinolyse und Funktion der Thrombocyten. Arzneimittelforsch. 17 1129 (1967).

446. Fischer, R., u. H. Berning: Über die Beeinflussung des Mineralhaushalte durch eine Plasmasubstitutionslösung. Med. Klin. 57, 1443 (1962).

447. Fisher, B., and E. R. Fisher: Experimental studies of factors influencin hepatic metastases. XVI. Rheologic alterations. Cancer Res. 26, 183 (1966)

447a. Fitts, W. T., jr., and M. J. Orloff: Blood transfusion and Jehovah' witnesses. Surg. Gynec. Obstet. 108, 502 (1959).

447b. Fitzgerald, P.: Symposium on shock. Don Salford Assoc., Dublin, 1966.

448. Flanagan, J. P., G. P. Steinmetz, E. W. Crawford, and K. A. Merendino: Observations on blood volume with special attention to loss an replacement in cardiac surgery. Surgery 56, 925 (1964).

449. Fleming, J. W., W. H. Cargill, and W. L. Bloom: Effects of intravenou administration of dextran on renal function. Proc. Soc. exp. Biol. 79, 60 (1952).

450. Flemma, R. J., A. J. Acinapura, D. Silver, and W. G. Anlyan: Effects o heparin, plasmin, dextran and low molecular weight dextran on electrically induced thromboses. Amer. Surg. 32, 17 (1966).

451. Fletcher, F., L. E. Martin, and A. Ratcliffe: Interaction of macromolecule and fibrinogen. Nature (London) 170, 319 (1952).

452. Flotte, C. T., and E. F. Cox: Dextran in the treatment of thrombophlebitis Trans. sth. surg. Ass. 74, 114 (1963).

453. —, and R. W. Buxton: Reduction of serum cholesterol by dextran. Circulation 28, 721 (1963).

454. — — Reduction of serum cholesterol and lipids by dextran. Circulation 32 suppl. 2, 85 (1965).

455. Folse, R., and J. G. Cope: A comparison of the peripheral and central hemodynamic effects of regular and low molecular weight dextran in patient with ischemic limbs. Surgery 58, 779 (1965).

456. Foster, L. L., and D. H. Brown: Prospects of low molecular weight dextran in cerebral infarction. Marquette med. Rev. 27, 180 (1962).

457. Foster, J. H., A. D. Killen, P. C. Jolly, and J. H. Kirtley: Low molecular weight dextran in vascular surgery: Prevention of early thrombosis following arterial reconstruction in 85 cases. Ann. Surg. 163, 764 (1966).

458. Fountain, S. S., and P. R. Schloerb: The dynamics of post-traumatic intestinal fluid sequestration. Surg. Gynec. Obstet. 123, 1237 (1966).

459. Fowler, N. O., R. H. Franch, and W. L. Bloom: Hemodynamic effects of anemia with and without plasma volume expansion. Circulat. Res. 4, 319 (1956).

460. —, W. L. Bloom, and J. A. Ward: Hemodynamic effects of hypervolemia with and without anemia. Circulat. Res. 6, 163 (1958).

461. — Plasma substitutes. Handbook of Physiology, section 2; Circulation, vol. 1, 63 (1962). Washington, D. C.: Amer. Physiol. Soc.

462. Fox, L., jr., J. M. Winfield, L. B. Slobody, C. M. Swindler, and J. K. Lattimmer: Electrolyte solution approximating plasma concentrations with increased potassium for routine fluid and electrolyte replacement. J. Amer. med. Ass. 147, 827 (1952).

463. Frank, H. A., A. M. Seligman, and J. Fine: Traumatic shock. X. The treatment of hemorrhagic shock irreversible to replacement of blood volume deficiency. J. clin. Invest. **24**, 435 (1945).
464. Frawly, J. P., C. P. Artz, and J. M. Howard: Plasma retention and urinary excretion of dextran and modified fluid gelatin in combat casualties. Surgery **37**, 784 (1955).
465. Freedman, S. O., J. Q. Bliss, J. L. Hutchison, and A. S. V. Burgen: Cutaneous and systemic reactions to human plasma. J. Allergy **31**, 134 (1960).
466. Freeman, J.: Physiological effects of haemorrhage. Ann. roy. Coll. Surg. Engl. **33**, 138 (1963).
467. Freiesleben, E.: Der hämolytische Transfusionszwischenfall. Bibl. haemat. fasc. 20, 9 (1965).
468. Freesen, O., u. H. Weese: Das gewebliche Bild nach Infusion verschiedener Kollidon-Fraktionen (Periston N, Periston, hochvisköses Periston) beim Tier. Beitr. path. Anat. **112**, 47 (1952).
469. Freuchen, I., A. Trostmann, and J. Østergaard: Haemaccel—a new plasma substitute. Acta anaesth. scand. suppl. **15**, 147 (1964).
470. Freysz, T., u. G. Hossli: Ein neuartiges Gerät zur raschen Aufwärmung von Blutkonserven. Anaesthesist **13**, 104 (1964).
471. Freytag, G., J. Lindner, and K. Ebert: New histochemical and autoradiographical findings on capillary permeability. Bibl. anat. **7**, 172 (1965).
472. — Autoradiographische Ergebnisse bezüglich der Permeabilität unter normalen und pathologischen Bedingungen. Vortr. 4. Mikrozirkulationskongr., Cambridge 1966.
473. Friberg, U., W. Graf, and B. Åberg: On the histochemistry of partly hydrolysed, bacterial dextran. Scand. J. clin. Lab. Invest. **3**, 221 (1951).
474. Friedman, E., E. Grable, and J. Fine: Central venous pressure and direct serial measurements as guides in blood-volume replacement. Lancet **II**, 609 (1966).
475. Friedman, E. A., and G. E. Thomson: Hepatitis complicating chronic haemodialysis. Lancet **II**, 675 (1966).
476. Friedrich, H. W., R. Schantz, u. H. L. du Mont: Klinische und experimentelle Untersuchungen über Dextran. Anaesthesist **1**, 144 (1952).
477. — — — Tierexperimentelle Untersuchungen nach Dextranapplikation. Anaesthesist **4**, 68 (1955).
478. Fries, C. C., and M. R. Golding: Evaluation of hydroxyethyl starch in the treatment of shock in pigs: A preliminary report. In: Third Conference on Artifical Colloidal Agents, p. 163. Washington, D. C.: Nat. Acad. Sci. 1965.
479. Froeschlin, W.: Schocktherapie mit Haemaccel, einem neuen Plasmaexpander. Dtsch. med. Wschr. **87**, 811 (1962).
480. Fry, W. J., and G. W. Parker: The influence of low molecular weight dextran on occlusive vascular disease. Surg. Gynec. Obstet. **123**, 531 (1966).
481. Fuchsig, P.: Erkennung und Behandlung hämolytischer Transfusionszwischenfälle. Bibl. haemat. fasc. **11**, 247 (1960).
482. — Die Dosierung der Transfusion in der operativen Medizin. Wien. klin. Wschr. **76**, 201 (1964).
483. Gabr, Y.: Studies on gelatin as a blood substitute. Arzneimittelforsch. **16**, 572 (1966).
484. Gadboys, H. L., R. Slonim, and R. S. Litwak: Homologous blood syndrome: I. Preliminary observations on its relationship to cardiopulmonary bypass. Ann. Surg. **156**, 793 (1962).

485. Gadboys, H. L., A. R. Jones, R. Slonim, B. G. Wisoff, and R. S. Litwak: The homologous blood syndrome: III. Influence of plasma, buffy coat and red cells in provoking its manifestations. Amer. J. Cardiol. **12**, 194 (1963).
486. — Blood volume changes during homologous blood exchange. Amer. Surg. **30**, 353 (1964).
487. —, R. S. Litwak, J. Ishiguro, and M. Kahn: Experimental large-volume hemodilution. Circulation **32**, suppl. 1, 121 (1965).
488. — —, M. Kahn, S. Kochwa, and W. E. Buerger: Experimental large-volume hemodilution with plasma. Circulation **32**, suppl. 2, 92 (1965).
489. — —, H. W. Wallace, M. Kahn, S. Kochwa, and W. Buerger: Experimental large-volume hemodilution with plasma. J. thorac. cardiovasc. Surg. **52**, 112 (1966).
490. Gall, E. A., W. A. Altemeier, L. Schiff, D. L. Hamilton, H. Braunstein, J. Giuseffi, and D. G. Freiman: Liver lesions following intravenous administration of polyvinylpyrrolidone (PVP). Amer. J. clin. Path. **23**, 1187 (1953).
491. Gann, D. S., and H. K. Wright: Augmentation of sodium excretion in postoperative patients by expansion of the extracellular volume. Surg. Gynec. Obstet. **118**, 1024 (1964).
492. — — Increased renal sodium reabsorption after depletion of the extracellular or intravascular fluid volumes. J. surg. Res. **6**, 196 (1966).
493. Garzon, A. A., H. L. Fink, G. W. Shaftan, and K. E. Karlson: Blood loss associated with administration of low molecular weight dextran. J. thorac. cardiovasc. Surg. **48**, 873 (1964).
494. Gasanov, S. G.: Changes in the volume of the circulating blood after infusion of polyglucin to dogs after lethal exsanguination. Probl. hemat. **5**, 560 (1960).
495. Gauer, O. H.: Die Wirkungen von Aderlaß und Transfusion auf die wichtigsten Kreislaufabschnitte. Bibl. haemat. fasc. **6**, 61 (1957).
496. —, and J. P. Henry: Circulatory basis of fluid volume control. Physiol. Rev. **43**, 423 (1963).
497. Gelin, L.-E.: Macrodex and oxygen in the primary treatment of extensive burns. Acta chir. scand. **103**, 351 (1952).
498. — Studies in anemia of injury. Acta chir. scand. suppl. **210**, 1 (1956).
499. — The significance of intravascular aggregation following injury. Bull. Soc. int. Chir. **18**, 4 (1959).
500. —, and B. Zederfeldt: Low molecular weight dextran—a rheologic agent counteracting capillary stagnation. Acta chir. scand. **119**, 168 (1960).
501. —, and O. K. A. Thorén: Influence of low viscous dextran on peripheral circulation in man. Acta chir. scand. **122**, 303 (1961).
502. —, and B. Ingelman: Rheomacrodex—a new dextran solution for rheological treatment of impaired capillary flow. Acta chir. scand. **122**, 294 (1961).
503. —, K. Korsan-Bengtsen, J. Ygge, and B. Zederfeldt: Influence of low vicous dextran on the hemostatic mechanism. Acta chir. scand. **122**, 324 (1961).
504. — Disturbance of the flow properties of blood and its counteraction in surgery. Acta chir. scand. **122**, 287 (1961).
505. —, L. Sölvell, and B. Zederfeldt: The plasma volume expanding effect of low viscous dextran and Macrodex. Acta chir. scand. **122**, 309 (1961).
506. — Effect of low viscous dextran in the early postoperative period. Acta chir. scand. **122**, 333 (1961).

507. Gelin, L.-E., and B. Zederfeldt: Experimental evidence of the significance of disturbances in the flow properties of blood. Acta chir. scand. 122, 336 (1961).
508. —, E. Persson, and B. Zederfeldt: Influence of low viscous dextran on the electrolyte balance in healthy subjects. Acta. chir. scand. 122, 329 (1961).
509. —, and W. C. Shoemaker: Hepatic blood flow and microcirculatory alterations induced by dextran of high and low viscosity. Surgery 49, 713 (1961).
510. —, and B. Zederfeldt: Low viscous dextran as a therapeutic agent against capillary stagnation. Bibl. anat. 1, 265 (1961).
511. — Rheologic disturbances and the use of low viscosity dextran in surgery. Rev. Surg. 19, 385 (1962).
512. — A method for studying the aggregation of blood cells, erythrostatis and plasma skimming in branching capillary tubes. Bibl. anat. 4, 362 (1964).
513. — Pathophysiologie und Klinik der Blutströmung in den kleinen Gefäßen. Anaesthesist 13, 333 (1964).
514. —, and C.-M. Rudenstam: The influence of intravascular aggregation on the spread and growth of experimental tumors. Bibl. anat. 4, 131 (1964).
515. — —, and B. Zederfeldt: The rheology of red cell suspension. Bibl. anat. 7, 368 (1965).
516. — Rheological disturbances following tissue injury. In: A. L Copley: Proc. 4th Intern. Congr. Rheology, part 4, p. 299. New York: Interscience 1965.
517. —, and C.-M. Rudenstam: Trauma, microcirculation and tumor spread. In: Swedish Cancer Soc. Yearbook 4, 55 (1965).
518. — Bruk och missbruk av Rheomacrodex. Svensk. Läk. Tidn. 63, 1377 (1966).
519. Gersmeyer, E. F.: Der Kreislaufkollaps. Berlin-Göttingen-Heidelberg: Springer 1961.
520. Gianelli, S., jr., J. R. Navarre, D. R. Mahajan, and G. H. Pratt: Use of vasopressor agents in hemorrhagic shock: Effect on posthemorrhagic hemodilution. Ann. Surg. 156, 41 (1962).
521. —, S. M. Ayres, R. A. Goldstone, P. Varriale, and M. E. Buehler: The effects of low molecular weight dextran infusion in humans. J. surg. Res. 5, 404 (1965).
522. Gibbs, C. E., and H. R. Misenhimer: The use of blood transfusion in obstetrics. Amer. J. Obstet. Gynec. 93, 26 (1965).
523. Giebel, O.: Zur Problematik der Blutvolumenbestimmung mit Hilfe von Radioisotopen. Anaesthesist 15, 173 (1966).
523a. —, und K. Horatz: Blutvolumenbestimmung mit Hilfe radioaktiver Isotope. Bruns Beitr. klin. Chir. 214, 491 (1967).
524. Giebisch, G., H. D. Lauson, and R. F. Pitts: Renal excretion and volume of distribution of various dextrans. Amer. J. Physiol. 178, 168 (1954).
525. Gillet, D. J., and D. F. J. Halmagyi: Result and limitations of blood volume measurements in sheep. J. surg. Res. 6, 211 (1966 a).
526. — — Blood volume in reversible and irreversible posthemorrhagic shock in sheep. J. surg. Res. 6, 259 (1966 b).
527. Gilmore, J. P.: Cardiovascular changes of the burned dog following the infusion of intravenous solutions. Amer. J. Physiol. 190, 513 (1957).
528. Giomini, M. L., e P. Giannotti: Studio clinico di un nuovo plasmaexpander. Minerva anest. 29, 364 (1963).
528a. Glenert, J., and S. N. Pedersen: Albumin transfer from blood to small intestine in dogs during exsanguination hypotension. Acta chir. scand. 133, 95 (1967).

529. GLIEDMANN, M. L., R. E. GIRARDET, M. KAPLITT, J. R. STUCKEY, and K. E. KARLSON: Inferior vena cava pressure gradient in the homologous blood syndrome. Circulation **28**, 727 (1963).
530. GLOOR, B.: Tierexperimentelle Untersuchungen über Morphologie, Pathogenese und funktionelle Bedeutung der Zuckerspeicherniere. Z. ges. exp. Med. **139**, 33 (1965).
531. GLYNN, L. E., E. J. HOLBOROW, and G. D. JOHNSON: The relationship of polymer size and sulphation to the haptenic specificity of dextrans. J. Path. Bact. **68**, 205 (1954).
532. GOEDDE, H. W.: Genetisch bedingte Reaktionen auf Pharmaka. Arch. Pharm. **299**, 184 (1966).
533. GOLDBERG, M., and J. FINE: Traumatic shock. XI. Intestinal absorption in hemorrhagic shock. J. clin. Invest. **24**, 445 (1945).
534. GOLDENBERG, M., R. D. CRANE, and H. POPPER: Effect of intravenous administration of dextran, a macromolecular carbohydrate, in animals. Amer. J. clin. Path. **17**, 939 (1947).
535. GOLLUB, S., and C. P. BAILEY: Management of major surgical blood loss without transfusion. J. Amer. med. Ass. **198**, 1171 (1966).
535a. —, C. SCHAEFER, and B. S. SQUITIERI: The bleeding tendency associated with plasma expanders. Surg. Gynec. Obstet. **124**, 1203 (1967).
536. GÖLTNER, E., u. F. LANG: Blutmenge und Diurese nach Gelatineinfusionen. Med. Welt, 1276, 1964.
537. —, H. ZITZMANN u. C. FUCHS: Die Kreislauf-, Blut- und Diurese-Verhältnisse nach Dextraninfussion. Med. Welt, 594, 1965.
538. GOMEZ, O. A., and W. F. HAMILTON: Functional cardiac deterioration during development of hemorrhagic circulatory deficiency. Circulat. Res. **14**, 327 (1964).
539. GOODWIN, J. F., J. M. KAY, and D. HEATH: Clinical pathologic conference. Amer Heart J. **70**, 239 (1965).
539a. GOODYER, A. V. N.: Left ventricular function and tissue hypoxia in irreversible hemorrhagic and endotoxin shock Amer. J. Physiol. **212**, 444 (1967).
540. GORDON, H., L. J. HOGE, and H. LAWSON: Gelatin as substitute for blood after experimental hemorrhage. Amer. J. med. Sci. **204**, 4 (1942).
541. GORLIN, R.: Regulation of intravascular volume in chronic congestive failure. Brit. med. J. **I**, 1128 (1961).
541a. GOULIAN, D., JR.: The use of bromphenol blue in the assay of Rheomacrodex effects on flap viability. Plast. reconstr. Surg. **39**, 227 (1967).
542. GOVIER, W. M., and G. C. COLOVOS: An animal survival method for the evaluation of agents designed to restore plasma volume. Ann. N.Y. Acad. Sci. **55**, 491 (1952).
543. GÖZSY, B., and L. KATO: Investigations into the mechanism of dextran-induced edema in rats. Canad. J. Biochem. **41**, 1855 (1963).
544. GRABLE, E.: Plasma volume measurements using the Volemetron. Anesthesiology **24**, 403 (1963).
545. —, J. ISRAEL, J. WILLIAMS, and J. FINE: Blood volume in experimental endotoxin and hemorrhagic shock. Ann. Surg. **157**, 361 (1963).
546. — Measurements of blood volume in patients and experimental animals. Amer. Surg. **30**, 379 (1964).
547. GRACEY, L.: Rheomacrodex in clinical Practice. In: Symposia on Rheomacrodex vol. 1, p. 50. London: Pharmacia 1964.

548. GRADY, G. F., T. C. CHALMERS, and the Boston Inter Hospital Liver Group: Risk of post transfusion viral hepatitis. New Engl. J. Med. 271, 337 (1964).

549. GRAF, H., S. RIEMANN, W. SPIELMANN u. W. WAGNER: Therapeutische und serologische Erfahrungen mit einem Plasmaexpander auf Polypeptidbasis (Haemaccel). Münch. med. Wschr. 105, 725 (1963).

550. GRAHAM-STEWART, C. W.: A clinical survey of blood transfusion. Lancet II, 421 (1960).

551. GRANATH, K., u. R. STRÖMBERG: Physikalisch-chemische Daten über einige in der Infusionstherapie verwendete Polymere. Anaesthesist 17, 224 (1968).

552. GRANT, J.: Complications of blood transfusion. Practitioner 195, 179 (1965).

553. GRANT, R. T., and E. B. REEVE: Observations on the general effects of injury in man. Medical Res. Counc., Special Rep. Ser. 277, 1. London: H. M. Stationery Office 1951.

554. GRAY, I., and G. P. HIGHLAND: Metabolism of plasma expanders studied with carbon-14-labeled dextran. Amer. J. Physiol. 174, 462 (1953).

555. GREEFF, K., K. SCHARNAGEL, R. LÜHR u. H. STROBACH: Die Abnahme des Kininogengehaltes des Plasmas beim toxischen, anaphylaktischen und anaphylaktoiden Schock. Arch. exp. Path. Pharmakol. 253, 235 (1966).

556. GREEN, H. D.: Shock and circulatory homeostasis. Josian Macy jr. Found., 1.—5. Conf. New York: Corlies, Macy 1952, 1953, 1954, 1955, 1957.

557. GREENFIELD, L., and A. BLALOCK: Effect of low molecular weight dextran on survival following hemorrhagic shock. Surgery 55, 684 (1964).

558. GREEP, J. M., S. B. LITWIN, and G. L. NARDI: Comparative study of new device for measuring blood volume. Arch. Surg. 86, 164 (1963).

559. GREGERSEN, M. I.: Physiological contributions to the problem of shock. Fed. Proc. 3, 354 (1946).

560. —, and R. A. RAWSON: Blood volume. Physiol. Rev. 39, 307 (1959).

561. —, B. FERIC, S. USAMI, S. CHIEN, C. CHANG, and D. G. SINCLAIR: Studies on blood viscosity at low shear rates: Effects of low and high molecular dextrans. Fed. Proc. 22, 641 (1963).

562. — — — — Relation of molecular size of dextran to its effects on the rheological properties of blood. Proc. Soc. exp. Biol. 112, 883 (1963).

563. — — — — Relation of molecular weight of dextran to its effects on viscosity and sedimentation rate of blood. Bibl. anat. 4, 58 (1964).

564. GRIEM, W., G. CZOK, u. K. LANG: Histologische und physiologische Untersuchungen an Ratten nach Verabreichung des Plasmaexpanders Gelifundol. Anaesthesist 13, 321 (1964 a).

565. — — — Histologische und physiologische Untersuchungen an Ratten nach Haemaccel- und Rattenserum-Injektionen. Anaesthesist 13, 324 (1964 b).

566. — — — Histologische und physiologische Untersuchungen an Ratten nach Verabreichung des Plasmaexpanders Plasmagel. Anaesthesist 13, 330 (1964 c).

567. — — Tierexperimentelle Untersuchungen über morphologische Veränderungen durch Plasmaexpander. In: K. LANG, R. FREY u. M. HALMAGYI: Infusionstherapie, p. 205. Berlin-Heidelberg-New York: Springer 1966.

568. GRIFFEN, W. O., JR., and J. B. AUST: Low molecular weight dextran and metastatic tumor. Surg. Forum 15, 338 (1964).

569. GRODINS, F. S.: Gelatin as a blood substitute in shock due to limb trauma. Fed. Proc. 2, 17 (1943).

570. GRÖNWALL, A., och B. INGELMAN: Några nya kolloidlösningar för infusionsändamål. Nord. Med. 21, 247 (1944 a).

571. GRÖNWALL, A., u. B. INGELMAN: Untersuchungen über Dextran und sein Verhalten bei parenteraler Zufuhr. Acta physiol. scand. **7**, 97 (1944 b).
572. — — Untersuchungen über Dextran und sein Verhalten bei parenteraler Zufuhr. II. Acta physiol. scand. **9**, 1 (1945 a).
573. — — Dextran as a substitute for plasma. Nature (London) **155**, 45 (1945 b).
574. — Erfahrungen mit einer kolloidalen Infusionslösung von Dextran (Macrodex). Dtsch. med. Wschr. **76**, 1023 (1951).
575. — Dextran and its use in colloidal infusion solutions. Uppsala: Almqvist & Wiksell 1957.
576. — Antigenicity of Swedish clinical dextran (Macrodex). Acta soc. med. upsalien. **64**, 244 (1959).
577. — Dextran: Plasma volume expanders—chemistry and biological activities. Med. postgrad. **4**, 1 (1966).
578. GROPPER, A. L., E. W. COCHRELL, L. G. RAISZ, and E. J. PULASKI: A comparison of dextran and oxypolygelatin in the treatment of hemorrhagic hypotension. Amer. J. Physiol. **169**, 749 (1952).
579. —, L. G. RAISZ, and W. H. AMSPACHER: Plasma expanders. Surg. Gynec. Obstet. **95**, 521 (1952).
580. GROTH, C. G., and H. G. R. THORSÉN: Effect of Rheomacrodex on factors of importance for the flow properties of blood. Bibl. anat. **7**, 267 (1965).
581. —, and O. MURUK: Changes in blood plasma viscosity in experimentally induced erythrocyte aggregation. Bibl. anat. **7**, 385 (1965).
582. —, and G. THORSÉN: The effect of Rheomacrodex and Macrodex on factors governing the flow properties of the human blood. Acta chir. scand. **130**, 507 (1965).
583. —, B. LÖFSTRÖM, and O. MURUK: The effect of infused thrombin on the tissue oxygen tension. I. An experimental study on the rabbit. Acta chir. scand. **132**, 1 (1966 a).
584. — The effect of infused thrombin on the tissue oxygen tension. II. The possible role of 5-hydroxytryptamine and histamine. An experimental study in the rabbit. Acta chir. scand. **132**, 15 (1966 b).
585. —, and B. LÖFSTRÖM: The effect of infused high and low molecular weight dextrans on the tissue oxygen tension. An experimental study in the rabbit. Acta chir. scand. **131**, 275 (1966 c).
586. — The effect of infused albumin and Rheomacrodex on factors governing the flow properties of the human blood. Acta chir. scand. **131**, 290 (1966 d).
587. — The effect of infused plasma expanders and blood on the tissue oxygen tension. With special reference to the significance of the flow properties of the blood. An experimental study in the rabbit. Acta chir. scand. **132**, 233 (1966 e).
588. GROTTE, G.: Passage of dextran molecules across the blood-lymph barrier. Acta chir. scand. suppl. **211** (1956).
589. GRUBER, U. F., u. J. SIEGRIST: Der Volumeneffekt verschiedener Plasmaersatzstoffe. Arch. klin. Chir. **301**, 128 (1962).
590. — Herstellung und Verwendung von $RI^{131}HSA$, im besonderen zur Blutvolumenbestimmung. Anaesthesist **12**, 227 (1963).
591. —, u. M. ALLGÖWER: Verbrennungen. Ther. Umsch. **20**, 259 (1963).
592. — — Indikationen für Plasmaexpander. In: K. HORATZ u. R. FREY: Schock und Plasmaexpander, p. 137. Berlin-Göttingen-Heidelberg: Springer 1964.
593. — — The use of the Volemetron for blood volume measurements. A critical analysis. Bull. Soc. int. Chir. **23**, 218 (1964).

594. GRUBER, U. F.: Indications des nouveaux expanders plasmatiques. Méd. Hyg. 22, 719 (1964).
595. — Neuere Resultate der Schockforschung und therapeutische Konsequenzen. Vjschr. schweiz. San. Off. 41, 194 (1964).
596. —, E. GERBER, S. GRASS, and M. ALLGÖWER: Volume effect of new plasma expanders in hypovolemic subjects. Xth Congr. int. Soc. Blood Transf., abstr. P4 : 1. Stockholm 1964.
597. —, und M. ALLGÖWER: Infusionsprobleme in der Chirurgie. Berlin-Göttingen-Heidelberg: Springer 1965.
598. — Sofortmaßnahmen bei Schockpatienten. Fortschr. Med. 83, 293 (1965).
599. —, S.-E. BERGENTZ, and L.-E. GELIN: Thrombus preventing effect of plasma expanders. Scand. J. clin. Lab. Invest. 17, suppl. 86, 143 (1965).
600. —, S. GRASS, E. MEILI-GERBER u. M. ALLGÖWER: Die Beeinflussung der Diurese durch Verabreichung verschiedener Blutersatz- und Plasmapräparate beim leicht hypovolämischen Menschen. Helv. chir. Acta 32, 610 (1965).
601. —, E. GERBER, S. GRASS, and M. ALLGÖWER: Volume effects of new plasma expanders in hypovolemic subjects. Bibl. haemat. 23, 1116 (1965).
602. — Clinical application of blood volume measurements in shock. Bibl. haemat. 23, 1079 (1965).
603. — Sind Blutvolumenbestimmungen in der klinischen Praxis wirklich nötig? Anaesthesist 14, 314 (1965).
604. —, S.-E. BERGENTZ, and Å. FRITJOFSSON: Recent advances in the clinical uses of dextran. Symp. on Rheomacrodex 1, 13. London: Pharmacia 1965.
605. — Therapie der Mikrozirkulationsstörungen. In: O. H. JUST u. H. LUTZ: Genese und Therapie des hämorrhagischen Schocks, p. 91. Stuttgart: Thieme 1966.
606. — Aktuelle Probleme der venerischen Krankheiten. Med. Neuh. 72, 51 (1966).
607. — Plasmaersatzstoffe. Actuelle Chir. 1, 71 (1966).
608. —, och S.-E. BERGENTZ: Den trombosprofylaktiska effekten av dextran. Nord. Med. 75, 762 (1966).
609. — Den volymexpanderande effekten av homolog plasmainfusion. Nord. Med. 75, 749 (1966).
610. — Die Abhängigkeit der Blutviskosität vom Hämatokrit. Z. prakt. Anästh. 1, 141 (1966).
611. —, u. C. BURRI: Tierexperimentelle Untersuchungen mit Plasmaexpandern. In: K. LANG, R. FREY u. M. HALMAGYI: Infusionstherapie, p. 214. Berlin-Heidelberg-New York: Springer 1966.
612. —, u. S.-E. BERGENTZ: Der Volumeneffekt von autologen und homologen Frischplasmatransfusionen bei hypovolämischen Individuen. Arch. klin. Chir. 316, 636 (1966).
613. —, u. M. ALLGÖWER: Entgegnung auf die Arbeit von A. HÄSSIG: Schockprobleme und Blutersatz unter besonderer Berücksichtigung der Expanderfrage. Anaesthesist 15, 332 (1966).
614. —, and S.-E. BERGENTZ: The antithrombotic effect of dextran. J. surg. Res. 6, 379 (1966).
615. — — Autologous and homologous fresh human plasma as a volume expander in hypovolemic subjects. Ann. Surg. 165, 41 (1967).
616. — Die chirurgische Behandlung der amerikanischen Kriegsverletzten in Vietnam. Vjschr. schweiz. San. Off. 44, 217 (1966).
617. — Bericht über das Verbrennungssymposium der N.Y. Academy of Sciences. Anaesthesist 16, 116 (1967).

618. GRUBER, U. F.: Intestinale Faktoren im Schock: Darmtoxine. Arch. klin. Chir. **319**, 909 (1967).
618a. —, u. S.-E. BERGENTZ: Neue Wege in der Thromboembolie-Prophylaxe. Helv. chir. Acta **34**, 14 (1967).
619. GRÜNERT, R. D., K. OEFF u. H. SCHULZE: Eigenschaften und Indikationen von Rheomacrodex. Anaesthesist **11**, 302 (1962).
620. GRÜNING, W. U., u. H. ROTH: Das Verhalten des Blutvolumens beim Menschen nach Infusion von Blutersatzflüssigkeiten. Klin. Wschr. **32**, 351 (1954).
621. GSELL, O., P. MIESCHER, M. ALLGÖWER u. L. HOLLÄNDER: Die Lebensdauer transfundierter, mit $Na_2Cr^{51}O_4$ markierter Erythrozyten bei verschiedenen Formen der Anämie. V. Kongr. europ. Ges. Hämatol., Freiburg i. Br., 1955, p. 55. Berlin-Göttingen-Heidelberg: Springer 1956.
622. GUERRINI, O., e G. SERIO: Primi risultati sull'impiego clinico di un nuovo sostituto plasmatico. Minerva anest. **29**, 377 (1963).
623. GUNNAR, R. M., R. J. PIETRAS, C. STAVRAKOS, H. S. LOEB, and J. R. TOBIN: The physiologic basis for treatment of shock associated with myocardial infarction. Med. Clin. N. Amer. **51**, 69 (1967).
624. GURD, F. N., and C. McG. GARDNER: Reappraisal of the treatment of hemorrhagic shock. Amer. J. Surg. **89**, 725 (1955).
625. —, L. G. HAMPSON, B. J. M. INNES, W. J. GIBSON, and D. S. MULDER: The value of a clinical shock study protocol in the management of refractory shock. J. Trauma **6**, 157 (1966).
626. GUYTON, A. C., A. W. LINDSEY, B. N. KAUFMANN, and J. B. ABERNATHY: Effect of blood transfusion and hemorrhage on cardiac output and on the venous return curve. Amer. J. Physiol. **194**, 263 (1958).
627. — A concept of negative interstitial pressure based on pressures in implanted perforated capsules. Circulat. Res. **12**, 399 (1963).
628. — Interstitial fluid pressure: II. Pressure-volume curves of interstitial space. Circulat. Res. **16**, 452 (1965).
629. —, K. SCHEEL, and D. MURPHREE: Interstitial fluid pressure. III. Its effect on resistance to tissue fluid mobility. Circulat. Res. **19**, 412 (1966).
630. HÄBERLI, R. H.: Über die Häufigkeit von Brucellosen bei den Schweizern des Jahrganges 1943. Schweiz. med. Wschr. **93**, 911 (1963).
631. HAEGER, K. H. M., and S. R. B. NORDQVIST: Intramyocardial perfusion with oxygenated blood or low-molecular-dextran in experimental infarction in dogs. Vasc. Dis. **2**, 247 (1965).
632. HAHN, F.: Zur Pharmakologie und Toxikologie körperfremder kolloidaler Blutersatzmittel. Bibl. haemat. **12**, 137 (1961).
633. HAIMOVICI, H., and J. FINE: The antithrombotic action of gelatin. New. Engl. J. Med. **233**, 8 (1945).
634. HALL, J. E., and L. M. HELLMAN: Transfusion reactions in obstetrics. Obstet. Gynec. **9**, 250 (1957).
635. HALMÁGYI, M., u. K. UEBERLA: Experimentelle Untersuchungen mit kolloidalen Volumenersatzlösungen. In: K. LANG, R. FREY u. M. HALMAGYI: Infusionstherapie, p. 232. Berlin-Heidelberg-New York: Springer 1966.
636. HAMILTON, J. I., W. S. HOAR, and R. E. HAIST: A comparison of the efficacy of different infusion media in shock. Canad. J. Res. **24**, 31 (1946).
637. HAMIT, H. F.: Current trends of therapy and research in shock. Surg. Gynec. Obstet. **120**, 835 (1965).
638. HAMMARSTEN, J. E., and B. I. HELLER: The effects of dextran in subjects with normal blood volumes and in subjects after bleeding. J. lab. clin. Med. **40**, 807 (1952).

639. HAMMARSTEN, J. E., B. I. HELLER, and R. V. EBERT: The effects of dextran in normovolemic and oligemic subjects. J. clin. Invest. **32**, 340 (1953).
640. HAMPSON, L. G., H. J. SCOTT, and F. GURD: A comparison of intraarterial and intravenous transfusion in normal dogs and in dogs with experimental myocardial infarction. Ann. Surg. **140**, 56 (1954).
641. HANSSON, L. O.: The influence of thrombocyte aggregation on renal circulation. Acta chir. scand. suppl. **345** (1965).
641a. HARA, M., M. MARIS, J. CRUMPLER, B. CORN, and W. H. PERKINS: Effect of various priming solutions upon red cell mass, plasma volume, and extracellular fluid volume of dogs following hemodilution technique of extracorporeal circulation. J. thorac. cardiovasc. Surg. **53**, 353 (1967).
642. HARDAWAY, R. M.: New cncepts of shock. J. occup. Med. **5**, 426 (1963).
643. —, M. J. ELOVITZ, W. R. BREWSTER, D. N. HOUCHIN, N. L. RENZI, and D. R. JACKSON: Influence of vasoconstrictors and vasodilators on disseminated intravascular coagulation in irreversible hemorrhagic shock. Surg. Gynec. Obstet. **119**, 1053 (1964).
644. —, B. CHUN, and R. B. RUTHERFORD: Coagulation in shock in various species including man. Acta chir. scand. **130**, 157 (1965).
645. —, C. BYUNGKYU, and R. B. RUTHERFORD: Histologic evidence of disseminated intravascular coagulation in clinical shock. Vasc. Dis. **2**, 254 (1965).
646. —, D. G. JOHNSON, D. N. HOUCHIN, E. B. JENKINS, J. W. BURNS, and D. R. JACKSON: The influence of extracorporeal handling of blood in hemorrhagic shock in dogs. Exp. Med. Surg. **23**, 28 (1965).
647. — Microcoagulation in shock. Amer. J. Surg. **110**, 298 (1965).
648. — Intravascular coagulation in irreversible shock. In: L. C. MILLS, and J. H. MOYER: Shock and hypotension, p. 621. New York: Grune & Stratton 1965.
649. —, W. R. BREWSTER, and M. J. ELOVITZ: The influence of vasoconstriction and acidosis on disseminated intravascular coagulation. Surgery **59**, 804 (1966).
649a. —, P. M. JAMES JR., R. W. ANDERSON, C. E. BREDENBERG, and R. L. WEST: Intensive study and treatment of shock im man. J. Amer. med. Ass. **199**, 779 (1967).
650. HARDIN, C., T. H. HENDREN, A. A. PARIS, and C. M. POSER: Pathogenesis of hemorrhagic infarction of the brain. Arch. Neurol. **9**, 473 (1963).
651. HARJOLA, P. T., and A. SIVULA: Gastric ulceration following experimentally induced hypoxia and hemorrhagic shock. Ann. Surg. **163**, 21 (1966 a).
652. — — Prevention of acute gastric shock ulcerations in rabbits with low molecular weight dextran, hydrocortisone, metaraminol and phenoxybenzamine. Acta chir. scand. **132**, 166 (1966 b).
653. HARKINS, H. N.: Recent advances in the study and management of traumatic shock. Surgery **9**, 231, 447, 607 (1941).
654. HARRFELDT, H. P.: Oxypoly-Gelatine, ein neuer Plasmaexpander; seine Eigenschaften. Med. Welt 1297 (1960).
655. —, u. G. HIERHOLZER: Probleme beim Schockpatienten und dessen Behandlung. Med. Klin. **60**, 1781 (1965).
655a. HARRIS, J. M., D. K. LUSCOMBE, and R. H. POYSER: The influence of molecular weight and structure on the vascular permability responses induced by glucose polymers in rat skin. Brit. J. Pharmacol. Chemother. **29**, 16 (1967).
656. HARRIS, L., JR., B. KIRIMLI, and P. SAFAR: Exsanguination treated with dextran, oxygen and controlled hyperventilation. Fed. Proc. **23**, 416 (1964).

656a. Harris, L. C., B. Kirimli, and P. Safar: Augmentation of artificial circulation during cardiopulmonary resuscitation. Anesthesiology **28**, 730 (1967).
657. Harrison, J. H.: Dextran as a plasma substitute with plasma volume anc excretion studies on control patients. Ann. Surg. **139**, 137 (1954)
658. —, W. F. Durden, and A. S. Kellum: Hydrodextran in the treatment oi hemorrhagic shock: With plasma volume, blood volume, protein anc excretion studies. Ann. Surg. **142**, 824 (1955).
659. Harrison, W., and A. A. Liebow: The effects of massive intravenous in fusions with special reference to pulmonary congestion and edema. Yal J. Biol. Med. **26**, 372 (1954).
659a. Hartman, F. W.: Tissue changes following the use of plasma substitutes Arch. Surg. **63**, 728 (1951).
660. — Fate and disposal of plasma substitutes. Ann. N.Y. Acad. Sci. **55**, 50 (1952).
661. Hascher, H., u. M. Hascher: Beitrag zur Therapie des Schocks unter beson derer Berücksichtigung der flüssigen Gelatine als Plasmaexpander Anaesthesist **9**, 236 (1960).
662. Hässig, A., B. v. Rütte u. K. Vettiger: Zur Frage der Hepatitisübertragung durch Blut- und Plasmatransfusionen. Schweiz. med. Wschr. **83**, 437 (1953)
663. — Der Blutspendedienst des Schweizerischen Roten Kreuzes. Ein Rückblid und Ausblick. Schweiz. Apoth.-Ztg. **92**, 736 (1954).
664. — Zur Frage der Hepatitisübertragung durch Blut- und Plasmatransfusio nen. Bibl. haemat. **2**, 127 (1955).
665. —, S. Barandun u. K. Stampfli: Zur therapeutischen Verwendung vo Plasmafraktionen. Bibl. haemat. **9**, 42 (1959).
666. — Hämotherapie mit Plasmafraktionen. Ciba-Filmabend, Bern 1962.
667. — Hämotherapie mit Plasmafraktionen. Triangel **5**, 238 (1962).
668. — Militärmedizinische Aspekte der Schocktherapie mit Blut, Plasma un Plasmaersatzpräparaten. 25. Sess. int. offices doc. méd. mil., 3. 9. 1963.
669. — Zur Verhütung von Krankheitsübertragungen durch die Transfusion vo Blut, Plasma und Plasmafraktionen. Bibl. haemat. **16**, 270 (1963).
670. — Diskussionsbemerkung betr. febrile Transfusionsreaktionen und anti leukocytäre Isoimmunisierungen. Bibl. haemat. **16**, 388 (1963).
671. — Schockprobleme und Blutersatz unter besonderer Berücksichtigung de Expanderfrage. Basel: Med. Ges. 1965.
672. — Zur Prüfung der serologischen Verträglichkeit bei Bluttransfusionen. Arc klin. Chir. **313**, 64 (1965).
673. — Plasmaexpander. Helv. chir. Acta **33**, 335 (1966).
674. — Schockprobleme und Blutersatz unter besonderer Berücksichtigung de Expanderfrage. Anaesthesist **15**, 271 (1966).
675. — Aktuelle Probleme der Bluttransfusion. Fortschr. Med. **84**, 239 (1966).
676. — Zur Verhütung von Transfusionszwischenfällen. In: K. Hutschenreu ter: Anaesthesie und Notfallmedizin, p. 180. Berlin-Heidelberg-Ne York: Springer 1966.
677. Hatcher, J. D., F. A. Sunhara, O. G. Edholm, and J. M. Woolner: Th circulatory adjustments to post-hemorrhagic anemia in dogs. Circulat. Re **2**, 499 (1954).
677a. Haussmann, H. G.: Prophylaxe der Transfusionshepatitis. Bibl. haemat. **2** 309 (1967).
678. Havens, W. P., jr., and J. R. Paul: Infectious hepatitis and serum hepatiti In: T. M. Rivers, and F. L. Horsfall jr.: Viral and rickettsial infectio of man. p. 570. Philadelphia: Lippincott 1959.

679. Havers, L., I. v. Borgstede u. H. Breuer: Klinisch experimentelle Untersuchungen mit einem neuen Plasmaexpander. Dtsch. med. Wschr. **87**, 730 (1962).

680. Hayasaka, H., and J. M. Howard: Septic shock. Experimental and clinical studies. Springfield, Ill.: Thomas 1964.

681. Haynes, B. W., and M. C. de Bakey: Evaluation of plasma substitutes in clinical shock. Dextran. Surg. Forum **2**, 631 (1952).

682. — Dextran therapy in severe burns. Amer. J. Surg. **88**, 684 (1960).

683. — Effect of glyco-algin on blood volume following hemorrhage in the dog; in Second Conference on Artificial Colloidal Agents, p. 130. Washington, D. C.: Nat. Acad. Sci. 1963.

683a. Heberer, G.: Makromolekulare Stoffe als Blut- und Gewebeersatz. Klin. Wschr. **45**, 874 (1967).

684. Hecht, G., u. H. Weese: Periston, ein neuer Blutflüssigkeitsersatz. Münch. med. Wschr. **90**, 11 (1943).

685. —, u. W. Scholtan: Über die Ausscheidung von Polyvinylpyrrolidon durch die normale Niere. Z. exp. Med. **130**, 557 (1959).

686. Heckner, F., u. F. Gehlmann: Cytologische Beobachtungen zur Kollidon-Speicherung. Z. ges. exp. Med. **127**, 213 (1956).

686a. Hegarty, J. C., and W. M. Stahl: Homologous blood syndrome. J. thorac. cardiovasc. Surg **53**, 415 (1967).

687. Hehre, E. J., and Y. Sugg: Serologically reactive polysaccharides produced through the action of bacterial enzymes. J. exp. Med. **75**, 339 (1942).

688. —, and J. M. Neill: Formation of serologically reactive dextrans by streptococci from subacute bacterial endocarditis. J. exp. Med. **83**, 147 (1946).

689. —, and D. M. Hamilton: Bacterial conversion of dextran into a polysaccharide with the serological properties of dextran. Proc. Soc. exp. Biol. **71**, 336 (1949).

690. —, and Y. Sugg: Serological reactivity of dextran plasma substitute. Fed. Proc. **9**, 383 (1950).

691. — —, and J. M. Neill: The serological activity of dextran. Ann. N.Y. Acad. Sci. **55**, 467 (1952).

692. Heidelberger, M., and A. C. Aisenberg: Serological reactivity of synthetic polyglucoses. Proc. nat. Acad. Sci., Wash. **39**, 453 (1953).

692a. Heidland, A., K. Klütsch, K. W. Schneider u. A. G. Gathof: Die Wirksamkeit verschiedener Plasmaexpander auf Nierenhämodynamik und Blutvolumen. Proc. 10th Congr. Soc. Haemat. europ. II, 1530 (1967).

693. Heim, W., u. W. Osten: Beitrag zur Therapie des Wundschockes mit Blut und einigen Blutflüssigkeitsersatzmitteln. Arch. klin. Chir. **278**, 453 (1954).

694. — — Zur Klinik und Physiologie der Plasmaexpander-Anwendung. Bibl. haemat. **12**, 173 (1961).

695. Heistø, H., and I. Lund: Studies on allergic reactions following administratiton of dextran. J. Oslo City Hosp. **3**, 159 (1953).

696. — Overföring av hepatitt ved blodtransfusjon. T. norske Laegeforen. **78**, 631 (1958).

697. Heiz, R.: A year's experience in the production of lyophilized single donor plasma. Vox Sang. **1**, 273 (1956).

698. Hellem, A. J.: The adhesiveness of human blood platelets in vitro. Scand. J. clin. Lab. Invest. **12**, suppl. 51 (1960).

699. HELLEM, A. J., A. E. OEDEGAARD, and B. A. SKÄLHEGG: Investigation adenosine diphosphate (ADP) induced platelet adhesiveness in vitro. I. ADP-platelet reaction in varius experimental conditions. Thromb. Di

699a. HELLFRITZ, H.: Kennzeichnung makromolekularer Stoffe. Kunststoffe 502 (1960).

700. HELLSTRÖM, G., and V. O. BJÖRK: Hemodilution with Rheomacrodex du total body perfusions. J. thorac. cardiovasc. Surg. **45,** 395 (19

701. HENDREN, T. H., and C. A. HARDIN: Low molecular dextran effect on porary renal ischemia. Arch. Surg. **88,** 206 (1964).

702. HENEGAR, G. C.: Introduction symposium on blood volume. Amer. Surg. 347 (1964).

703. HENRY, C. L., G. C. NELSON, and W. F. PIPES: Fatal rebleeding indices dogs following administration of blood, plasma, dextran and crystal solutions. Amer. Surg. **22,** 93 (1956).

704. HERSHEY, S. G.: Shock. Boston: Little Brown 1964.

705. HEYL, J. T., J. G. GIBSON II, and C. A. JANOWAY: Studies on the pla proteins. V. The effect of concentrated solutions of human and bo serum albumin on blood volume after acute blood loss in man. J. Invest. **22,** 763 (1943).

706. HEYMANN, W., G. NASH, C. GILLKEY, and M. LEWIS: Studies on the ca role of hypoalbuminemia in experimental nephrotic hyperlipemia clin. Invest. **37,** 808 (1958).

707. HIGGINS, A. R., H. A. HARPER, J. R. KIMMEL, T. W. BURNS, R. E. JONES T. W. D. SMITH, and C. L. KLEIN: A study of oxypolygelatin in hu subjects. J. appl. Physiol. **4,** 776 (1952).

708. HILDEBRANDT, F.: Untersuchungen über Dextran als Blutflüssigkeitsers Ärztl. Wschr. **5,** 141 (1950).

709. HILL, G. C.: Homologous serum jaundice and its transfer in whole bl transfusion. J. nat. med. Ass. **57,** 112 (1965).

710. HILL, J. M., E. E. MUIRHEAD, C. T. ASHWORTH, and W. D. TIGERTT: The of desiccated plasma with particular reference to shock. J. Amer. Ass. **116,** 395 (1941).

711. HILLMAN, R. S.: Pooled human plasma as a volume expander. New Eng Med. **271,** 1027 (1964).

712. HINSHAW, J. R., W. J. PORIES, P. D. HARRIS, T. P. DAVIS, and S. T. SCHWA Effect of the molecular size of dextran on liver and kidney oxygen sion. Surg. Forum **11,** 360 (1960).

713. HINT, H. C.: The flow properties of erythrocyte suspensions in isol rabbit's ear; the effects of erythrocyte aggregation, hematocrit and fusion pressure. Bibl. anat. **4,** 112 (1964).

714. — The relationship between the molecular weight of dextran and its eff in Symposia on Rheomacrodex I, p. 2. London: Pharmacia 1964.

715. — Colloid osmotic effect in isolated perfused rabbit's ear. Bibl. anat. **7,** (1965).

716. HIRSH, B. D.: Responsibilities in blood transfusion. Medicoleg. Dig. **1,** (1960).

717. HISSEN, W., R. L. SWANK, L. LINO, and G. V. F. SEAMAN: Physicochem changes in circulating canine blood on exsanguination or administra of histamine. Surg. Gynec. Obstet. **122,** 1003 (1966).

718. HOFFMAN, W. S., and D. D. KOZOLL: Fate of intravenously injected gel in human subjects. J. clin. Invest. **25,** 575 (1946).

719. HOGEN, J. J.: The intravenous use of colloidal gelatin solutions in shock. J. Amer. med. Ass. **54**, 721 (1915).
720. HOLLAND, P. V., R. M. RUBINSON, A. G. MORROW, and P. J. SCHMIDT: Gamma globulin in the prophylaxis of posttransfusion hepatitis. J. Amer. med. Ass. **196**, 471 (1966).
721. HOLLÄNDER, L. P., u. H. WILLENEGGER: Technisch bedingte Gefahren bei der Übertragung von Blut und Blutersatzmitteln. Bibl. haemat. **16**, 231 (1963).
722. HOLM, I., and J. WETTERFORS: Some aspects of the behaviour of plasma albumin on saline infusion. An experimental study in dogs. Acta chir. scand. **132**, 33 (1966).
723. HOLMES, J. H., and E. E. PAINTER: The role of extracellular fluid in traumatic shock in dogs. Amer. J. Physiol. **148**, 201 (1947).
724. HOPKINS, R. W., G. SABGA, J. PENN, and F. A. SIMEONE: Hemodynamic aspects of hemorrhagic and septic shock. J. Amer. med. Ass. **191**, 731 (1965).
725. HORATZ, K., u. R. LANGER: Probleme der Schockbekämpfung im Verteidigungsfalle. Wehrmed. Mitt. **9**, 129 (1963).
726. —, u. R. FREY: Schock und Plasmaexpander. Berlin-Göttingen-Heidelberg: Springer 1964.
727. HORSEY, P. J.: Osmolar and electrolyte changes in haemorrhagic shock. Lancet I, 603 (1963).
728. HORVATH, S. M., L. H. HAMILTON, G. B. SPURR, E. B. ALLBAUGH, and B. K. HUTT: Plasma expanders and bleeding time. J. appl. Physiol. **7**, 614 (1955).
729. HOSSLI, G.: Prophylaxe und Therapie des posttraumatischen Schockes. Praxis **48**, 1130 (1959).
730. HOWARD, J. M: Battle casualties in Korea. Studies of the Surgical Research Team, vol. I, II, III. Washington, D. C.: U.S. Army Med. Serv. Graduate School 1955.
731. —, J. P. FRAWLEY, C. P. ARTZ, and Y. SAKO: The fate of dextran and modified gelatine in casualties with renal insufficiency. Surg. Gynec. Obstet. **100**, 207 (1955).
732. —, C. T. TENG, and R. K. LOEFFLER: Studies of dextrans of various molecular sizes. Ann. Surg. **143**, 369 (1956).
733. —, R. V. EBERT, W. L. BLOOM, and M. H. SLOAN: The present status of dextran as a plasma expander. Amer. J. Surg. **97**, 593 (1959).
734. — Fluid replacement in shock and hemorrhage. J. Amer. med. Ass. **173**, 516 (1960).
735. HOWLAND, W. S., O. SCHWEIZER, and C. P. BOYAN: Physiological alterations with massive blood replacement. Surg. Gynec. Obstet. 101, 478 (1955).
736. —, C. P. BOYAN, and O. SCHWEIZER: Ventricular fibrillation during massive blood replacement. Amer. J. Surg. **92**, 356 (1956).
737. —, J. W. BELLVILLE, M. B. ZUCKER, C. P. BOYAN, and E. E. CLIFTON: Massive blood replacement. V. Failure to observe citrate intoxication. Surg. Gynec. Obstet. **105**, 529 (1957).
738. —, R. G. JACOBS, and H. H. GOULET: Evaluation of calcium administration during rapid blood replacement. Anaesth. Analg. **39**, 557 (1960).
739. —, and O. SCHWEIZER: Acid base lesion of bank blood. Anesthesiology **25**, 102 (1964).
740. — —, and C. P. BOYAN: Massive blood replacement without calcium administration. Surg. Gynec. Obstet. **118**, 814 (1964).
741. — — — The effect of buffering on the mortality of massive blood replacement. Surg. Gynec. Obstet. **121**, 777 (1965).

742. HOWLAND, W. S., and O. SCHWEIZER: Diagnosis and therapy of the physiolog changes occurring during shock and massive transfusion. In: L. R. ORKI Management of the patient in shock. Clin. Anesth. **2**, 25 (1965).

743. HOXWORTH, P. I., W. E. HAESLER JR., and H. SMITH JR.: The risk of hepatit from whole blood and stored plasma. Surg. Gynec. Obstet. **109**, 38 (195

744. HOYE, R. C., A. S. KETCHAM, and N. I. BERLIN: Total red cell and plasn volume alterations occurring with extensive surgery in humans. Su Gynec. Obstet. **123**, 27 (1966).

745. HOYT, R. K., E. DOMANIG, P. HAHNLOSER, N. A. DELIN, and W. G. SCHEN Blood viscosity alteration following hemorrhage and after volume restit tion with saline, plasma, dextrans, or shed blood. Surg. Forum **15**, (1964).

746. HUDSPETH, A. S., and A. R. CORDELL: Cardiovascular responses to induc hypervolemia. Ann. Surg. **164**, 183 (1966).

747. HÜGIN, W.: Plasma-Expander. Anaesthesist **8**, 280 (1959).

748. HUGGINS, C. E.: Frozen blood—clinical experience. Surgery **60**, 77 (1966).

749. HUGGINS, R. A., E. L. SMITH, and S. DEAVERS: Some effects of autologous a homologous blood or plasma overtransfusions in the dog. Amer. Physiol. **209**, 673 (1965).

750. HUGUENARD, R.: Etude clinique du dextran de bas poids molécula (d.b.p.m.) „Rheoslug-Rhéomacrodex". Ann. Anesth. **5**, 767 (1964).

751. HULME, B., and L. J. LAWSON: Renal failure and low molecular weight de tran. Brit. med. J. **II**, 1455 (1966).

752. HUME, R.: Blood volume expansion effect of Rheomacrodex. In: Symposia Rheomacrodex vol. **2**, p. 38. London: Pharmacia 1964.

753. HUMMEL, K., u. T. HALSE: Theoretische Grundlagen der blutstillenden Wi kung von Kolloiden. Klin. Wschr. **30**, 688 (1952).

753a. HUNT, P. S., and T. S. REEVE: Arterial thrombus prevention and dissoluti after low molecular weight dextran infusion in sheep. Med. J. Aust **I**, 539 (1967).

754. HUNZINGER, W. A., H. WILLENEGGER u. A. L. MEIER: Blutvolumetrie m $I^{131}$-Albumin nach Infusion von Plasmaersatzmitteln. Klin. Wschr. **32**, 7 (1954).

755. HUEPER, W. C.: Experimental carcinogenic studies on macromolecular chem cals. Cancer **10**, 8 (1957).

756. — Bioassay on polyvinylpyrrolidones with limited molecular weight rang J. nat. Cancer Inst. **26**, 229 (1961).

757. HÜSSELMANN, H.: Speicherungserscheinungen beim Menschen nach Peristo Klin. Wschr. **33/34**, 801 (1952).

758b. —, L. I. PENA, and A. E. LENHERT: Thrombophlebitis in pregnancy. Amer. Obstet. Gynec. **97**, 901 (1967).

758a. HUSNI, E. A.: The edema of arterial reconstruction. Circulation **36/3** suppl. **1**, 169 (1967).

758b. —, L. I. PENA, and A. E. LENHERT: Thrombophlebitis in pregnancy. Amer. Obstet. Gynec. **97**, 901 (1967).

759. HUTCHISON, J. L., S. O. FREEDMAN, B. A. RICHARDS, and A. S. V. BURGE Plasma volume expansion and reactions after infusion of autologous a nonautologous plasma in man. J. lab. clin. Med. **56**, 734 (1960).

760. —, and A. S. V. BURGEN: Infusion of non-autologous plasma, effects of chlo pheniramine, prednisolone and adrenaline. Brit. med. J. **II**, 904 (1963).

761. Hyde, G. M., N. I. Berlin, R. J. Parsons, and B. Whittington: The blood volume expansion produced by gelatin, serum albumin, and plasma. Surg. Gynec. Obstet. **95**, 657 (1952).
762. Ingelman, B., and K. Siegbahn: An electron-microscopic study of dextran molecules. Ark. Kemi **18 b**, 1 (1944 a).
763. — — Dextran and levan molecules studied with the electron microscope. Nature (London) **154**, 237 (1944 b).
764. — Dextran and its use as a plasma substitute. Acta chem. scand. **1**, 738 (1947).
765. — Investigations on dextran and its application as a plasma substitute. Upsala Läk. Fören. Förh. **54**, 107 (1949).
766. — The chemistry of dextran and properties of low molecular weight dextran and other dextran preparations. In: Conference on Evaluation of Low Molecular Weight Dextran, p. 2. Washington, D. C.: Nat. Acad. Sci 1963.
767. Ingraham, R. C., and H. C. Wiggers: Alkalinizing agents and fluid priming in hemorrhagic shock. Amer. J. Physiol. **144**, 505 (1945).
768. Intaglietta, M., and B. W. Zweifach: Indirect method for measurement of pressure in blood capillaries. Circulat. Res. **19**, 199 (1966).
769. Ivy, A. C., H. Greengard, I. F. Stein, F. S. Grodins, and D. F. Dalton: Effect of various blood substitutes in resuscitation after otherwise fatal hemorrhage. Surg. Gynec. Obstet. **76**, 85 (1943).
770. Jacobaeus, U., L. Troell, and B. Åberg: Erfarenheter av lågmolekylärt dextran. Nord. Med. **53**, 666 (1955).
771. — Studies on the effect of dextran on the coagulation of blood. Acta med. scand. **157**, suppl. 322 (1957).
772. Jacobellis, P., and M. Vitelli: L'uso dell'Emagel nella pratica ospedaliera. Minerva chir. **21**, 31 (1966).
773. Jacobsson, L.: Intravenous infusion of clinical B 512 dextran in normal human subjects with dextran-reacting antibodies in serum. Acta Soc. Med. upsalien. **63**, 196 (1958).
774. —, and R. Wikström: The detection of dextran-reacting antibodies in human serum. Acta Soc. Med. upsalien. **63**, 180 (1958).
775. —, and J. Zsiga: Dextran-reacting antibodies in human serum. Acta Soc. Med. upsalien. **63**, 165 (1958).
776. — — The effect of intravenous infusion of dextran on blood pressure in Leuconostoc-immunized rabbits. Acta Soc. Med. upsalien. **63**, 188 (1958).
777. Jahnke, E. J., jr., and S. F. Seeley: Acute vascular injuries in the Korean war. Ann. Surg. **138**, 158 (1953).
778. James, J. D., and E. J. Stokes: Effect of temperature on survival of bacteria in blood for transfusion. Brit. med. J. **II**, 1389 (1957).
779. Jaenike, J., and C. Waterhouse: Metabolic and hemodynamic changes induced by the prolonged administration of dextran. Circulation **11**, 1 (1955).
780. Janota, M., H. Necheles, R. E. Weston, V. Weissman, and O. Levinson: Gelatin infusion in hemorrhagic shock. Exp. Med. Surg. **1**, 298 (1943).
781. Jansonius, N. J., and W. G. Zijlstra: Various factors influencing rouleaux formation of erythrocytes studied with the aid of syllectometry. Proc. kon. nederl. Akad. Wet. **68**, 121 (1965).
782. Janzarik, H., u. H. G. Lasch: Plasmaersatzstoffe beim akuten Blutverlust des Kaninchens. Helv. chir. Acta **33**, 302 (1966).
783. Jeanes, A.: Dextran, a selective bibliography. U.S. Dept. of Agriculture AIC, 288, 1952.

784. JEANES, A.: Preparation of dextrans from growing Leuconostoc cultures. In: R. WHISTLER: Methods in carbohydrate chemistry **5**, 118. New York: Acad. Press 1965.

785. JECKELN, E.: Über gewebliche Äußerungen des Säuglingsorganismus nach wiederholten Periston-Gaben. Virchows Arch. path. Anat. **322**, 529 (1952).

786. JENKINS, M. T., A. H. GIESECKE JR., and G. T. SHIRES: Electrolyte therapy in shock: Management during anesthesia. Clin. Anesth. **2**, 40 (1965).

787. JENKINS, W. J.: Blood groups and blood transfusion. Practitioner **195**, 159 (1965).

788. JENKNER, F. L.: Orientierende Untersuchung über die hämodynamischen Verhältnisse an „durchblutungsgestörten" Extremitäten peripher von Gefäßverschlüssen. Z. Kreisl.-Forsch. **54**, 300 (1965).

788a. JOHANSEN, S. H., and M. B. LAVER: Cardiovascular effects of severe anemic hypoxia. Acta anaesth. scand. suppl. **24**, 63 (1966).

789. JOHNSTON, E. V., and J. S. LUNDY: Use of dextran (Macrodex) in burns. Amer. J. Surg. **85**, 713 (1953).

790. JOHNSTON, G. S., W. T. PEARSON, and G. P. MURPHY: The hemodynamic alterations induced by low molecular weight dextran in normotension and hypotension. I. Simultaneous direct measurement of cardiac and renal hemodynamics. Invest. Urol. **1**, 566 (1964).

791. JÓZSA, L., L. SAJTOS, M. PERNECZKY u. G. LUSZTIG: Chemische Untersuchung der Aortenwand in experimenteller und durch Dextran gehemmter Cholesterinsklerose. Z. ges. inn. Med. **16**, 935 (1961).

792. —, M. PERNECZKY u. G. LUSZTIG: Histologische Beobachtungen bei Behandlung mit Dextran und bei experimenteller Cholesterinsklerose. Zbl. allg. Path. path. Anat. **103**, 200 (1962).

793. —, L. SAJTOS, M. PERNECZKY, J. PATAKI, L. SZIKULAI u. G. LUSZTIG: Dextran und Histaminwirkung. Z. ges. inn. Med. **17**, 173 (1962).

794. JUDD, D., T. HARENDEEN, and H. B. SHUMACKER JR.: Influence of mannitol and low molecular weight dextran upon renal blood flow. Surgery **56**, 529 (1964).

795. JULLIARD, J., P. H. BONNEL, J. LASSNER, and M. HASCHER: Clinical study of modified fluid gelatin. Bibl. haemat. **7**, 282 (1958).

796. JUST, O. H., u. H. LUTZ: Genese und Therapie des hämorrhagischen Schocks. Stuttgart: Thieme 1965.

797. JUST-VIERA, J. O., and G. H. YEAGER: Prevention of thrombosis in the inferior vena cava. Surg. Gynec. Obstet. **117**, 271 (1963).

798. — — Protection from thrombosis in large veins. Surg. Gynec. Obstet. **118**, 354 (1964).

799. —, W. B. STAUFER, and G. H. YEAGER: Antithrombogenic properties of dextran. Clin. Med. 31 (1966).

800. KABAT, E. A., and D. BERG: Production of precipitine and cutaneous sensitivity in man by injection of small amounts of dextran. Ann. N.Y. Acad. Sci. **55**, 471 (1952).

801. — — Dextran—an antigen in man. J. Immunol. **70**, 514 (1953).

802. — Some configurational requirements and dimensions of the combining site on an antibody to a naturally occurring antigen. J. Amer. chem. Soc. **76**, 3709 (1954).

803. —, D. BERG, D. RITTENBERG, L. PONTECORVO, M. EIDENOFF, and L. HELLMAN: Precipitation of $C^{14}$-labelled dextran by human anti-dextran. J. Amer. chem. Soc. **76**, 564 (1954).

804. Kabat, E. A.: Heterogeneity in extent of the combining regions of human antidextran. J. Immunol. 77, 377 (1956).
805. —, G. M. Turino, A. B. Tarrow, and P. H. Maurer: Studies on the immunochemical basis of allergic reactions to dextran in man. J. clin. Invest. **36,** 1160 (1957).
806. —, and A. E. Bezer: The effect of variation in molecular weight on the antigenicity of dextran in man. Arch. Biochem. **78,** 306 (1958).
807. Kahn, D. R., J. C. Cerny, R. W. S. Lee, and H. Sloan: The effect of dextran and mannitol on renal function during open-heart surgery. Surgery **57,** 676 (1965).
808. Kalra, S. L., G. Singh, M. Ram, and S. O. Waller: A modified gelatin as a plasma expander. Experiments on haemorrhaged dogs. Indian J. med. Res. **46,** 171 (1958).
809. —, G. Singh, M. Ram, and S. O. Waller: A modified gelatin as a plasma expander. Indian J. med. Res. **46,** 179 (1958).
810. Karlson, K. E., and L. Y. Senn: Simultaneous determination of red cell mass and plasma volume with $Cr^{51}$ and $I^{131}$ using a pulse height analyzer. Ann. Surg. **158,** 309 (1963).
810a. — A. A. Garzon, G. W. Shaftan, and C. J. Chu: Increased blood loss associated with administration of certain plasma expanders: Dextran 75, dextran 40 and hydroxyethyl starch. Surgery **62,** 670 (1967).
811. Katz, R., H. Ducci, H. Bennett, and J. Rodriguez: Incidence of hepatitis following transfusions of whole blood. Amer. J. clin. Path. **27,** 406 (1957).
812. Keddie, N. C., J. L. Provan, and W. G. Austen: Central venous pressure, blood volume determinations, and the effects of vasoactive drugs in hypovolemic shock. Surgery **60,** 427 (1966).
813. Keith, N. M., L. G. Rowntree, and J. T. Geraghty: A method for the determination of plasma and blood volume. Arch. intern. Med. **16,** 547 (1915).
814. Keler-Bačoka, M., Z. Pučar, and A. Benaš: A paper strip electrophoretic examination of the action of dextran in colloidal solution on human serum. Experientia **16,** 488 (1960).
815. — Die Wirkung von Dextran in kolloider Lösung auf Serumlipide verschiedener Tiergattungen. Zbl. Vet. Med. **9,** 46 (1962).
816. — The characteristic specificity of plasmocytoma lipids concerning their resistance to form DL-fractions with colloidal dextran. Experientia **21,** 338 (1965).
816a. Kho, L. K., and W. C. Shoemaker: Cardiorespiratory changes in acute hemorrhage. Surg. Gynec. Obstet. **124,** 826 (1967).
817. Kief, H., u. K. Engelbart: Reabsorptive Vacuolisation der gewundenen Nierenhauptstücke. Frankf. Z. Path. **75,** 53 (1966).
818. Killian, R.: Haemaccel, ein neuer Expander, zugleich ein Beitrag zur Steuerung einer Infusion. Med. Klin. **58,** 560 (1963).
819. Killman, S.-Å.: Leucocyte agglutinins. Oxford: Blackwell 1960.
820. Kilman, J. W., and J. A. Waldhausen: Failure of low molecular weight dextran to increase peripheral flow in the face of controlled cardiac output. Surg. Forum **16,** 36 (1965).
820a. —, J. A. Waldhausen, and H. B. Shumacker: Effects of low molecular weight dextran on peripheral blood flow with controlled cardiac output. Ann. Surg. **166,** 190 (1967).
821. Kinney, J. M.: Lecture Outlines; Postgraduate course on pre- and postoperative care. Chicago: Amer. Coll. Surg. 1966

822. KIRCHNER, E., u. H. OEHMIG: Schock und Kollaps. In: H. BÜRKLE DE LA CAMP u. M. SCHWAIGER: Hb. d. ges. Unfallheilk., 3. Aufl., p. 309. Stuttgart: Enke 1963.
823. —, H. HUNDESHAGEN u. E. H. GRAUL: Über die Fehlerbreite der „Blutvolumenbestimmung" mit RISA im Volemetron. Atompraxis **9**, 373 (1963).
824. — Bluttransfusion und Schocktherapie. Arch. klin. Chir. **313**, 119 (1965).
825. —, I. LIETZ u. A. WÜRTERLE: Zur Therapie der „akuten tonischen Kreislaufinsuffizienz". Z. Geburtsh. Gynäk. **164**, 282 (1965).
826. KIVIKOSKI, J., S. LUNDBOM, and J. T. AIRAKSINEN: The dextran concentration in the umbilical cord of a newborn infant. Acta anaesth. scand. suppl. **24**, 33 (1966).
827. KLASSEN, G. A., and R. A. MILCH: Extraction of aortic wall lipids by high molecular weight dextran. J. surg. Res. **6**, 312 (1966).
828. KLEINBERG, W., J. W. REMINGTON, W. J. EVERSOLE, R. R. OVERMAN, and W. W. SWINGLE: The effectiveness of plasma, gelatin and saline transfusions in preventing shock induced by leg muscle trauma and tourniquets. Amer. J. Physiol. **140**, 197 (1943).
829. KLIMAN, A.: Presently useful plasma volume expanders. Anaesthesiology **27**, 417 (1966).
830. KLÜTSCH, K. VON, A. HEIDLAND u. H. KAMMERER: Nierenfunktion nach Infusion von niedermolekularem Dextran. Med. Klin. **60**, 464 (1965).
831. KNIGHT, C. P. F.: A blood heater for use in transfusion. Lancet **II**, 862 (1962).
832. KNISELEY, M. H.: Experimental separation of quite different types of circulatory shock. In: L. C. MILLS, and G. H. MOYER: Shock and hypotension, p. 295. New York: Grune & Stratton 1965.
833. KNUTSON, R. C., J. L. BOLLMAN, and J. S. LUNDY: Comparative effectiveness of certain volemic substances in maintaining plasma volume after blood loss. Surg. Forum **2**, 637 (1952).
834. KOEKENBERG, L. J. L.: Experimental use of Macrodex as a prophylaxis against post-operative thrombo-embolism. Bull. Soc. int. Chir. **21**, 501 (1962).
835. KOLETSKY, S., and G. E. GUSTAFSON: Reversibility of tourniquet shock with massive saline therapy. Amer. J. Physiol. **182**, 439 (1955).
836. KOOP, C. E., and L. BULLITT: Gelatin as plasma substitute; effect of gelatin infusion on subsequent typing and crossmatching of blood with method of eliminating phenomenon of pseudoagglutination. Amer. J. med. Sci. **209**, 28 (1945).
837. KORTH, J., u. H. HEINLEIN: Vergleichende experimentelle Untersuchungen über die kreislaufauffüllende Wirkung verschiedener Blutersatzmittel. Arch. klin. Chir. **278**, 36 (1954).
838. KØSTER, K. H., M. SCHWARTZ, V. SELE, and E. SINDRUP: Blood-volume changes after infusion of dextran solutions. Lancet **II**, 262 (1957).
839. KREBS, J.-J., u. P. SCHARENBERG: Serumhepatitis nach Bluttransfusionen. Dtsch. med. Wschr. **84**, 1376 (1959).
840. KRØLL, J., and R. DYBKJAER: In vitro—precipitations in plasma by low molecular weight dextran. Scand. J. clin. Lab. Invest. **16**, 31 (1964).
841. — Studies on the effect of low molecular weight dextran upon the clotting process in vitro. Scand. J. clin. Lab. Invest. **17**, 51 (1965).
842. KUHN, L. A., H. WEINRAUCH, T. JACOBSON, R. APTER, and L. MELTZER: Hemodynamic effects of low molecular weight dextran in experimental myocardial infarction with shock. Clin. Res. **11**, 169 (1963).
843. KUNIN, C. .M: Serum hepatitis from whole blood: Incidence and relation to source of blood. Amer. J. med. Sci. **237**, 293 (1959).

844. KWAK, H. H., H. B. MANDELL, and D. R. WILSON: Beneficial effect of low molecular weight dextran on acute ischemic limb. Surg. Forum **15**, 230 (1964).

845. LAAFF, H., H. GIERTZ, F. HAHN u. B. WIRTH: Zum Mechanismus der Dextranwirkung bei der Ratte. Arch. int. Pharmacodyn. **162**, 30 (1966).

845a. LAFRANCE, L., and J. LE BLANC: Effects of compound 48/80, chlorpromazine, dextran, and reserpine in rabbits fed a 1% cholesterol diet. Canad. J. Physiol. Pharmacol. **45**, 215 (1967).

846. LAMBERT, J., G. JOHNSON, and R. M. PETERS: Cardiovascular response to electrolyte fluid overload. Surg. Forum **17**, 52 (1966).

847. LAMPE, W. T.: Interstitial nephritis. Angiology **16**, 281 (1965).

848. LAMPERT, H.: Die Verhütung des Kreislaufkollapses durch Blutersatzflüssigkeiten. Hippokrates **22**, 264 (1951).

849. LAMSON, P. D., and W. E. DE TURK: Studies on shock induced by hemorrhage. XI. A method for the accurate control of blood pressure. J. Pharmacol. exp. Ther. **38**, 250 (1945).

850. LANDIS, E. M., and J. R. PAPPENHEIMER: Exchange of substances through the capillary walls. In: Handbook of physiology, section 2, p. 961. Washington, D. C.: Amer. Physiol. Soc. 1963.

851. LANG, K., u. H. SCHWIEGK: Blutersatzmittel. Wien. klin. Wschr. **39/40**, 579 (1943).

852. —, R. FREY u. M. HALMÁGYI: Infusionstherapie. Anaesth. Resusc. **13**, Berlin-Heidelberg-New York: Springer 1966.

853. LANGDELL, R. D., E. ADELSON, F. W. FURTH, and W. H. CROSBY: Dextran and prolonged bleeding time. Results of a sixty-gram, one-liter infusion given to one hundred sixty-three normal human subjects. J. Amer. med. Ass. **166**, 346 (1958).

854. LANGSJOEN, P. H.: Electrocardiographic changes in acute myocardial infarction treated with low molecular dextran. J. lab. clin. Med. **60**, 993 (1962).

855. —, S. A. SANCHEZ, and N. C. HIGHTOWER: Laboratory observations in acute myocardial infarction treated with low molecular dextran. Clin. Res. **11**, 55 (1963).

856. — The use of low molecular weight dextran in acute myocardial infarction. In: Conf. on Evaluation of Low Molecular Weight Dextran in Shock, p. 113. Washington, D. C.: Nat. Acad. Sci. 1963.

857. —, H. S. FALCONER, S. A. SANCHEZ, and D. J. LYNCH: Observations in treatment of acute myocardial infarction with low molecular dextran. Angiology **14**, 465 (1963).

858. — Use of low molecular dextran in acute myocardial infarction. Texas St. J. Med. **61**, 92 (1965).

859. — Obervations in the excretion of low molecular dextran. Angiology **16**, 148 (1965).

860. — Blood viscosity changes in acute myocardial infarction. Postgrad. Med. **36**, A-42 (1966).

861. LANGSTON, H. T., G. MILLES, and W. DALESSANDRO: Further experiences with autogenous blood transfusions. Ann. Surg. **158**, 333 (1963).

862. LARCAN, A., M. CALAMAI et B. GENETET: Emploi clinique d'un dextran de poids moléculaire faible. Thérapie **20**, 1265 (1965).

863. —, G. RAUBER, P. MATHIEU, P. MASSE et M. CALAMAI: Le syndrome métabolique gravissime secondaire aux révascularisations trop tardives après ischémies prolongées. Presse méd. **73**, 1819 (1965).

864. LARCAN, A., F. STREIFF, A. PETERS et B. GENETET: Détermination de la viscosité de substituts du plasma. Agressologie 7, 229 (1966).

865. LARENG, L, G. VOURC'H et coll.: Le plasmagel. 15e Congr. français d'Anesthésie-Réanimation, Toulouse 1965.

865b. —, J. DUCOS, L. BOISSON, C. VIRENQUE, F. LEPERT et J.-C. QUILICI: Incidence d'un soluté de dextran de bas poids moléculaire sur les mécanismes de l'hémostase en période post-opératoire. Presse méd. 75, 341 (1967).

866. LARSEN, O. A.: The plasma volume in man. Scand. J. clin. Lab. Invest. 17, suppl. 86, 63 (1965).

867. LAURELL, A.: Influence of dextran on the conversion of fibrinogen to fibrin. Scand. J. clin. Lab. Invest. 3, 262 (1951).

868. LAURENT, T. C.: The interaction between polysaccharides and other macromolecules. V. The solubility of proteins in the presence of dextran. Biochem. J. 89, 253 (1963).

869. LAVER, M. B.: Sauerstofftransport, Erythrocytenkonservierung und extrakorporale Zirkulation. Anaesthesist 13, 110 (1964).

870. —, and H. H. BENDIXEN: Atelectasis in the surgical patient, recent conceptual advances. Progr. Surg. 5, 1 (1966).

871. LAWRENCE, A. C. K., and G. WALTERS: The extraction of Evans Blue (T 1824) from plasma and the measurement of plasma volume. J. clin. Path. 12, 123 (1959).

872. LAWSON, H., and W. S. REHM: The relation value of various fluids in replacement of blood lost by hemorrhage, with special reference to the value of gelatin solutions. Amer. J. Physiol. 140, 431 (1943).

873. LEDERMANN, K. L.: Zur Frage der Hepatitisübertragung durch menschliche Plasmafraktionen. Praxis 49, 273 (1960).

874. LEE, W. H., JR.: Red blood cell envelope in intravascular hemagglutination. In: Conf. on Evaluation of Low Molecular Weight Dextran in Shock, p. 40. Washington, D. C.: Nat. Acad. Sci 1963.

875. —, and N. S. WALSH: Effect of low molecular weight dextrans on blood sludging. In: L. C. MILLS, and J. H. MOYER: Shock and hypotension, p. 655. New York: Grune & Stratton 1965.

876. LEHANE, D., C. M. S. KWANTES, M. G. UPWARD, and D. R. THOMSON: Homologous serum jaundice. Brit. med. J. II, 572 (1949).

877. LEHMANN, W.: Osmo- und Onkotherapie, insbesondere bei Hirndruck und Hirnödem. Med. Klin. 60, 1555 (1965).

878. LEPLEY, D., JR., C. J. MANI, and E. H. ELLISON: Influence of low molecular weight dextran on acute occlusion of the mesenteric vein. Surg. Forum 12, 328 (1961).

879. — — — Superior mesenteric venous occlusion. A study using low molecular weight dextran to prevent infarction. J. surg. Res. 2, 403 (1962).

880. —, M. WEISFELDT, A. S. CLOSE, R. SCHMIDT, J. BOWLER, R. C. KORY, and E. H. ELLISON: Effect of low molecular weight dextran on hemorrhagic shock. Surgery 54, 93 (1963).

881. LEVEEN, H. H., H. S. PASTERNACK, J. LUSHIN, R. SHAPIRO, E. BECKER, and A. H. HELFT: Hemorrhage and transfusion as major cause of cardiac arrest. J. Amer. med. Ass. 173, 720 (1960).

882. —, B. SCHATMAN, and G. FALK: The consequence of repeated infusions of potassium in acute compensated hypovolemia. Surgery 47, 364 (1960).

882a. LEVINSON, S. O., M. JANOTA, F. ARIMOTO, and H. NECHELES: Gelatin solution in the treatment of shock from graded hemorrhage. Surg. Gynec. Obstet. 84, 925 (1947).

883. LEVY, S. W., and R. L. SWANK: Relationship of native heparin to clearing of an alimentary lipemia. Proc. Soc. exp. Biol. 82, 553 (1953).
884. LEWIS, D. H., and S. MELLANDER: Competitive effects of sympathetic control and tissue metabolites on resistance and capacitance vessels and capillary filtration in skeletal muscle. Acta physiol. scand. 56, 162 (1962).
885. LEWIS, J. H., I. L. F. SZETO, W. L. BAYER, M. TAKAORI, and P. SAFAR: Severe hemodilution with hydroxyethyl starch and dextrans. Arch. Surg. 93, 941 (1966).
886. LEWIS, L. A., I. H. PAGE, and O. GLASSER: Plasma proteins (electrophoretic technique) in normal and shocked dogs. Amer. J. Physiol. 161, 101 (1950).
887. LIECHTI, R.: Lues bei Blutspendern. Praxis 53, 1174 (1964).
888. LILJEDAHL, S. O., B. OLHAGEN, L. O. PLANTIN, and G. BIRKE: Studies on burns. VII. Acta chir. scand. suppl. 309 (1963).
889. LILLEHEI, R. C., J. K. LONGERBEAM, J. H. BLOCH, and W. G. MANAX: The nature of irreversible shock. Ann. Surg. 160, 682 (1964).
890. — — — — The modern treatment of shock based on physiologic principles. Clin. Pharmacol. Ther. 5, 63 (1964).
891. — — — — Experimental irreversible shock. In: S. G. HERSHEY: Shock, p. 181. Boston: Little Brown 1964.
892. LINDÉN, L.: Myocardial infarction treated with low molecular weight dextran. Lancet II, 759 (1964).
892a. LINDÉN, L.: Reomacrodex-behandling vid hjärtinfarkt. Nord. Med. 78, 954 (1967).
893. LINDENSCHMIDT, T. O.: Traumatischer Schock. Chirurg 36, 145 (1965).
894. LINDNER, J.: Experimentelle Untersuchungen zum Abbau von Polysacchariden in Lymphknoten. Verh. dtsch. Ges. Path. 37, 197 (1953).
895. — Über das Schicksal des Dextrans im menschlichen Organismus. Verh. dtsch. Ges. Path. 38, 162 (1954).
896. — Histochemische Untersuchungen über das Schicksal von Blutflüssigkeitsersatzmitteln im menschlichen und tierischen Organismus. Bibl. haemat. 5, 190 (1955).
897. — Über die Bedeutung und das Schicksal makromolekularer Stoffe im menschlichen Organismus mit besonderer Berücksichtigung des Dextran. Ärztl. Forsch. 10, 275 (1956).
898. — Zur Pathologie des Blutflüssigkeitsersatzes. Arzneimittelforsch. 8, 569 (1958).
899. — Stoffwechsel des Dextrans aus der Sicht des Pathologen. Anaesthesist 8, 55 (1959).
900. — Die Pathologie der geschädigten Niere (und die Verwendung von Plasmaexpandern). Anaesthesist 9, 254 (1959).
901. —, u. W. GUSEK: Elektronenmikroskopische Untersuchungen an Lymphknoten nach Dextranzufuhr. Frankf. Z. Path. 70, 367 (1960).
902. — Tierexperimentelle Untersuchungen zum Problem der sog. Polymerkrebse. Verh. dtsch. Ges. Path. 44, 272 (1960).
903. — Morphologische Untersuchungen über das Schicksal von Plasmaexpandern. In: K. HORATZ u. R. FREY: Schock und Plasmaexpander, p. 23. Berlin-Göttingen-Heidelberg: Springer 1964.
904. LISTER, J., I. F. MCNEILL, V. C. MARSHALL, L. F. PLZAK, F. J. DAGHER, and F. D. MOORE: Transcapillary refilling after hemorrhage in normal man: Basal rates and volumes; effect of norepinephrine. Ann. Surg. 158, 698 (1963).

905. LISTER, J., M. S. WIN, and R. P. ALTMAN: Factors influencing homeostati responses to hemorrhage. Surgery 60, 43 (1966).

906. LITTLE, J. M., and H. S. WELLS: Capillary permeability to intravenously ac ministered gelatin. Amer. J. Physiol. 138, 495 (1943).

907. —, J. LOEWENTHAL, and F. H. MILLS: Venous thromboembolic disease. Bri J. Surg. 53, 657 (1966).

908. LITWAK, R. S., R. SLONIM, B. G. WISOFF, and H. L. GADBOYS: Homologoı blood syndrome during extracorporeal circulation in man. II. Phenomer of sequestration and desequestration. New Engl. J. Med. 268, 1377 (1963

909. — Late volumetric alterations after clinical extracorporeal circulation. Ame Surg. 30, 349 (1964).

910. —, H. L. GADBOYS, M. KAHN, B. G. WISOFF, and H. PICKHOLTZ: High flo total body perfusion utilizing diluted perfusate in a large prime syster J. thorac. cardiovasc. Surg. 49, 74 (1965).

911. LITWIN, M. S., L. L. SMITH, and F. D. MOORE: Metabolic alkalosis followi massive transfusion. Surgery 45, 805 (1959).

912. —, C. W. WALTER, P. EJARQUE, and E. D. REYNOLDS: Synergistic toxicity gram-negative bacteria and free colloidal hemoglobin. Ann. Surg. 157, 4 (1963).

913. —, S.-E. BERGENTZ, A. CARSTEN, L.-E. GELIN, C.-M. RUDENSTAM, and B. S DERHOLM: Hidden acidosis following intravascular red blood cell aggr gation in dogs. Ann. Surg. 161, 532 (1965).

914. LÖFSTRÖM, B.: Induced hypothermia and intravascular aggregation. Ac anaesth. scand. suppl. 3 (1959).

915. LOMONACO, F.: Lo shock ed il riprissino della massa liquida circolan (esperienze cliniche con plasmaexpander). Minerva anest. 29, 379 (1963).

916. LONG, D. M., L. SANCHEZ, R. L. VARCO, and C. W. LILLEHEI: The use of lo molecular weight dextran and serum albumin as plasma expanders extracorporeal circulation. Surgery 50, 12 (1961).

917. — The status of plasma expanders in open heart surgery. Dis. Chest. 41, 5 (1962).

918. —, M. W. MYER, E. B. BROWN, JR., and C. W. LILLEHEI: Myocardial necro and electrocardiographic changes related to microcirculatory abnormaliti Amer. J. Cardiol. 10, 695 (1962).

919. — Pharmacology of low molecular weight dextran and its effect on clotti and crossmatching. Conf. on Evaluation of Low Molecular Weight De tran in Shock, p. 26. Washington, D. C.: Nat. Acad. Sci 1963.

920. LOENNECKEN, S. J.: Diskussionsbemerkung. Anaesthesist 8, 42 (1959).

921. LOSTUMBO, M. M., P. V. HOLLAND, and P. J. SCHMIDT: Isoimmunization af multiple transfusion. New Engl. J. Med. 275, 141 (1966).

922. Low Molecular Weight Dextran (Rheomacrodex). Symposium held at t Roy. Soc. Med., London. Uppsala: Pharmacia 1963.

923. LUND, J., H. HEISTØ, and C. MÜLLER: Observations on adjustments of blo volume and circulation following infusion of whole blood and dextran blood depleted dogs. J. Oslo City Hosp. 4, 101 (1954).

924. LUNDSGAARD-HANSEN, P.: Zum Vergleich von Dextran- und Gelatine-E pandern. Méd. Hyg. 746, 840 (1966).

925. —, A. v. GRAFFENRIED u. H. RIEDWYL: Die therapeutische Wirkung von Bl Macrodex, Physiogel und Ringer-Lösung in einem standardisierten häm rhagischen Schock. Helv. chir. Acta 33, 558 (1966).

925a. — Zur Expanderfrage. Schweiz. Z. Militärmed. 44, 9 (1967).

925b. LUNDSGAARD-HANSEN, P., H. RIEDWYL u. A. HÄSSIG: Vergleich von Dextran und Gelatine als Plasmaersatzmittel. Anaesthesist **16**, 206 (1967).

926. LUNDY, J. S., E. B. TUCHY, R. D. ADAMS, L. H. MOUSEL, T. H. SELDON, and J. W. PENDER: Annual Report for 1946 of the section on Anesthesiology: Including data and remarks concerning blood transfusion and the use of blood substitutes. I. Proc. Mayo Clin. **22**, 357 (1947).

927. —, and H. K. GRAY: Dextran in supportive therapy with comments on Periston and gelatin. Arch. Surg. **61**, 55 (1950).

928. — New solutions. Minnesota Med. **34**, 21 (1951).

929. LÜSCHER, E. F., u. B. TSCHIRREN: Nebeneffekte von Plasmaexpandern. Anaesthesist **9**, 211 (1960).

930. LUSKY, L. M., and A. A. NELSON: Fibrosarcoma induced by multiple subcutaneous injections of carboxy-methylcellulose (CM), polyvinylpyrrolidone (PVP) and polyoxyethylene sorbitan monostearate. Fed. Proc. **16**, 318 (1957).

931. LUSZTIG, G., L. SAJTOS, J. PATAKY, L. JOSZA u. M. PERNECZKY: Die Wirkung von Dextran im Spiegel der hämochemischen Untersuchungen. Z. ges. inn. Med. **16**, 807 (1961).

932. —, L. JOZSA, M. PERNECZKY, L. SAJTOS, P. PATAKY u. L. SZIKULAI: Die Frage des antiatherogenen Effekts und Wirkungsmechanismus des Dextrans. Z. ges. inn. Med. **17**, 114 (1962).

933. — — — — Hemmung der experimentellen Cholesterinsklerose mit Dextran. Z. ges. inn. Med. **17**, 152 (1962).

934. LUTZ, J., u. W. SCHEGA: Plasmavolumenbestimmungen nach Verwendung partiell hydrolisierter Gelatine als Plasmaersatzmittel. Anaesthesist **8**, 273 (1959).

935. LUTZ, H.: Sauerstoffbindung unter Verwendung von Blutersatzmitteln. Anaesthesist **13**, 136 (1964).

936. — Zu: Tierexperimentelle Untersuchungen mit Plasmaexpandern. In: K. LANG, R. FREY u. M. HALMAGYI: Infusionstherapie, p. 226. Berlin-Heidelberg-New York: Springer 1966.

937. — Experimentelle Untersuchungen über den Volumeneffekt kolloidaler Infusionsmittel auf der Basis von Dextran und Gelatine. Z. prakt. Anaesth. **2**, 40 (1967).

938. MACLEAN, L. D., and A. VAN TYN: Ventricular fibrillation. J. Amer. med. Ass. **175**, 471 (1961).

939. — Blood volume versus central venous pressure in shock. Surg. Gynec. Obstet. **118**, 594 (1964).

940. —, J. H. DUFF, H. M. SCOTT, and D. I. PERETZ: Treatment of shock in man based on hemodynamic diagnosis. Surg. Gynec. Obstet. **120**, 1 (1965).

941. — The clinical management of shock. Brit. J. Anaesth. **38**, 255 (1966).

941a. —, G. W. MULLIGAN, A. P. H. MCLEAN, and J. H. DUFF: Alkalosis in septic shock. Surgery **62**, 655 (1967).

942. MADSEN, S.: Incidence of hepatitis after use of blood and serum transfusions. J. Amer. med. Ass. **155**, 1331 (1954).

943. MAIER, C.: Indikation und Kontraindikation der Bluttransfusion. Schweiz. med. Wschr. **95**, 54 (1965).

944. MAILLOUX, L. U., R. L. CAPIZZI, C. D. SWARTZ, G. ONESTI, O. RAMIREZ, and A. N. BREST: Acute renal shutdown following low molecular weight dextran infusion: Clinical and experimental evidence. Circulation **34**, suppl. 3, 161 (1966).

945. MAINARDI, L. C., K. BHANGANDADA, J. D. MACK, and C. W. LILLEHEI: Hem dilution in extracorporeal circulation: Comparative study of low mol cular weight dextran and 5 percent dextrose. Surgery **56,** 349 (1964).
946. MAKK, L., P. C. JOHNSON, J. D. MCMURREY, and A. C. BEALL: Effects traumatic hypovolemic shock on coronary blood flow and cardiac outp in man. Amer. J. Surg. **108,** 757 (1964).
947. MALINOW, M. R., A. A. PELLEGRINO, and E. H. RAMOS: Prevention of aort atherosclerosis in rabbit by intravenous microcrystallized estradi benzoate and dextran. Proc. Soc. exp. Biol. **97,** 446 (1958).
948. MALM, J. R., W. M. MANGER, S. F. SULLIVAN, E. N. PAPPER, and G. G. NAHA The effect of acidosis on sympatho-adrenal stimulation. J. Amer. me Ass. **197,** 121 (1966).
949. MALONEY, J. V., C. McC. SMYTHE, J. P. GILMORE, and S. W. HANDFOR Intra-arterial and intravenous transfusion. A controlled study of the effectiveness in the treatment of experimental hemorrhagic shock. Sur Gynec. Obstet. **97,** 529 (1953).
950. MANSBERGER, A. R., JR., R. M. OLLODART, S. ATTAR, A. COWLEY, and R. BUXTON: Therapy of refractory shock. Ann. Surg. **161,** 955 (1965).
951. MANSBERGER, A. R., E. F. COX, C. T. FLOTTE, and R. W. BUXTON: "Washou acidosis following resection of aortic aneurysms: Clinical metabolic stu of reactive hyperemia and effect of dextran on excess lactate and p Ann. Surg. **163,** 778 (1966).
952. MARKLEY, K., M. BOCANEGRA, A. BAZAN, R. TEMPLE, M. CHIAPPORI, G. MOR LES, and A. CARRION: Clinical evaluation of saline solution therapy burn shock. II. Comparison of plasma therapy with saline solution ther py. J. Amer. med. Ass. **170,** 1633 (1959).
953. MARSHALL, L. H., and C. H. HANNA: Differences of T-1824 and cell conce tration of venous blood of dogs after dextran. Amer. J. Physiol. **176,** 3 (1954).
954. MARSHALL, R. J., and T. D. DARBY: Shock, pharmacological principles treatment. Springfield, Ill.: Thomas 1966.
955. MARSHALL, V. C.: Shock and haemorrhage. Med. J. Austr. **52,** 384 (1965).
956. — Blood volume monitoring in surgical patients with a semi-automat machine: Clinical experience. Med. J. Austr. **52,** 414 (1965).
957. — Circulatory refilling after surgery. I. Austr. NZ J. Surg. **35,** 245 (1966).
958. —, H. ROSS, and D. E. YOFFA: Circulatory refilling and renal haemodynami after surgery. II. Effects of replacement with dextrans and mannit Austr. NZ J. Surg. **36,** 96 (1966).
959. MARSTON, N.: Cross-matching of blood in the presence of dextran. Lanc **II,** 688 (1954).
960. MARTI, W. K.: Intraarterielle Langzeitinfusionen mit Vasodilatatoren u niedrigmolekularem Dextran in der Behandlung peripherer arteriell Durchblutungsstörungen. Schweiz. med. Wschr. **93,** 1746 (1963).
961. MARTINOVIC, D., and D. G. MELROSE: The use of low molecular weig dextran in extracorporeal circulation. J. cardiovasc. Surg. **4,** 610 (1963).
962. MATHESON, N. A., T. T. IRVIN, and A. J. HEDLEY: The renal response to lo molecular-weight dextran. Lancet **II,** 501 (1962).
963. —, T. T. IRVIN, and A. J. HEDLEY: The renal response to low-molecula weight dextran. Lancet **II,** 501 (1964).
964. —, D. R. HARPER, A. J. HEDLEY, and T. T. IRVIN: Effect of low-molecul weight dextran on postoperative renal function. Lancet **I,** 779 (1965).
965. — Effects of dextran 40 on urine flow. Postgrad. Med. J. **42,** 457 (1966).

966. Matheson, N. A.: Renal failure with low-molecular-weight dextran. Brit. med. J. II, 1198 (1966).
967. —, and J. W. Robertson: Effects of dextran 40 on postoperative renal haemodynamics. Lancet II, 251 (1966).
967a. — Renal effects of low molecular weight dextran. Monogr. surg. Sci. 3, 303 (1966).
968. Matthews, D. N.: Recent advances in the surgery of trauma. London: Churchill 1963.
969. Maunsbach, A. B., S. C. Madden, and H. Latta: Light and electron microscopic changes in proximal tubules of rats after administration of glucose, mannitol, sucrose or dextran. Lab. Invest. 11, 421 (1962).
970. Maurer, G.: Zur Verhütung einer Virushepatitis bei der Blutübertragung. Arch. klin. Chir. 313, 101 (1965).
971. Maurer, P. H.: Dextran, an antigen in man. Proc. Soc. exp. Biol. 83, 879 (1953).
972. —, F. J. Dixon, and W. Dukstein: Effect of infusion of polyvinylpyrrolidone on the immune response in rabbits. Proc. Soc. exp. Biol. 88, 550 (1955).
973. —, and Lebovitz, H.: Studies on the antigenicity of modified fluid gelatin. J. Immunol. 76, 335 (1956).
974. —, and H. C. Mansmann: On non-antigenicity of polysaccharides in guinea pigs. Proc. Soc. exp. Biol. 99, 378 (1958).
975. — Immunologische Untersuchungen mit Plasmaersatzmitteln. Klin. Wschr. 38, 417 (1960).
976. — Antigenicity of gelatin in rabbits and other species. J. exp. Med. 100, 515 (1964).
977. — Immunogenicity studies with hydroxyethyl starch. In: Third Conference on Artificial Colloidal Agents, p. 26. Washington, D. C.: Nat. Acad. Sci. 1965.
978. Maycock, W. d'A.: The infusion of dextran solutions. Lancet I, 1081 (1952).
979. — British experience with dextran. Bibl. haemat. 7, 272 (1958).
980. —, and C. R. Ricketts: Stability of dextran during prolonged storage. Nature (Lond.) 192, 174 (1961).
981. — The national blood transfusion service. Practitioner 195, 147 (1965).
982. —, and C. R. Ricketts: Stability of dextran during prolonged storage. Nature (Lond.) 213, 88 (1967).
983. Mayerson, H. S., C. G. Wolfram, H. R. Shirley jr., and K. Wasserman: Regional differences in capillary permeability. Amer. J. Physiol. 198, 155 (1960).
984. McCarthy, M. D., and J. W. Draheim: Survival of thermally injured rats infused with saline, polyvinylpyrrolidone, dextran and oxypolygelatin. Proc. Soc. exp. Biol. 79, 346 (1952).
984a. McClelland, R. N., G. T. Shires, C. R. Baxter, C. D. Coln, and J. Carrico: Balanced salt solution in the treatment of hemorrhagic shock. J. Amer. med. Ass. 199, 830 (1967).
985. McClenahan, J. B., N. Yamauchi, and B. B. Roe: Blood volume studies in cardiac surgery patients. J. Amer. med. Ass. 195, 356 (1966).
986. McDermott, W. V., jr., R. D. Adams, and A. G. Riddell: Ammonia levels in blood and cerebrospinal fluid. Proc. Soc. exp. Biol. 88, 380 (1955).
987. McEntegart, M. G.: Dangerous contaminants in stored blood. Lancet II, 909 (1956).
988. McGowan, G. K.: Osmolar and electrolyte changes in haemorrhagic shock. Lancet I, 775 (1963).

989. McGowan, G. K., and G. Walters: The value of measuring central ven pressure in shock. Brit. J. Surg. **I**, 821 (1963).

990. — — Central venous pressure in oligaemic shock. Lancet **I**, 1390 (1964).

991. — — A clinical study of surgical shock. Lancet **I**, 611 (1966).

992. McMurrey, J. D., H. E. Garrett, and M. E. de Bakey: Blood volume m surements in patients receiving cardiovascular surgical treatment. Card vasc. Res. Center Bull. **1**, 51 (1962/63).

993. McNeill, I. F., J. P. Williams, and F. D. Moore: The effects of hemorrh and hormones on the partition of body water. I. A method for measur small sequential increases in the volume of the extracellular fluid. J. su Res. **3**, 322 (1963).

994. —, J. P. Dixon, and F. D. Moore: The effects of hemorrhage and hormo on the partition of body water. II. The effects of acute single and multi hemorrhage and adrenal corticosteroids in the dog. J. surg. Res. **3**, : (1963).

995. — — — The effects of hemorrhage and hormones on the partition of bc water. III. The effects of hemorrhage and corticosteroids on fluid partit on the adrenalectomized dog. J. surg. Res. **3**, 344 (1963).

996. McPherson, R. C., and A. J. Haller: The comparative effects of blo saline and low molecular dextran on irreversible hemorrhagic sho J. Trauma **4**, 414 (1964).

997. Medical Science Publication No. 3: Symposium on Circulation and Hom stasis. Army Med. Serv. Graduate School, Walter Reed Army Med. Cen Washington, D. C. 1953.

998. Medical Science Publication No. 4: Recent Advances in Medicine and Surg based on Professional Medical Experiences in Japan and Korea 1950 1953, vol. I and II. Army Med. Serv. Graduate School, Walter R Army Med. Center, Washington, D. C. 1954.

999. Meili-Gerber, E.: Volumeneffekt und Reaktion nach Infusionen von Plasr pasteurisierter Plasmaprotein-Lösung, Gelatine- und niedrig molekula Dextranlösung. Diss. Zürich 1965.

999a. Meiselman, H. J., E. W. Merrill, E. W. Salzman, E. R. Gilliland, a G. A. Pelletier: Effect of dextran on rheology of human blood: L shear viscometery. J. appl. Physiol. 22, 480 (1967).

1000. Mellander, S., and D. H. Lewis: Effect of hemorrhagic shock on reactivity of resistance and capacitance vessels and on capillary filtrati transfer in cat skeletal muscle. Circulat. Res. **13**, 105 (1963).

1001. Melrose, D. G., R. Nahas, D. Alvarez, I. A. D. Todd, and W. J. Dempst Postoperative hypoxia after extracorporeal circulation—a possible gr against host reaction. Experientia **21**, 47 (1965).

1002. Mendlowitz, M.: The specific heat of human blood. Science **107**, 97 (194

1003. Merck, D. E., J. D. Hardy, and J. A. Grönwall: Hemodynamic a clotting problems of superior vena cava—right pulmonary arte anastomosis (Glenn operation). Clin. Res. **11**, 25 (1963).

1004. — —, R. H. Cannon, and J. A. Grönvall: Experimental pulmonary arter vena cava anastomosis (Glenn operation). Efficacy of low molecul weight dextran vs heparin in preventing thrombosis with notes on pr sure changes. J. thorac. cardiovasc. Surg. **47**, 367 (1964).

1005. Merrill, E. W., E. R. Gilliland, G. Cokelet, H. Shin, A. Britten, a R. E. Wells jr.: Rheology of blood and flow in the microcirculatic J. appl. Physiol. **18**, 255 (1963).

1006. Mertz, D. P.: Klinisch-experimentelle Untersuchungen über die Wirkung eines neuen Plasmaexpanders auf die Nierenhämodynamik und den Mechanismus der Harnkonzentrierung. Arzneimittelforsch. **12,** 489 (1962).

1007. Messmer, K.: Intestinale Faktoren im Schock: Intestinaler Kreislauf. Arch. klin. Chir. **319,** 890 (1967).

1008. —, W. Brendel, H. Holper u. L. Sunder-Plassmann: Extreme Blutverdünnung durch Volumensubstitution. Symp. Akute Elementargefährdung und Wiederbelebung, Mainz, 13. 10. 1967.

1009. Metcalf, W., L. M. Rousselot, J. M. Harmon, and F. E. Gilbertson: The determinants of the efficacy of various expanders in plasma volume expansion and maintenance in normal subjects. Surg. Forum **4,** 714 (1954).

1010. —, L. M. Rousselot, F. E. Gilbertson, and J. M. Harmon: A clinical method for the determination of the molecular weights and the molecular weight distribution of plasma expanders. Surg. Forum **4,** 719 (1954).

1011. —, E. L. Dargan, E. J. Hehre, S. Levitsky, and T. J. di Buono: Clinical physiological characterization of a new dextran. Surg. Gynec. Obstet. **115,** 199 (1962).

1011 a. Meyer, J. S., F. Gotoh, M. Akiyama, and S. Yoshitake: Monitoring cerebral metabolic disorder in stroke and some therapeutic trials in human volunteers. Circulation **36,** 197 (1967).

1012. Meyer, L. M., N. I. Berlin, G. M. Hyde, R. J. Parsons, and B. Whittington: Changes in blood volume following administration of dextran—determined by $P^{32}$ labeled red cells. Surg. Gynec. Obstet. **94,** 712 (1952).

1013. Meyer, W.: Alltägliche Schockprobleme, ihre Genese und therapeutischen Möglichkeiten. Praxis **11,** 362 (1964).

1014. Meznik, A.: Vaskulärer Volumenmangel beim Schock. Wien klin. Wschr. **14,** 303 (1966).

1015. Michaelson, S., and J. Howland: Combined effect of dextran and anticoagulants in the normal dog. Fed. Proc. **16,** 366 (1957).

1016. Michie, A. J., C. E. Koop, J. M. Walker, M. C. Ragni, and J. Tracy: Renal hemodynamics following i.v. administration of gelatin. J. appl. Physiol. **4,** 677 (1952)

1017. Miller, E. B., and L. H. Tisdall: Reactions to 10 000 pooled liquid human plasma transfusions. J. Amer. med. Ass. **128,** 863 (1945).

1018. Milles, G., H. Langston, and W. Dalessandro: Experiences with autotransfusions. Surg. Gynec. Obstet. **115,** 689 (1962).

1019. — — — Studies show a patient may be his own best donor. Mod. Hosp. **102,** 104 (1964).

1020. Millican, R. C., and M. S. Rosenthal: Physical agents and trauma. Mechanisms and therapy of traumatic shock. Ann. Rev. Med. **5,** 285 (1954).

1021. Mills, L. C., and J. H. Moyer: Shock and Hypotension, Pathogenesis and Treatment. New York: Grune & Stratton 1965.

1022. Miner, R. W., G. Shwartzman, and L. Salin: Hemorrhage. Ann. N. Y. Acad. Sci. **49,** art. 4, 483 (1948).

1023. Mioduszewski, J. Z.: Dextran „Polfa". Ciech Rev. **4,** 27 (1966).

1024. Mirick, G. S., R. Ward, and R. W. McCollum: Modification of post-transfusion hepatitis by gamma globulin. New Engl. J. Med. **273,** 59 (1965).

1025. Mohn, G.: Die Speicherung von Polyvinylpyrrolidon im Rattenorganism durch den direkten fluoreszenzmikroskopischen Nachweis. Acta hist chem. **9**, 76 (1960).

1026. Moeller, J., u. A. Iglhaut: Leucopenien nach Injection von Dextran l Nierenkranken und Gesunden. Dtsch. med. Wschr. **80**, 1736 (1955).

1027. —, u. A. Sykudes: Die Verträglichkeit von Haemaccel unter besonderer E rücksichtigung der Nierenfunktion. Dtsch. med. Wschr. **87**, 726 (1962).

1028. — Erfahrungen mit einem Polymerisat aus abgebauter Gelatine als Plasm expander. Pharmacotherapia **1**, 131 (1963).

1029. Mollison, A. W., and J. B. Rennie: Treatment of renal oedema with de tran. Brit. med. J. **I**, 893 (1954).

1030. Mollison, P. L.: Investigation of haemolytic transfusion reactions. Brit. me J. **I**, 528 (1943).

1031. — Blood transfusion in clinical medicine, 4. Aufl. Oxford: Blackwell 19(

1032. Moncrief, J. A., J. C. Darin, P. C. Canizaro, and R. B. Sawyer: Use dextran to prevent arterial and venous thrombosis. Ann. Surg. **158**, 5 (1963).

1033. — Dextran vs heparin in thrombophlebitis. J. Amer. med. Ass. **192**, 4 (1965).

1034. — Effect of various fluid regimens and pharmacologic agents on the c culatory hemodynamics of the immediate postburn period. Ann. Su **164**, 723 (1966).

1035. Monkhouse, F. C., and S. Milojevic: Changes in thrombin generation a antithrombin titer following massive bleeding and transfusion in do Canad. J. Biochem. **38**, 475 (1960).

1036. Moens, R. S., R. Busset, R. A. Collet et R. S. Mach: Utilisation l'albumine-$I^{131}$ (RIHSA) pour la détermination du volume plasmatic et du volume sanguin chez le sujet normal. Schweiz. med. Wschr. 1660, 1697 (1962).

1037. Moon, V. H.: Shock: Its dynamics, occurrence and management. Philad phia: Lea & Febiger 1942.

1038. Moore, F. D.: Metabolic care of the surgical patient. Philadelphia: Sau ders 1959.

1039. — Tris buffer, mannitol and low viscous dextran. Three new solutions old problems. Surg. Clin. N. Amer. **43**, 577 (1963).

1040. — Irreversible shock. New Engl. J. Med. **268**, 108 (1963).

1041. —, K. H. Olesen, J. D. McMurrey, H. V. Parker, M. R. Ball, and C. Boyden: The body cell mass and its supporting environment. Philac phia: Saunders 1963.

1042. — The effects of hemorrhage on body composition. New Engl. J. M **273**, 567 (1965).

1043. — Terminal mechanisms in human injury. Amer. J. Surg. **110**, 317 (1965).

1044. —, F. J. Dagher, C. M. Boyden, C. J. Lee, and J. H. Lyons: Hemorrhage normal man: I. Distribution and dispersal of saline infusions follow acute blood loss. Ann. Surg. **163**, 485 (1966).

1044a. —, and G. T. Shires: Editorial-Moderation. Ann. Surg. **166**, 300 (1967).

1045. Moore, R. C., P. L. Canizaro, R. B. Sawyer, J. C. Darin, and J. A. M( crief: An evaluation of methods for measuring operative blood l Anaesth. Analg. **44**, 130 (1965).

1045a. Moraes, I., E. Teixeira, J. Arbit, and J. J. Bergan: Augmentation arterial collateral blood flow. Arch. Surg. **95**, 49 (1967).

1046. MOREHEAD, R. P., and J. M. LITTLE: Morphological study following intravenous administration of gelatin solutions to dogs. Amer. J. Path. **21**, 233 (1945).
1047. MORGAN, T. O., J. M. LITTLE, and W. A. EVANS: Renal failure associated with low-molecular-weight dextran infusion. Brit. med. J. II, 737 (1966).
1047a. — — Renal failure and low-molecular-weight dextran. Brit. med. J. **I**, 635 (1967).
1048. MORRISON, A. E., JR., J. S. LUNDY, and H. E. ESSEX: An evaluation of replacement fluids in laboratory animals following control hemorrhage. Circulation **5**, 208 (1952).
1049. MORRISON, A. B.: The effect of dextran on serum proteins and serum cholesterol. Quart. J. exp. Physiol. **41**, 51 (1956).
1050. MORSE, D. P.: The management of shock in cardiac surgery. Amer. J. Cardiol. **12**, 624 (1963).
1051. MORTON, J. H.: An evaluation of blood transfusion practices on a surgical service. New Engl. J. Med. **263**, 1285 (1960).
1052. MOSLEY, J. W., and H. B. DULL: Transfusion-associated viral hepatitis. Anesthesiology **27**, 409 (1966).
1053. MOWRY, R. W., J. B. LONGLEY, and R. C. MILLICAN: Histochemical demonstration of intravenously injected detran in kidney and liver of the mouse. J. lab. clin. Med. **39**, 211 (1952).
1054. MOYER, C. A., H. W. MARGRAF, and W. W. MONAFO JR.: Burn shock and extravascular sodium deficiency; treatment with Ringer's solution with lactate. Arch. Surg. **90**, 799 (1965).
1055. MUDD, S., and W. T. THALHIMER: Blood substitutes and blood transfusion. Springfield, Ill.: Thomas 1942.
1056. MUIR, I. F. K.: The treatment of the severely burned patient. Brit. J. Anaesth. **38**, 267 (1966).
1057. MULDER, D. G., E. A. MAZZEI, and R. N. MACALPIN: Ball-valve replacement for aortic valvular disease. A follow-up evaluation. J. thorac cardiovasc. Surg. **52**, 76 (1966).
1058. MULDOWNEY, F. P., and B. FLANAGAN: The body-haematocrit: Venous haematocrit ratio in normal human pregnancy. Clin. Sci. **27**, 329 (1964).
1059. MÜLLER, W., and L. L. SMITH: Changes in the hepatic circulation with graded hemorrhage, retransfusion and blood volume overexpansion; an experimental study in the dog. Surg. Forum **12**, 73 (1961).
1060. — — Hepatic arterial and portal venous circulatory changes following acute hemorrhage in the dog. Surg. Gynec. Obstet. **117**, 753 (1963).
1061. MUNDTH, E. D., R. B. BROWN, and E. HARDENBERGH: The protective effect of low molecular weight dextran against tissue injury from freezing. Fed. Proc. **22**, 224 (1963).
1062. —, D. M. LONG, and R. B. BROWN: Treatment of experimental frostbite with low molecular weight dextran. J. Trauma **4**, 246 (1964).
1063. MUNGIBÌ, S.: L'uso di un nuovo plasmaexpander nella prevenzione e nella terapia dello shock chirurgico. Minerva anest. **29**, 414 (1963).
1064. MURPHY, G. P., J. A. GAGNON, R. L. MUNDY, B. MEHLMAN, and R. A. EWALD: The physiological properties of glyco-alginate, a new Japanese plasma volume expander. In: Second Conference on Artificial Colloidal Agents, p. 131. Washington, D. C.: Nat. Acad. Sci. 1963.
1065. — — The hemodynamic alterations induced by low molecular weight dextran in normotension and hypotension. II. Observed alterations in renal clearances and transport. Invest. Urol. **1**, 574 (1964).

1066. MURPHY, G. P.: The renal effects of acute hemodilution with hydroxyetl starch, dextran, or saline. Surg. Gynec. Obstet. **121**, 1325 (1965).

1067. MURPHY, W. P., JR., and W. G. WORKMAN: Serum hepatitis from poo irradiated dried plasma. J. Amer. med. Ass. **152**, 1421 (1953).

1068. MURRAY, J. F., P. H. GOLD, and B. L. JOHNSON: Systemic oxygen transp in induced normovolemic anemia and polycythemia. Amer. J. Phys. **203**, 720 (1962).

1069. MUSCHAWECK, R., u. W. BENOIT: Zur Pharmakologie eines neuen kolloida Plasmaersatzmittels. Arzneimittelforsch. **12**, 380 (1962).

1069a. MYERS, M. B., and G. CHERRY: Design of skin flaps to study vascular sufficiency. Failure of Dextran 40 to improve tissue survival in vascularized skin. J. Surg. Res. **7**, 399 (1967).

1070. MYHRE, E., and H. RUSTAD: Blood volume determination with $Cr^{51}$ label red cells. Acta chir. scand. **125**, 197 (1963).

1070a. NAGEL, W., G. WOLFF, J. P. GIGON u. F. ENDERLIN: Zur Bestimmung Inulinclearance in Gegenwart von Dextran. Klin. Wschr. **45**, 1 (1967).

1071. NAHAS, G. G., and A. ESTIME: Etude expérimentale des gélatines flui modifiées dans le traitement des hémorrhagies massives (40% volume sanguin total). Rev. hémat. **10**, 725 (1955).

1072. NASTORG, G.: Essai de traitement des artérites des membres inférieurs des perfusions de dextran à faible poids moléculaire. Diss. Paris 1965.

1073. NASTUCK, W. L., and C. H. BEATTY: Standardization of hemorrhagic sh in the dog. Amer. J. Physiol. **156**, 202 (1949).

1074. Nat. Acad. Sci., Nat. Res. Counc.: Criteria of satisfactory plasma volu expanders. Washington, D. C. 1963.

1074 a. NECHELES, H., S. O. LEVINSON, M. JANOTA, and F. ARIMOTO: Preinfusion a study in the prevention of hemorrhagic shock. Surg. Gynec. Obstet. 499 (1947).

1075. NEILL J. M., E. J. HEHRE, Y. SUGG, and E. JAFFE: Serological studies sugar. I. Reaction between solutions of reagent sucrose and Type II an pneumococcus serum. J. exp. Med. **70**, 427 (1939).

1076. —, J. Y. SUGG, E. JAFFE, and E. J. HEHRE: Influence of sucrose upon p duction of serologically reactive material by certain streptococci. Pr Soc. exp. Biol. **47**, 339 (1941).

1077. —, and I. ABRAHAMS: Reaction of dextrans with antiserums of rabb immunized with S. typhi. Proc. Soc. exp. Biol. **78**, 537 (1951).

1078. —, and A. H. PINKES: Antipneumococcal cross reactions of antigens Leuconostoc mesenteroides. Proc. Soc. exp. Biol. **87**, 553 (1954).

1079. NELSON, A. H., and L. M. LUSKY: Pathologic changes in rabbits from peated injections of PVP or dextran. Proc. Soc. exp. Biol. **76**, 765 (195

1080. NENCI, G., e E. MIGLIORINI: Ricerche clinico-sperimentali su di un nuo plasmaexpander. Minerva anest. **29**, 387 (1963).

1081. NEPTUNE, W. B., and J. A. BOUGAS: Results of open heart surgery witho donor blood prime in pump-oxygenator. Dis. Chest **42**, 79 (1962).

1082. NIALL, J. F., and J. C. DOYLE: Renal failure associated with dextran i fusions. Int. Congr. Nephrol., abstr. II, p. 248. Washington, D. C. 196

1082a. NICK, W. V., and M. C. DODD: DNA-Antibody in the serum of patients shock. Ann. Surg. **166**, 357 (1967).

1083. NIEPOTH, G., u. N. NIKOLAI: Wirksamkeit der Elektrolytlösungen bei Bl verlusten. Arch. klin. Chir. **293**, 84 (1959).

1084. NILSSON, I. M., and O. EIKEN: Further studies on the effect of dextran of various molecular weight on the coagulation mechanism. Thromb. Diath. haemorrh. **11**, 38 (1964).
1085. NITSCHMANN, H., P. KISTLER, H. R. RENFER, A. HÄSSIG, and A. JOSS: A heat stable human plasma protein solution obtained by desalting. Vox Sang. **1**, 183 (1956).
1086. — — Large scale production of human plasma fractions. Vox Sang. **7**, 414 (1962).
1087. —, u. H. R. GYGAX: Eine einfache Methode zur Messung der relativen onkotischen Wirksamkeit von kolloidalen Plasmaersatzlösungen. Path. Microbiol. **27**, 548 (1964).
1088. — —, P. MOSER, and H. R. STOLL: A simple concentration osmometer and its application to the determination of the oncotic efficiency of plasma substitutes. Vox Sang. **12**, 106 (1967).
1089. NITTIS, S., C. LADOPOULOS, and M. SCHWIMMER: Effect of dextran infusion on bleeding time. Bull. N.Y. med. Coll. **16**, 86 (1953).
1090. NOBLE, R. P., and M. I. GREGERSEN: Blood volume in clinical shock. II. The extent and cause of blood volume reduction in traumatic, hemorrhagic and burn shock. J. clin. Invest. **25**, 172 (1946).
1091. NOEL, P. R. B., L. E. MAWDESLEY-THOMAS, and A. E. STREET: Rheomacrodex administration by intravenous transfusions to pedigree dogs. Final Report, Huntingdon Res. Center, Engl. 1966.
1092. NORBÄCK, B.: Effect of blood substitution on the cerebral metabolic rate of oxygen. Acta chir. scand. suppl. **364**, 33 (1966).
1093. NORGREN, L., L. Å. NILSSON och L. RYTTINGER: Posttransfusion hepatit. Svensk. Läk. Tidn. **63**, 2996 (1966).
1094. NORLANDER, O.: Total hemoglobin, blood volume and circulatory changes in surgical patients. Acta chir. scand. suppl. **199** (1955).
1095. NUNN, J. F., and J. FREEMAN: Problems of oxygenation and oxygen transport during hemorrhage. Anaesthesia **19**, 206 (1964).
1096. NUSSBAUMER, P.-A., et P. AMACKER: Les substituants du plasma. Schweiz. Apoth. Ztg. **104**, 321 (1966).
1096a. OBERMAN, H. A.: The indications for transfusion of freshly drawn blood. J. Amer. med. Ass. **199**, 93 (1967).
1097. OECHSLIN, R., W. SCHEITLIN u. P. FRICK: Schockzustände bei Sepsis mit gramnegativen Erregern. Schweiz. med. Wschr. **92**, 1151 (1962).
1098. ODIN, M.: Den akuta hepatitens symptom. Acta Univ. gotoburg. **6** (1954).
1099. OEFF, K.: Über den Wirkungsmechanismus von kolloidalen Plasmaersatzmitteln. Anaesthesist **8**, 45 (1959).
1100. OHLKE, R. F., and J. J. SCALES: Plasma augmenters in clinical surgery. Canad. med. Ass. J. **68**, 260 (1953).
1101. OLESEN, K. H.: Måling af det centrale venetryk. Nord. Med. **74**, 870 (1965).
1102. OLLODART, R., and A. R. MANSBERGER: The effect of hypovolemic shock on bacterial defense. Amer. J. Surg. **110**, 302 (1965).
1103. O'NEILL, J. A., JR., and J. H. FOSTER: The influence of low molecular weight dextran on lethal endotoxemia. Amer. Surg. **30**, 612 (1964).
1104. —, N. ENDE, I. S. COLLINS, and H. A. COLLINS: A quantitative determination of perfusion fibrinolysis. Surgery **60**, 809 (1966).
1105. ORKIN, L. R.: Clinical Management of the Patient in Shock. Clin. Anesth. **2**. Oxford: Blackwell 1965.
1106. OSTEN, W.: Die Behandlung des Schocks durch Plasmaexpander. Anaesthesist **8**, 33 (1959).

1107. OTT, VON: Über den Einfluß der Kochsalzinfusion auf den verblutete Organismus im Vergleich mit anderen zur Transfusion verwendeten Flü: sigkeiten. Arch. path. Anat. **93,** 114 (1883).

1108. OZINSKY, J.: The need of warming stored blood. S. Afr. med. J. **39,** 14 (1965).

1109. PANNACCIULLI, E., e G. C. SERRA: Azione sul circolo di un nuovo sostitut plasmatico costituito da polimerizzati di gelatina scissa. Minerva anes **29,** 369 (1963).

1110. —, ed F. AJMAR: Le variazioni della volemia in rapporto alla somministra zione di un sostituto plasmatico („Emagel"). Minerva chir. **21,** 67 (1966

1111. PAPPENHEIMER, J. R.: Passage of molecules through capillary walls. Physio Rev. **33,** 387 (1953).

1112. PAREIRA, M. D., K. D. SERKES, and S. LANG: Influence of mixing time o determination of red cell volume in normal and shocked rats. Proc. So exp. Biol. **101,** 233 (1959).

1113. — — — Plasma volume response to graded hemorrhage. Surgery **52,** 37 (1962).

1114. — — — Enhanced efficacy of plasma after aging in treatment of tourni quet shock. Proc. Soc. exp. Biol. **115,** 660 (1964).

1115. PARKINS, V. M., C. E. KOOP, C. RIEGEL, H. M. VARS, and J. S. LOCKWOOD Gelatin as plasma substitute with particular reference to experiment hemorrhage and burn shock. Ann. Surg. **118,** 193 (1943).

1116. —, J. H. PERLMUTT, and H. M. VARS: Dextran, modified fluid gelatin an other plasma volume expanders in hemorrhaged dogs. Fed. Proc. **11,** 11 (1952).

1117. — — — Dextran, oxypolygelatin and modified fluid gelatin as replace ment fluids in experimental hemorrhage. Amer. J. Physiol. **173,** 40 (1953).

1118. PATAKY, J., L. SZIKULAY, L. SAJTOS, L. JÓZSA, M. PERNECZKY u. G. LUSZTIG Klinische Beobachtungen bei Atherosklerose im Zusammenhang m der Verabreichung von Dextran. Z. ges. inn. Med. **16,** 854 (1961).

1119. —, L. DÉNES, G. JUHÁSZ u. G. LUSZTIG: Über die Möglichkeiten der Be handlung der senilen Atherosklerose mit Dextran. Z. ges. inn. Med. **1**, 973 (1962).

1120. PATTONO, R., e G. MARCHIARO: Nostre esperienze con un nuovo plasma expander. Minerva anest. **29,** 349 (1963).

1121. PAULI, H. G.: Flüssigkeits- und Elektrolyttherapie bei Schock. Ther. Umsd **20,** 255 (1963).

1122. PAYNE, R., and M. R. ROLFS: Further observations on leukoagglutinin trans fusion reactions. Amer. J. Med. **29,** 449 (1960).

1122a. PENNELL, R. B.: Communication. XIth Congr. int. Soc. Blood Transf Sydney, Aug. 1966 (Abstr. of papers, p. 22).

1123. PERKINS, A. H., M. R. ROLFS, A. V. MCBRIDE, and B. ROE: Low molecula weight dextran in open heart surgery: Effect on coagulation factors an on red cell antibody activity. Transfusion **4,** 10 (1964).

1124. PERNECZKY, M., G. LUSZTIG, L. JÓSZA, L. SAJTOS u. J. PATAKY: Weitere Bei träge zu den durch Dextran verursachten hämochemischen Veränderun gen (Serumeiweiß, Lipoidfraktion). Z. ges. inn. Med. **16,** 998 (1961).

1125. PERRY, J. F.: Hemorrhage and death in the receiving room. Surgery **60,** 77 (1966).

1126. PETRI, G., B. TANOS, and H. SZABO: Humoral transfer of experimenta ischaemic shock. Acta chir. Acad. Sci. hung. **7,** 159 (1966).

1127. Petropoulos, P. C., and N. G. Heijne: Comparative results of the cardiac function during perfusion of a main coronary artery with lower or higher molecular weight dextran under normal and hyperbaric oxygenation. J. thorac. cardiovasc. Surg. **47**, 651 (1964).

1128. Pettenkofer, H. J.: Zur Blutgruppenbestimmung nach Verabreichung von kolloidalen Plasmaersatzmitteln. Chirurg. **30**, 25 (1959).

1129. Pfeifer, G.: Blutersatz durch Plasmaexpander und die Reaktionen im Gerinnungssystem. Geburtsh. Frauenheilk. **26**, 720 (1966).

1130. Piccinino, F., e G. di Stasio: Assenza di movimento anticorpale (anticorpi devianti il complemento) in soggetti sottoposti a singole o ripetute somministrazioni per via endevenosa di soluzioni colloidali di polimerizzati di gelatina scissa. Minerva anest. **29**, 340 (1963).

1131. Pichlmayr, I., u. W. Stich: Der bilirubinostatische Ikterus, eine neue Ikterusform beim Zusammentreffen von Operation, Narkose und Bluttransfusion. Klin. Wschr. **40**, 665 (1962).

1132. Pickert, H.: Über Austauschvorgänge zwischen intra- und extravasalem Raum. Im Hinblick auf das Dextranverhalten als Beispiel für die Dynamik großmolekularer Stoffe. Anaesthesist **8**, 42 (1959).

1133. Pirani, C. L., R. Juster, D. F. Froeb, D. F. Consolazio, and R. C. Ingraham: Use of dextran in hemorrhagic shock. J. appl. Physiol. **8**, 193 (1955).

1134. Pittman, M.: A study of bacteria implicated in transfusion reactions and of bacteria isolated from blood products. J. lab. clin. Med. **42**, 273 (1953).

1135. Planque, B. A. de, G. C. Geyskes, R. van Dongen, and E. J. Dorthout Mees: Simultaneous determination of extracellular volume and blood volume with the Volemetron. Clin. chim. Acta **2**, 270 (1965).

1136. Pollock, J. H.: A survey of surgical shock with special reference to fluids, electrolytes and metabolites. Springfield, Ill.: Thomas 1966.

1137. Pomerat, C. .M, and R. R. Overman: Electrolytes and plasma expanders. I. Reaction of human cells in perfusion chambers with phase contrast, time-lapse cine records. Z. Zellforsch. **45**, 2 (1956).

1138. Ponder, E., and R. Ponder: The interaction of dextran with serum albumin, gamma globulin, and fibrinogen. J. gen. Physiol. **43**, 753 (1960).

1139. — — Age and molecular weight of dextrans, their coating effect and their interaction with serum albumin. Nature (Lond.) **190**, 277 (1961).

1140. Popper, H.: Symposium on hepatitis. Gastroenterology **49**, 718 (1965).

1141. Powell, N. A., jr., and D. G. Johnston: Criteria for blood transfusions. Calif. Med. **97**, 12 (1962).

1142. Powley, P. H.: Rheomacrodex in peripheral ischaemia. Lancet **I**, 1189 (1963).

1143. Prentice, T. C., J. M. Olney, C. P. Artz, and J. M. Howard: Studies of blood volume and transfusion therapy in the Korean battle casualty. Med. Sci. Publ. **4**, Vol. 1, 163 (1954).

1144. Price, H. L., S. Deutsch, B. E. Marshall, G. W. Stephen, M. G. Behar, and G. R. Neufeld: Hemodynamic and metabolic effects of hemorrhage in man, with particular reference to the splanchnic circulation. Circulat. Res. **18**, 469 (1966).

1145. Prochazka, J.: Serumhepatitis nach Transfusionen von Blut, Erythromasse und gemischtem Plasma. Z. ges. inn. Med. **12**, 276 (1957).

1146. Pučar, Z., and M. Keler-Bačoka: Effect of molecular weights of colloidal dextran on human serum lipids. Science **134**, 1369 (1961).

1147. Pulaski, E. J.: Discussion. Arch. Surg. **63**, 745 (1951).

1148. Pulaski, E.: The clinical status of dextran, PVP and gelatin products. Quart Rev. Med. **9**, 44 (1952).

1149. — War wounds. New Engl. J. Med. **249**, 890 (1953).

1150. Putnam, T. C., S. V. Kovy, and R. L. Replogle: Factors affecting the viscosity of blood. Surg. Forum **16**, 126 (1965).

1151. Rabelo, A., M. S. Litwin, M. P. Brady, and F. D. Moore: A comparison of the effects of several osmotic diuretic agents after acute hemorrhage in the dog. Surg. Gynec. Obstet. **115**, 657 (1962).

1152. —, M. P. Brady, M. S. Litwin, and F. D. Moore: A comparison of several osmotic diuretics in hydropenic and hydropenic-DOCA-pitressin treated dogs. J. surg. Res. **3**, 237 (1963).

1152a. Race, D., H. Dedichen, and W. G. Schenk, jr.: Regional blood flow during dextran-induced normovolemic hemodilution in the dog. J thorac. cardiovasc. Surg. **53**, 578 (1967).

1153. Raison, J. C. A.: A clinical report of the use of low-molecular-weight dextran in a rotating oxygenator. Thorax **17**, 338 (1962).

1154. — Bleeding after heart-lung operations using low-molecular-weight dextran. Lancet **I**, 1425 (1963).

1155. Raisz, L. G., and E. J. Pulaski: A comparison of efficacy of dextran, oxypolygelatin, plasma and saline as plasma volume expanders. Amer. J Physiol. **169**, 475 (1952).

1156. —, and I. T. Stinson: Dextran and oxypolygelatin as plasma volume expanders: Renal excretion and effects on renal function. J. lab. clin Med. **40**, 880 (1952).

1157. Ramgren, O., och J.-E. Tengberg: Kliniska synpunkter på blodtransfusion Svensk. Läk. Tidn. **57**, 1904 (1960).

1158. Ratliff, A. H. C.: Low-molecular-weight dextran (Rheomacrodex) in the treatment of severe vascular insufficiency after trauma. Lancet **I**, 118[illegible] (1963).

1159. Ravdin, I., and W. Fitts: The so-called "blood substitutes". Amer. J. Surg **80**, 744 (1950).

1160. — Plasma expanders. J. Amer. med. Ass. **150**, 10 (1952).

1161. Ravin, H. A., A. M. Seligman, and J. Fine: Polyvinylpyrrolidone as a plasma expander. New Engl. J. Med. **247**, 921 (1952).

1162. —, and J. Fine: Current concepts and controversies on traumatic shock Progr. Surg. **3**, 102 (1963).

1163. Rawson, A., S. H. V. Chien, M. T. Pong, and R. J. Dellenbach: Determination of residual blood volume required for survival in rapidly hemorrhaged splenectomized dogs. Amer. J. Physiol. **196**, 179 (1959).

1164. Redeker, A. G., C. E. Hopkins, B. Jackson, and P. Peck: A controlled study of the safety of pooled plasma stored in the liquid state at 30—32° C for six month. Transfusion **8**, 60 (1968) and personal communication.

1165. Reeve, E. B.: The contribution of $I^{131}$-labeled proteins to measurements of blood volume. Ann. N.Y. Acad. Sci. **70**, 137 (1957).

1166. —, T. H. Allen, and J. E. Roberts: Blood volume regulation. Ann. Rev Physiol. **22**, 349 (1960).

1167. — Development of knowledge of traumatic shock in man. Fed. Proc. **20**, 1[illegible] (1961).

1168. Reeve, T. S., P. S. Hunt, and S. Argall: Venous thrombosis: A clinical study of 40 cases. Med. J. Austr. **52**, 168 (1966).

1169. Regan, T. J., M. J. Frank, P. H. Lehan, J. G. Galante, and H. K. Hellems: Myocardial blood flow and oxygen uptake during acute red cell volume increments. Circulat. Res. **13**, 172 (1963).
1170. Rehn, J.: Verbrennungen und Plasmaersatzmittel. Anaesthesist **8**, 264 (1959).
1171. Rehn, J.: Neuere Ergebnisse der Schockforschung und ihre therapeutischen Schlußfolgerungen. Arch. klin. Chir. **301**, 109 (1962).
1172. — Kreislaufdynamik und Schock. Arch. klin. Chir. **313**, 78 (1965).
1173. Reinert, M.: Die Wirkung hypertonischer Kochsalzlösung im irreversiblen hämorrhagischen Schock der Ratte. Z. Kreisl.-Forsch. **55**, 134 (1966).
1174. Reissigl, H.: Zur Gefahr der Serumhepatitis — Übertragung durch Bluttransfusionen. Zbl. Chir. **81**, 233 (1956).
1175. — Die Bluttransfusion. Wien: Maudrich 1961.
1176. — Zweckmäßige Schockbekämpfung. Med. Welt 232, 1964.
1177. Remington, J. W., W. F. Hamilton, N. Wheeler, and W. F. Hamilton jr.: Validity of pulse contour method for calculating cardiac output in the dog, with notes on effect of various anesthetics. Amer. J. Physiol. **159**, 379 (1949).
1178. —, and C. H. Baker: Plasma volume changes accompanying reactions to infusions of blood or plasma. Amer. J. Physiol. **197**, 193 (1959).
1179. Renkin, E. M.: Transport of large molecules across capillary walls. Physiologist **7**, 13 (1965).
1180. Replogle, R. L., H. Kundler, and R. E. Gross: Studies on the hemodynamic importance of blood viscosity. J. thorac. cardiovasc. Surg. **50** 658 (1965).
1180a. —, H. J. Meiselman, and E. W. Merrill: Clinical implications of blood rheology studies. Circulation **36**, 148 (1967).
1181. Reymond, C., C. Hahn et J. J. Livio: Place des dextrans en chirugie humaine. Praxis **49**, 114 (1960).
1182. Reynolds, M.: Cardiovascular effects of large volumes of isotonic saline infused intravenously into dogs following severe hemorrhage. Amer. J. Physiol. **158**, 418 (1949).
1183. Rhoads, J. E., and J. M. Howard: The Chemistry of Trauma. Springfield, Ill.: Thomas 1963.
1184. —, and S. J. Dudrick: Hypovolemic shock. Current clinical concepts of diagnosis and management. Postgrad. Med. **39**, 3 (1966).
1185. Richards, D. W., jr.: The circulation in traumatic shock in man. Harvey Lectures, ser. **39**, 217. Lancaster, Pa.: Science Press 1944.
1186. Richter, W.: Suspension stability of horse blood as a function of the molecular weight of added dextran. Acta chir. scand. **128**, 7 (1964).
1187. — Lowest molecular weight of dextran fraction with aggregating effect on human erythrocytes. Acta chir. scand. **129**, 457 (1965).
1188. — Normalizing effect of low molecular weight dextran fractions on the reduced suspension stability of human erythrocytes in vitro. Acta chir. scand. **131**, 1 (1966).
1189. — Relative aggregation tendency of erythrocytes from man and various animal species. Acta chir. scand. **132**, 601 (1966).
1190. Ricketts, C. R., L. Lorenz, and W. d'A. Maycock: Molecular composition of dextran solutions for intravenous use. Nature (Lond.) **165**, 770 (1950).
1191. — Interaction of dextran and fibrinogen. Nature (Lond.) **169**, 970 (1952).
1192. — The chemistry of dextran. In: J. W. Cook, and W. Carruthers: Progress in organic chemistry, vol. 5, p. 73. London: Butterworth 1961.
1193. — Molecular composition of transfusion dextran. Brit. med. J. **II**, 1423 (1966).

1194. RICKETTS, C. R.: Isotopically labelled macromolecules in biological researc Dextran labelled with radioactive iodine. Nature (Lond.) **210**, 113 (196

1194a. —, E. COPE, and J. THOMLINSON: Dextran and the placental barrier. Br med. J. **I**, 1050 (1966).

1195. RIEGER, Å., and S.-O. LILJEDAHL: Inverkan av olika substitut på restit tionen av blodvolym och plasmaprotein efter standardiserad blödni på hund. Nord. Med. **75**, 251 (1966).

1195a. — — Restitution av plasma-proteiner via ductus-thoracicus-lymfan eft blödning och substitution. Nord. Med. **78**, 1138 (1967).

1196. RITTMANN, W. W., and L. L. SMITH: Effect of treatment agents on cerebr blood flow following hemorrhage. Surg. Forum **16**, 411 (1965).

1197. ROBB, H. J.: The role of micro-embolism in the production of irreversib shock. Ann. Surg. **158**, 685 (1963).

1198. ROBBINS, L. B., B. B. CARLISLE, and J. H. FOSTER: Assessment of an thrombogenic properties of dextran solutions. Amer. Surg. **32**, 798 (196

1199. ROBERTS, M., and J. N. PAGONES: Preliminary tests of hydroxyethyl star solution in animals. In: Third Conference on Artifical Colloidal Agen p. 120. Washington, D. C.: Nat. Acad. Sci. 1965.

1200. ROBERTSON, J. D.: The effect of hemorrhage of varying degree on blood a plasma volume, on blood sugar and on arterial blood pressure. J. Physi **84**, 393 (1935).

1201. ROBERTSON, H. R., and A. D. MCKENZIE: Plasma, plasma expanders, bloo transfusions and blood fractions. Surg. Clin. N. Amer. **34**, 1219 (1954).

1202. ROBINSON, B. R., S. E. EPSTEIN, R. L. KAHLER, and E. BRAUNWALD: Circul tory effects of acute expansion of blood volume: Studies during maxim exercise and at rest. Circulat. Res. **19**, 26 (1966).

1203. ROBINSON, D. S., P. M. HARRIS and C. R. RICKETTS: The lipolytic activi of rat plasma after the intravenous injection of various dextran sulphate Biochem. J. **69**, 11P (1957).

1203 a. ROBSCHEIT-ROBBINS, R. S., L. L. MILLER, and G. H. WHIPPLE: Gelatin — i usefulness and toxicity. J. exp. Med. **80**, 145 (1944).

1204. ROCHE, P., JR., R. A. DODELIN, and W. BLOOM: Effect of dextran on bloo typing and crossmatching. Blood **7**, 373 (1952).

1205. RODBARD, S.: Biophysical principles governing the flow of blood in t vascular system. In: L. C. MILLS, and J. H. MOYER: Shock and hyp tension, p. 69. London: Grune & Stratton 1965.

1206. ROE, B. B., S. A. HEPPS, and E. E. SWENSON: Hemodiluation with and wit out low-molecular dextran: Laboratory studies and clinical experienc Circulation **28**, 792 (1963).

1207. —, E. E. SWENSON, S. A. HEPPS, and D. L. BRUNS: Total body perfusion cardiac operations. Arch. Surg. **88**, 128 (1964).

1208. —, J. C. HUTCHINSON, and E. E. SWENSON: High-flow body perfusion wi calculated hemodilution. Ann. thorac. Surg. **1**, 581 (1965).

1209. ROE, C. F., M. J. GOLDBERG, C. S. BLAIR, and J. M. KINNEY: The influence body temperature on early postoperative oxygen consumption. Surge **60**, 85 (1966).

1210. ROSENQVIST, H.: The primary treatment of extensive burns. Acta chir. scan **95**, suppl. 124 (1947).

1211. —, and G. THORSÉN: Macrodex in the treatment of extensive burns. Arc Surg. **62**, 524 (1951).

1212. Rosenthal, A.: Der Verbrennungsschock. Koblenz: Verlag Ziviler Luftschutz Dr. Ebeling KG 1960.
1213. Rosenthal, S. M., and H. Tabor: Electrolyte changes and chemotherapy in experimental burn and traumatic shock and hemorrhage. Arch. Surg. **51**, 244 (1945).
1214. —, and R. C. Millican: The role of fluids, electrolytes and plasma proteins in experimental traumatic shock and hemorrhage. Pharmacol. Rev. **6**, 489 (1954).
1215. Ross, S., and R. Ebert: Microelectrophoresis of blood platelets and the effects of dextran. J. clin. Invest. **38**, 155 (1959).
1216. Rossano, C.: Un polimerizzato di polipeptidi della gelatina proposto come nuovo sostituto del plasma. Minerva anest. **29**, 383 (1963).
1217. Rothman, S., E. Adelson, A. Schwebel, and R. D. Langdell: Adsorption of carbon-14-dextran to human blood platelets and red blood cells in vitro. Vox Sang. **2**, 104 (1957).
1218. Rothschild, M. A., M. Oratz, E. Wimer, and S. S. Schreiber: Effects of dextran on cortisone-induced hyperlipemia in rabbits. Proc. Soc. exp. Biol. **104**, 478 (1960).
1219. Rowe, D. S.: Colloid osmotic pressures of dextran, serum and dextran-serum mixtures. Nature (Lond) **175**, 554 (1955).
1219a. Royster, T. S.: Thrombophlebitis after vena caval clipping. Amer. J. Surg. **113**, 754 (1967).
1220. Rozenberg, G. Y., A. A. From, T. V. Polushina, E. A. Chernysheva, and R. I. Lavrova: Optimal molecular weight for the blood substitute polyglucin. Fed. Proc. **25**, T805 (1966).
1221. Rozenfeld, E. L.: The enzymic splitting of dextrans by extracts of the spleen. Biohimija **21**, 84 (1956); ref.: Chem. Abstr. **50**, 10 148d (1956).
1222. —, and I. S. Lukomskaya: The hydrolysis of 1 : 6 bonds of dextran by animal tissues. Biohimija **21**, 312 (1956); ref.: Chem. Abstr. **50**, 16 906 a (1956).
1223. —, A. I. Shubina, and A. A. Kuznetsov: Cleavage of dextran by spleen extracts. Doklady Akad. nauk. S.S.S.R. **104**, 115 (1955); ref.: Chem. Abstr. **50**, 5806f (1956).
1224. —, and I. S. Lukomskaya: The splitting of dextran and isomaltose by animal tissues. Clin. chim. Acta **2**, 105 (1957).
1225. —, and A. S. Saienko: Metabolism in vivo of clinical dextran. Clin. chim. Acta **10**, 223 (1964).
1226. Rubinson, R. M., F. Holland, P. J. Schmidt, and A. G. Morrow: Serum hepatitis after open-heart operations. J. thorac. cardiovasc. Surg. **50**, 575 (1965).
1226a. Rudenstam, C. M.: Experimental studies on trauma and metastasis formation. Acta Chir. Scand. Suppl. 391 (1968).
1227. Rudin, C. L.: Das Dextran (Macrodex) im Rahmen der Plasmaersatzfrage. Diss. Basel, 1953.
1228. Rügheimer, E., u. R. Leutschaft: Kalt- oder Warmblutinfusion beim hämorrhagischen Schock? Experimentelle und klinische Untersuchungen. Arch. klin. Chir. **301**, 135 (1962).
1229. —, u. H. Grimm: Kalt- oder Warmtransfusion im haemorrhagischen Schock. Bibl. haemat. **20**, 101 (1965).
1229a. Rush, B. F.: Treatment of experimental shock: Comparison of the effects of norepinephrine, dibenzyline, dextran, whole blood, and balanced saline solutions. Surgery **61**, 938 (1967).

1229b. Rush, B. F., and B. Eiseman: Limits of non-colloid solution replacement in experimental hemorrhagic shock. Ann. Surg. **165,** 977 (1967).

1229c. —, and R. Morehouse: Volume replacement following acute bleeding compared to replacement after hemorrhagic shock: Effectiveness of dextran and buffered saline. Surgery **62,** 88 (1967).

1230. Rushmer, R. F., R. L. Van Citters, and D. L. Franklin: Some axioms, popular notions, and misconceptions regarding cardiovascular control. Circulation **27,** 118 (1963).

1231. Russell, H. E., R. R. Bradham, and W. H. Lee: Evaluation of infusion therapy for venous thrombosis. Circulation **32,** suppl. **2,** 184 (1965).

1232. —, R. R. Bradham, and W. H. Lee: An evaluation of infusion therapy (including dextran) for venous thrombosis. Circulation **33,** 839 (1966).

1233. Rustad, H.: Gangrene of the lower extremity of venous origin. J. cardiovasc. Surg. **4,** 357 (1963).

1234. — Factors affecting blood volume determination in surgical patients. Acta chir. scand. **131,** 9 (1966).

1235. —, P. Bjornstad, B. Fretheim, H. N. Haugen, J. Kofstad, R. Nesbakken, and S. C. Sommerfelt: Changes in blood volume, plasma volume, and red cell volume following gastric resection. Acta chir. scand. suppl. **357,** 127 (1966).

1236. Safar, P., L. Harris, B. Kirimli, and M. Takaori: Treatment of exsanguinating hemorrhage. Acta anaesth. scand. suppl. **15,** 142 (1964).

1237. Saegesser, M.: Der hypovolämische Schock. Praktisch-klinische Beobachtungen. Schweiz. med. Wschr. **95,** 95 (1965).

1238. Sajtos, L., L. Józsa, M. Perneczky u. G. Lusztig: Chemische Untersuchungen bei der durch Dextran gehemmten Cholesterinsklerose. Z. ges. inn. Med. **17,** 13 (1962).

1239. Sakai, Y., and F. J. Lewis: A study on platelet aggregation and blood velocity in vitro. J. thorac. cardiovasc. Surg. **49,** 982 (1965).

1240. Salsbury, A. J.: Transfusion of blood fractions. Practitioner **195,** 193 (1965).

1241. Sapirstein, L.: Macromolecular exchanges in capillaries. In: S. R. M. Reynolds, and B. W. Zweifach: Microcirculation: Symposium on factors influencing exchange of substances across capillary wall, p. 47. Urbana: Univ. of Illinois Press 1959.

1242. Sawyer, R. B., J. A. Moncrief, and P. C. Canizaro: Dextran therapy for thrombophlebitis. J. Amer. med. Ass. **188,** 450 (1964).

1243. — — — Dextran therapy in thrombophlebitis. J. Amer. med. Ass. **191,** 740 (1965).

1244. — — Dextran specificity in thrombus inhibition. Arch. Surg. **90,** 562 (1965).

1245. Sayers, M. A., G. Sayers, and C. N. H. Long: Standardization of hemorrhagic shock in rats. Amer. J. Physiol. **147,** 155 (1946).

1246. Sayman, W. A., R. L. Gauld, S. A. Star, and J. G. Allen: Safety of liquid plasma—statistical appraisal. J. Amer. med. Ass. **168,** 1735 (1958).

1247. —, and G. J. Allen: Blood plasma and expanders of plasma volume in the treatment of hemorrhagic shock. Surg. Clin. N. Amer. **39,** 133 (1959).

1248. Sborov, V. M., B. Giges, and J. D. Mann: Incidence of hepatitis following use of pooled plasma. Follow-up study in 587 Korean casualties. Arch. intern. Med. **92,** 678 (1953).

1249. Scatchard, G.: Some physical chemical aspects of plasma extenders. Ann. N. Y. Acad. Sci. **55,** 455 (1952).

1250. SCHALLOCK, G.: Anatomische Untersuchungen über das Schicksal von Blutersatzmitteln im Empfängerorganismus und der durch sie ausgelösten Reaktionen. Beitr. path. Anat. **108**, 405 (1943).
1251. SCHECHTER, I., and S. HESTRIN: Use of levan as an expander of blood-volume. Vox Sang. **8**, 82 (1963).
1252. — — Levulan as a blood expander: Relationship of polymer size and behavior in the organisms. J. lab. clin. Med. **61**, 962 (1963).
1253. SCHEGA, H. W.: Das Oedem der Magen- und Darmwand nach intravenösen Infusionen. Arch. klin. Chir. **276**, 478 (1953).
1254. — Eine Methodik zur fortlaufenden Registrierung postinfusioneller Oedembildung am Magen-Darm-Kanal des lebenden Versuchstieres. Z. ges. exp. Med. 122, 387 (1953).
1255. — Die Oedembildungen in den Wandungen des Magen-Darm-Kanals nach intravenösen Infusionen. Bruns Beitr. klin. Chir. **188**, 109 (1954).
1256. — Experimentelle Untersuchungen zur Frage der osmotherapeutischen Beeinflußbarkeit des Oedems. Arch. klin. Chir. **280**, 479 (1955).
1257. SCHENK, W. G., JR., F. A. CAMP, K. B. KJARTANSSON, and L. POLLOCK: Hemorrhage without hypotension. Ann. Surg. **160**, 7 (1964).
1258. —, N. A. DELIN, E. DOMANIG, P. HAHNLOSER, and R. K. HOYT: Blood viscosity as a determinant of regional blood flow. Arch. Surg. **89**, 783 (1964).
1259. SCHERER, F. u. K. H. WUNSCH: Klinische Erfahrungen mit einem neuen Plasmaexpander. Chirurg **34**, 356 (1963).
1260. SCHJELDERUP, H.: Traume og Rheomacrodex. Nord. Med. **75**, 247 (1966).
1261. SCHLUETER, T. M., and T. R. KELLY: Effect of low molecular weight dextrans and fibrinolysins on hemorrhagic shock. Surg. Forum **15**, 32 (1964).
1262. SCHMID, L.: Die Wirkung verschiedener Dextranfraktionen auf die Endotoxinresistenz der Maus. Helv. chir. Acta **35**, 378 (1968).
1263. SCHMIDT, G.: Der Arzt am Unfallort. Der Hannover-Vorschlag für einen Arzt-Unfall-Koffer. Dtsch. Ärztebl. **61**, 206 (1964).
1264. SCHMIDT, H. D., u. J. SCHMIER: Kontraktilitätsschädigung des Herzens im frühen hämorrhagischen Schock. Pflügers Arch. ges. Physiol. **285**, 241 (1965).
1265. SCHMIDT, K.: Herzzeitvolumensteigerung durch Volumenersatzmittel; in O. H. JUST und H. LUTZ: Genese und Therapie des hämorrhagischen Schocks, p. 68 (Thieme, Stuttgart 1965).
1265a. —, u. H. SCHMALZ: Zur Blutvolumenänderung nach Osmo-Onko-Therapie. Anaesthesist **16**, 201 (1967).
1266. SCHMIDT, W., V. STEINERT u. G. KLAPPACH: Experimenteller Beitrag zum therapeutischen Einsatz des Dextrans im Ileus. Pharmazie **21**, 304 (1966).
1267. SCHMIDT-THOMÉ, J., A. MAGER u. H. H. SCHÖNE: Zur Chemie eines neuen Plasmaexpanders. Arzneimittelforsch. **12**, 378 (1962).
1268. SCHMUTZER, K. J., E. RASCHKE, and J. V. MALONEY JR.: Intravenous l-norepinephrine as a cause of reduced plasma volume. Surgery **50**, 452 (1961).
1269. SCHNABEL, T. G., JR., H. ELIASCH, B. THOMASSON, and L. WERKÖ: The effect of experimentally induced hypervolemia on cardiac function in normal subjects and patients with mitral stenosis. J. clin. Invest. **38**, 117 (1959).
1270. SCHNEIDER, K. W.: Gefahren der Bluttransfusion in der inneren Medizin. Med. Welt 1899, 1960.
1271 —, u. L. PIPPIG: Der Einfluß von Humanalbumininfusionen auf die Hämodynamik. Dtsch. med. Wschr. **87**, 1291 (1962).
1272. — Diskussion. Bibl. haemat. **16**, 104 (1963).

1273. Schneider, K. W.: Der hämorrhagische Schock. In: Verh. VII. internat. Kongr. inn. Med. München, p. 398. Stuttgart: Thieme 1963.

1274. — Kurz- und langfristige Blutvolumenveränderungen nach Infusion von Erythrozytenkonzentrat und modernen Plasmaexpandern unter Verwendung des Volemetron-Gerätes. Bibl. haemat. **20,** 159 (1965).

1275. — Diskussion. Bibl. haemat. **20,** 181 (1965).

1276. —, K. Klütsch, A. Heidland, E. von Parish u. A. Gathof: Blutvolumen, Serum-Elektrolyte und Eiweiß nach Infusion von pasteurisierten Plasma. Bibl. haemat. **23,** 1120 (1965).

1277. — Fragekasten. Münch. med. Wschr. **107,** 347 (1965).

1278. — Volumenmangel als Elementargefährdung und als therapeutisches Problem in der Praxis. Therapiewoche **15,** 1047 (1965).

1279. — Die Wandlungen in der Lehre der Schockpathogenese und der Schocktherapie in den letzten 15 Jahren. Med. heute **15,** 133 (1966).

1280. Schneider, M.: Zur Pathophysiologie der verschiedenen Schockformen. Bibl. haemat. **16,** 10 (1963).

1281. — Zur Pathophysiologie des Schocks. In: K. Horatz u. R. Frey: Schock und Plasmaexpander, p. 1. Berlin-Göttingen-Heidelberg: Springer 1964.

1282. Schneider, W., u. H. J. Köster: Zur Beurteilung von Transfusionsreaktionen. Konsequenzen für die Praxis. Münch. med. Wschr. **108,** 1478 (1966).

1283. Schoch, T. J.: The chemistry of hydroxyethyl starch. In: Second Conference on Artificial Colloidal Agents, p. 121. Washington, D. C.: Nat. Acad. Sci. 1963.

1284. Scholer, H.: Das Blutvolumen, eine klinisch relevante, aber wesensmäßig unbekannte Betriebsgröße. Bull. schweiz. Akad. med. Wiss. **19,** 235 (1963).

1285. —, u. M. Schnös: Probleme des Blutvolumens in der Cardiologie. Hinweis auf ein neues Gerät auf Isotopen-Basis. Cardiologia **42,** 74 (1963).

1286. — Das Blutvolumen, Versuch einer Deutung seines Wesens. Med. Welt 182, 1964.

1287. Scholtan, W.: Über die Adsorptionsfähigkeit wasserlöslicher polymerer Verbindungen, insbesondere Polyvinylpyrrolidon. Makromol. Chemie **11,** 131 (1953).

1288. — Bestimmung der Molekulargewichtsverteilung von Polyvinylpyrrolidon mit kleinem und großem Molekulargewicht und von Albumin in der Ultrazentrifuge. Makromol. Chemie **36,** 162 (1960).

1289. Schoen, H.: Organveränderungen beim Säugling nach Zufuhr von Periston. Klin. Wschr. **27,** 463 (1949).

1290. Schubert, R.: Über die Ausscheidung an Periston gebundener Stoffe. (Bilirubin, Indigocarmin) und einiges über die Ausscheidung von Periston selbst. Klin. Wschr. **26,** 143 (1948).

1291. —, G. Seybold u. H. Wundt: Zellsanierung durch Kollidon. Versuche an Frosch und Meerschweinchen mit Diaminreinblau, Trypanblau und niedermolekularem Kollidon. Z. klin. Med. **147,** 513 (1951).

1292. — — Entfernung granulär gespeicherter Stoffe aus gewissen Zellsystemen durch Kollidon verschiedenen Molekulargewichts. Ärztl. Forsch. **6,** 1 (1952).

1293. —, D. Klaus u. U. Lutz-Dettinger: Klinische Erfahrungen beim Vergleich der Clearance von Inulin, PAH und Polyvinylpyrrolidon bei Nierengesunden und Nierenkranken. Medizinische **14,** 639 (1959).

1294. SCHÜLKE, K., u. W. HARTEL: Vergleichende Untersuchungen über das Verhalten der Plasmaviskosität und des Blutvolumens nach Gabe von hoch- und niedermolekularen Dextranen. Arch. klin. Chir. **316**, 623 (1966).

1295. SCHUMER, W.: Physiochemical and metabolic effects of low molecular weight dextran in oligemic shock. J. Trauma **7**, 40 (1967).

1296. SCHWAIGER, M., u. K. SCHMEISER: Zur Infusionstherapie nach Eingriffen am Magen. Chirurg **21**, 613 (1956).

1297. SCHWARTZ, S. I.: Blood-transfusion, coagulation, thrombosis and thrombolysis. In: W. F. BALLINGER: Research methods in surgery, p. 221. Boston: Little, Brown 1964.

1298. —, H. P. SHAY, H. BEEBE, and C. ROB: Effect of low molecular weight dextran on venous flow. Surgery **55**, 106 (1964).

1299. SCHWARTZKOPFF, W.: Zur Wirkung von Dextran als Plasmaexpander. Z. klin. Med. **157**, 156 (1962).

1300. — Determination of permeability of the abdominal capillary membranes with low and high molecular substances. Bibl. anat. **7**, 156 (1965).

1301. SCHWEIZER, O., and W. S. HOWLAND: Effect of citrated bank blood on acid-base balance. Surg. Gynec. Obstet. **114**, 90 (1962).

1302. SCHWENZER, A. W.: Neuzeitliche Sicherungen bei Bluttransfusionen. 3b. Hepatitis. Ergebn. inn. Med. Kinderheilk. **5**, 415 (1954).

1303. SCHWICK, G., u. U. FREUND: Immunologische Untersuchungen mit Haemaccel. Dtsch. med. Wschr. **87**, 737 (1962).

1304. SCHWIEGK, H.: Schock und Kollaps. Klin. Wschr. **21**, 741, 765 (1942).

1305. SCOTT, C. C., H. M. WORTH, and E. B. ROBBINS: Comparative value of some blood substitutes used for treatment of experimental shock. Arch. Surg. **48**, 315 (1944).

1306. SCOTT, J.: Blood coagulation failure in obstetrics. Brit. med. J. **II**, 290 (1955).

1307. SCUDDER, J.: Shock: Blood studies as a guide to therapy. Philadelphia: Lippincott 1940.

1308. SEAMAN, G. V. F., W. HISSEN, L. LINO, and R. L. SWANK: Physico-chemical changes in blood arising from dextran infusions. Clin. Sci. **29**, 293 (1965).

1308a. SEAMAN, A. J., C. L. LUTCHER, C. A. MOFFAT, and B. E. HUEBER: Induced intravascular thromboembolic phenomena. Arch. intern. Med. **119**, 600 (1967).

1309. SEAVERS, R., and P. B. PRICE: Effects and fate of blood transfusions in normal dogs. Arch. Surg. **59**, 275 (1949).

1310. SEEGERS, W. H., W. G. LEVINE, and S. A. JOHNSON: Inhibition of prothrombin activation with dextran. J. appl. Physiol. **7**, 617 (1955).

1311. SEELEY, S. F., and J. R. WEISINGER: Recent progress and present problems in the field of shock. Fed. Proc. suppl. 9 (Washington, D. C., 1961).

1312. SEGAL, A.: The clinical use of dextran solution. New York: Grune & Stratton 1964.

1313. SEMPLE, R.: The effects of single large infusions of various dextran solutions on hypovolemic dogs. Canad. J. Biochem. Physiol. **32**, 670 (1954).

1314. — Changes in protein fractions of dog plasma after bleeding and dextran infusion. J. lab. clin. Med. **45**, 61 (1955).

1315. SENIOR, J. R.: Post-transfusion hepatitis. Gastroenterology **49**, 315 (1965).

1316. SENN, L. Y., and K. E. KARLSON: Methodologic and actual error of plasma volume determination. Surgery **44**, 1095 (1958).

1317. SERKES, K. D., S. LANG, and M. D. PAREIRA: Efficacy of plasma and dextran compared to saline for fluid replacement following toruniquet shock. Surgery **45**, 623 (1959).
1318. — — — The time relationship in plasma-volume response to graded hemorrhage. Surgery **56**, 380 (1964).
1319. — — — Blood volume, methodology and applications. Monogr. surg. Sci. **2**, 69 (1965).
1320. — — — Enhanced protection with the use of gamma globulin proteins in the treatment of tourniquet shock with plasma expanders. Surgery **59**, 566 (1966).
1321. — — Changes in extracellular fluid volume after hemorrhage and tourniquet trauma. Surg. Forum **17**, 58 (1966).
1322. SEVESO, M.: Su di un nuovo sostituto del plasma. Minerva anest. **29**, 398 (1963).
1323. SEVITT, S.: The boundaries between physiology, pathology, and irreversibility after injury. Lancet **II**, 1203 (1966).
1324. SHANBROM, E., R. H. BERGER, and J. W. GRACELY: Observations on the inhibition of erythrocyte sedimentation by low molecular weight dextran. Amer. J. med. Sci. **246**, 289 (1963).
1325. SHERMAN, P. H., D. KRUMHAAR, T. TANAKA, L. R. BENNETT, and J. V. MALONEY, JR.: Measurement of intravascular erythrocyte sequestration by $Cr^{51}$: Effect of endotoxin in dogs and clinical status, extracorporeal circulation and rapid sampling in man. Ann. Surg. **164**, 23 (1966).
1326. SHILLING, D. A., E. H. GINN, W. R. RICHARDSON, and H. E. DUNLAP: A new approach to fluid therapy of the severly burned patient. Ann. Surg. **150**, 756 (1959).
1327. SHIMADA, N., T. FUKUDA, Y. ISHII, D. SEKIKAWA, M. OHTSUKI, M. MATSUA, K. KODEKI, G. OHYA, F. NAGAO, N. KIMURA, S. NAKANO, S. MURAKAMI, S. MIYAMOTO, and T. TSUCHIYA: Serum hepatitis in Japan. Bibl. haemat. **23**, 1066 (1965).
1328. SHIRES, G. T., J. WILLIAMS, and F. BROWN: Simultaneous measurement of plasma volume, extracellular fluid volume, and red blood cell mass in man utilising $I^{131}S^{35}O_4$, and $Cr^{51}$. J. lab. clin. Med. **55**, 776 (1960).
1329. —, F. T. BROWN, P. CANIZARO, and N. SOMERVILLE: Distributional changes in extracellular fluid during acute hemorrhagic shock. Surg. Forum **11**, 115 (1960).
1330. —, D. COLN, J. CARRICO, and S. LIGHTFOOT: Fluid therapy in hemorrhagic shock. Arch. Surg. **88**, 688 (1964).
1331. —, C. J. CARRICO, and D. COLN: The role of the extracellular fluid in shock. Int. Anesth. Clin. **2**, 435 (1964).
1332. — — Current status of the shock problem. In: M. M. RAVITCH: Current problems in surgery, p. 1. Chicago: Yearbook Med. Publ. 1966.
1333. SHOEMAKER, W. C.: Recent additions to the knowledge of the cause and management of shock. Surg. Clin. N. Amer. **42**, 3 (1962).
1334. — Measurement of rapidly and slowly circulating red cell volumes in hemorrhagic shock. Amer. J. Physiol. **202**, 1179 (1962).
1335. —, and F. IIDA: Studies on the equilibration of labeled red cells and T-1824 in hemorrhagic shock. Surg. Gynec. Obstet. **114**, 539 (1962).
1336. — Pathophysiologic mechanisms in shock and their therapeutic implications. Amer. J. Surg. **110**, 337 (1965).
1337. —, U. BRUNIUS, and L.-E. GELIN: Hemodynamic and microcirculatory effects of high and low viscosity dextrans. Surgery **58**, 518 (1965).

1337a. SHOEMAKER, W. C.: Shock, chemistry, physiology and therapy. Springfield, Ill.: Thomas 1967.

1338. SCHUMACKER, H. B., D. HAWTOF, T. HERENDEEN, D. JUDD, and M. K. WEBB: Osmotic diuresis and experimental renal ischemia. Surgery **55**, 687 (1964).

1339. SIEGEL, D. L., A. BILGUTAY, L. SANCHEZ, and C. W. LILLEHEI: Experience with an artificial plasma for use with extracorporeal circulation. J. Amer. med. Ass. **179**, 206 (1962).

1340. SILK, M. R.: The effect of dextran and hydroxyethyl starch on renal hemodynamics. J. Trauma **6**, 717 (1966).

1341. SILVAY, J., M. SCHNORRER, E. ŠUJANSKÝ u. J. STYK: Die Auswahl von Ersatzlösungen zur Füllung der Herz-Lungen-Maschine. Arch. klin. Chir. **316**, 630 (1966).

1342. SIMEONE, F. A.: Traumatic shock—the physiologic effects of blood loss. Bull. New Engl. Med. Center **10**, 112 (1948).

1343. — Shock and blood pressure. Surg. Gynec. Obstet. **108**, 740 (1959).

1344. — Hemorrhagic shock. Amer. J. Cardiol. **12**, 589 (1963).

1345. —, and F. J. DAGHER: Treatment of hemorrhagic shock in the dog with dextran and hydroxyethyl starch. In: Third Conference on Artificial Colloidal Agents, p. 150. Washington, D. C.: Nat. Acad. Sci. 1965.

1346. SIMON, E., et M. HASCHER: Un soluté de gélatine fluide modifiée: Plasmagel en pratique courante de réanimation. Bibl. haemat. **10**, 481 (1958).

1347. SIMON, S., and T. SIMON: The duration of the effect of polyvinylpyrrolidone and dextran preparations in hemorrhagic shock of the cat. Acta physiol. Acad. Sci. hung. **23**, 189 (1963).

1348. SINGER, A.: Low-molecular-weight dextran in the treatment of peripheral arterial insufficiency. Lancet **II**, 1050 (1965).

1349. SJOKK: Sjokksyndromenes patofysiologi, klinikk og terapi. T. norske Laegeforen. **86**, 579 (1966).

1350. SJÖSTRAND, T.: Volume and distribution of blood and their significance in regulating the circulation. Physiol. Rev. **33**, 202 (1953).

1351. — Blood volume. In: Handbook of physiology, section 2: Circulation, vol. 1, p. 51. Washington, D. C.: Amer. Physiol. Soc. 1962.

1352. SJÖSTRÖM, B.: Infusion therapy after controlled bleeding. An investigation by means of animal experiments. Acta Soc. Med. upsalien. **59**, 17 (1953).

1353. SKINSNES, O. K.: Gelatin nephrosis, renal tissue changes in man resulting from the intravenous administration of gelatin. Surg. Gynec. Obstet. **85**, 563 (1947).

1354. SMITH, B., M. AL OMERI, D. G. MELROSE, H. H. BENTALL, and S. ALLWORK: Blood-loss after cardio-pulmonary bypass. Lancet **II**, 273 (1964).

1355. SMITH, E. L., S. DEAVERS, R. A. HUGGINS, and G. STOLZOFF: Effects of time and volume of blood overtransfused on the loss of plasma and protein in the dog. Amer. J. Physiol. **196**, 1039 (1959).

1356. — — — Effects of autologous and homologous blood replacement in hypovolemic dogs. Proc. Soc. exp. Biol. **120**, 199 (1965).

1357. SMITH, L. L., and B. W. BRANSON: Refractory hypotension. Calif. Med. **95**, 150 (1961).

1358. —, and F. D. MOORE: Refractory hypotension in man—is this irreversible shock? New Engl. J. Med. **267**, 733 (1962).

1359. —, R. L. FOSTER, and W. MÜLLER: Intrinsic cardiac output variability in the anesthetized normal and splenectomized dog. Amer. J. Physiol. **202**, 1155 (1962).

1360. SMITH, L. L., W. MÜLLER, U. P. VERAGUT, and W. D. JOLLEY: Hemodynamik effects of acute salt depletion and hemorrhage in the dog. Surg. Gynec. Obstet. **118**, 1263 (1964).

1361. — Physiologic considerations in the diagnosis and management of shock. Med. Arts Sci. **19**, 29 (1965).

1362. SMITH, M. C.: The dextrans. Amer. J. Hosp. Pharmacy **22**, 273 (1965).

1363. SMITH, O. A., JR., S. J. JABBUR, R. F. RUSHMER, and E. P. LASHER: Role of hypothalamic structures in cardiac control. Physiol. Rev. **40**, suppl. 4, 136 (1960).

1364. SMYTHE, C. MCC., J. P. GILMORE, J. V. MALONEY, and S. W. HANDFORD: An analysis of the direct hydraulic effect of intra-arterial transfusion. Amer. J. Physiol. **178**, 412 (1954).

1365. SNEDDON, E.: Preoperative blood volumes. Amer. Surg. **30**, 370 (1964).

1366. SNYDER, H. E., B. B. CARLISLE, H. E. WOLLOWICK, and J. H. FOSTER: Protection of kidneys following experimental acute ischemia. Effect of intra-arterial Mannitol and low-molecular-weight dextran. Amer. Surg. **32**, 9 (1966).

1367. SOLYOM, A., G. CSEH, I. K. SZABÓ, and K. VILLANYI: The effect of polysaccharides not containing sulphur on fat metabolism. Acta physiol. Acad. Sci. hung. **26**, 73 (1965).

1368. SOMER, T.: The viscosity of blood, plasma and serum in dys- and paraproteinemias. Acta med. scand. **180**, suppl. 456 (1966).

1369. SPEAR, P. W., M. SASS, and J. J. CIUCOTTI: Ammonium levels in transfused blood. J. lab. clin. Med. **48**, 702 (1956).

1370. SPIELMANN, W.: Serologische und anaphylaktische Eigenschaften des Dextrans. Anaesthesist **8**, 41 (1959).

1371. — Können moderne Plasmavolumenexpander die Ergebnisse der serologischen Untersuchungen vor Bluttransfusionen stören? In: K. HORATZ u. R. FREY: Schock und Plasmaexpander, p. 152. Berlin-Göttingen-Heidelberg: Springer 1964.

1372. — Transfusionskunde. Stuttgart: Thieme 1967.

1373. SPINK, W. W.: Circulatory shock. A symposium on advances in the understanding of mechanisms and treatment. Calif. Med. **103**, 310 (1965).

1374. SPIRGI, E.: Über Blutbedarf bei chirurgischen Eingriffen. Méd Hyg. **22**, 589 (1964).

1375. SPOEREL, W. E., and F. C. HEAGY: Blood volume determination for evaluation of blood loss during operation. Canad. J. Surg. **5**, 25 (1962).

1376. SQUIRE, J. R., J. P. BULL, W. D'A. MAYCOCK, and C. R. RICKETTS: Dextran, its properties and use in medicine. Oxford: Blackwell 1955.

1377. STAIB, I., D. MAROSKE, P. DRINGS u. H. OEHMIG: Änderungen des Herzminutenvolumens (HMV) nach verschiedenen Medikamenten und Plasmaexpandern. Arch. klin. Chir. **308**, 848 (1964).

1378. STALKER, A. L.: Intravascular erythrocyte aggregation. Bibl. anat. **4**, 108 (1964).

1378a. STAMPFLI, K.: Posttransfusionelle Hepatitiden mit letalem Verlauf. Schweiz. med. Wschr. **97**, 1487 (1967).

1379. STARLING, E. H.: On the absorption of fluids from the connective tissue spaces. J. Physiol. **19**, 312 (1896).

1380. STEAD, E. A., JR., and R. V. EBERT: Studies on human albumin. In: S. MUDD, and W. THALHIMER: Blood substitutes and blood transfusion, p. 185. Springfield, Ill.: Thomas 1942.

1381. Steele, R., D. D. van Slyke, and J. Plazin: The fate of intravenously administered polyvinylpyrrolidone. Ann. N.Y. Acad. Sci. **55**, 479 (1952).

1382. Steinbrunn, W.: Einfluß verschiedener Plasmaersatzstoffe auf den Säure-, Basen- und Elektrolythaushalt beim normovolämischen Kaninchen. Z. ges. exp. Med. **140**, 1 (1966).

1383. Steinfeld, J. L., F. E. Greene, D. L. Tabern, R. R. Paton, and A. L. Flick: Degradation of iodinated human serum albumin prepared by various procedures. J. lab. clin. Med. **51**, 756 (1958).

1483a. Wangensteen, S. L., H. B. Hechtmann, L. R. Rose, and C. F. Vor der Bruegge: The army in surgical research. J. surg. Res. **7**, 239 (1967).

1384. Steinhausen, M. von, A. Loreth u. S. Olson: Tubuläre Harnstromstärken von Katzen, ihre Abhängigkeit vom arteriellen Druck und von experimentellen Änderungen der Harnviskosität. Pflügers Arch. ges. Physiol. **283**, R23 (1965).

1385. Stěrba, O., J. Horejši u. R. Petz: Experimentelle Schocktherapie mit den durch Glutathion verstärkten Blutplasmaersatzlösungen. Blut **12**, 236 (1966).

1386. Stern, K.: Effect of polyvinylpyrrolidone on reticuloendothelial storage. Proc. Soc. exp. Biol. **79**, 618 (1952).

1387. —, S. Busch, and A. Buznitsky: Experiences and experiments with crossmatching procedures. Bibl. haemat. **7**, 420 (1958).

1388. Stevens, A. R., J. S. Legg, B. S. Henry, J. M. Dille, W. M. M. Kirby, and C. A. Finch: Fatal transfusion reactions from contamination of stored blood by cold growing bacteria. Ann. intern. Med. **39**, 1228 (1953).

1389. Stewart, J. D., and G. M. Rourke: Intracellular fluid loss in hemorrhage. J. clin. Invest. **15**, 697 (1936).

1390. Stoeckel, H., S. J. Walter u. J. Voll: Die Rolle der Bluttransfusion für die Entstehung des postoperativen Ikterus. Arch. klin. Chir. **313**, 111 (1965).

1391. Stoner, H. B., and C. J. Threlfall: The biochemical response to injury. In: Lectures on the scientific basis of medicine. Oxford: Blackwell 1960.

1392. — Critical analysis of traumatic shock models. Fed. Proc. suppl. **9**, 38 (1961).

1393. Strawitz, J. G., H. Hift, R. L. Temple, A. Erhardt, and N. Rozansky: Irreversible hemorrhagic shock in rats: Method and critical bleeding volume. Amer. J. Physiol. **200**, 257 (1961).

1394. —, and N. Grossblatt: Septic shock. Washington, D. C.: Nat. Acad. Sci., Nat. Res. Counc. 1965.

1395. Streicher, H.-J., K. Eberhardt u. W. Kirmess: Hemmen Plasmaexpander die Leukocytenausschwemmung aus dem Knochenmark? Arch. klin. Chir. **311**, 252 (1965).

1396. Strumia, M. M., W. H. Crosby, J. G. Gibson, T. J. Greenwalt, and J. R. Krevans: General principles of blood transfusion. Transfusion **3**, 306 (1963).

1397. Sugg, J. Y., and E. J. Hehre: Reactions of dextran of Leuconostoc mesenteroides with the antiserum of Leuconostoc and of types 2, 20 and 12 pneumococcus. J. Immunol. **43**, 119 (1942).

1397a. Sundt, T. M., A. G. Waltz, and G. P. Sayre: Experimental cerebral infarction: Modification by treatment with hemodiluting, hemoconcentrating, and dehydrating agents. J. Neurosurg. **26**, 46 (1967).

1398. Suzuki, F., and W. C. Shoemaker: Effect of low viscosity dextran on red cell circulation in hemorrhagic shock. Surgery **55**, 304 (1964).

1399. Suzuki, F., R. J. Baker, and W. C. Shoemaker: Red cell and plasma volume alteration after hemorrhage and trauma. Ann. Surg. **160**, 263 (1964).
1400. —, W. C. Shoemaker, R. J. Baker and J. S. Carey: Use of labeled red cells and low viscosity dextran in the study of trapped blood. Surg. Gynec. Obstet. **121**, 51 (1965).
1401. Swan, H. J., J. Blavier, T. Marchioro, D. Jenkins, and V. Montgomery: Experimental hemorrhage. Arch. Surg. **79**, 176 (1959).
1402. Swan, H., V. Montgomery, D. Jenkins, and T. L. Marchioro: A method for the continuous measurement of plasma volume in the dog. Ann. Surg. **151**, 319 (1960).
1403. Swank, R. L.: Suspension stability of the blood after injections of dextran. J. appl. Physiol. **12**, 125 (1958).
1404. —, J. H. Fellman, and W. W. Hissen: Influence of aggregation of blood cells on screen filtration pressure and blood flow. Bibl. anat. **7**, 185 (1965).
1405. —, and E. Davis: Blood cell aggregation and screen filtration pressure. Circulation **33**, 617 (1966).
1406. —, G. V. F. Seaman, W. Hissen, and L. Lino: Physicochemical changes in blood induced by trauma. Surg. Gynec. Obstet. **123**, 251 (1966).
1407. Swingle, W. W., W. Kleinberg, and H. W. Hays: A study of gelatin and saline as plasma substitutes. Amer. J. Physiol. **141**, 329 (1944).
1408. — — Plasma, gelatin and saline therapy in experimental wound shock. Amer. J. Physiol. **141**, 713 (1944).
1409. Sykes, M. K.: Venous pressure as a clinical indication of adequacy of transfusion. Ann. roy. Coll. Surg. Engl. **33**, 185 (1963).
1410. —, B. Robinson, D. G. Melrose, and R. Nahas: Pulmonary changes after extracorporeal circulation in dogs. Brit. J. Anaesth. **38**, 432 (1966).
1410a. —, F. A. Neematallah, and P. M. Cooke: The effect of low molecular weight dextran and haemodilution on acid-base balance and lactate and pyruvate levels during cardiopulmonary bypass. Brit. J. Anaesth. **39**, 94 (1967).
1411. Symposia on Rheomacrodex, vol. I and II. London: Pharmacia G. B. 1964.
1412. Szabó, G., and Z. Magyar: Kapillarpermeabilität im ischämischen Schock. Acta med. hung. **8**, 287 (1955).
1413. Tabor, H., H. Kabat, and S. M. Rosenthal: The chemotherapy of burns and shock. VI. Standardized hemorrhage in the mouse. VII. Therapy of experimental hemorrhage. Publ. Hlth. Rep. (Wash.) **59**, 637 (1944).
1414. Takaori, M., and P. Safar: Adaptation to acute hemodilution with four blood volume expanders. In: Third Conference on Artificial Colloidal Agents, p. 170. Washington, D. C.: Nat. Acad. Sci 1965.
1415. — — Adaptation to acute severe hemodilution with dextran 75 in dogs. Arch. Surg. **92**, 743 (1966).
1416. — — Treatment of massive hemorrhage with colloid and crystalloid solutions. J. Amer. med. Ass. **199**, 297 (1965).
1417. — — Acute, severe hemodilution with lactated Ringer's solution. Arch. Surg. **94**, 67 (1967).
1418. Takayama, T.: Glyco-algin as a transfusion solution. Bibl. haemat. **7**, 287 (1958).
1419. Tarrow, A. B., and E. J. Pulaski: Reactions in man from infusion with dextran. Anesthesiology **14**, 359 (1953).
1420. Tatooles, C. J., N. S. Braunwald, and A. G. Morrow: Prosthetic replacement of the tricuspid valve. Surg. Forum **16**, 171 (1965).
1421. Taylor, N. B., and E. T. Waters: Isinglass as transfusion fluid in haemorrhage. Canad. med. Ass. J. **44**, 547 (1941).

1422. TERRY, R., and C. L. YUILE: Fate of intravenous $C^{14}$-labeled dextran in dogs. Fed. Proc. **11**, 430 (1952).
1423. — — Reports to Nat. Res. Counc. Washington, D. C.: Nat. Acad. Sci., Nat. Res. Counc. 1952—53.
1424. — —, A. GOLODETZ, C. E. PHILIPS, and R. R. WHITE: Metabolism of dextran—a plasma volume expander. Studies of radioactive carbonlabeled dextran in dogs. J. lab. clin. Med. **42**, 6 (1953).
1425. THAL, A. P.: Shock and metabolism. Surg. Gynec. Obstet. **122**, 283 (1966).
1426. THAUER, R., und K. WEGLER: Die Kreislaufwirkung der gebräuchlichsten tierexperimentellen Narkotika. Arch. exp. Path. Pharmakol. **200**, 84 (1942).
1427. THEYL, R. A., and G. F. TUOHY: Hemodynamics and blood volume during operation with ether anesthesia and unreplaced blood loss. Anesthesiology **25**, 6 (1964).
1428. THOMAS, J. P., and C. F. BARTTER: Blood volume measurements in normal subjects and in patients with cirrhosis or cardiac disease. Clin. Sci. **21**, 301 (1961).
1429. THOMAS, K., u. F. HOFMANN: Herstellung einer albuminreichen pasteurisierbaren und damit hepatitissicheren Plasmaproteinlösung (PPL-D). Dtsch. GesundhWes. **21**, 1168 (1966).
1430. THOMPSON, W. L.: Plasma substitutes. A review. J. Sth Carolina med. Ass. **56**, 456 (1960).
1431. —, J. J. BRITTON, and R. P. WALTON: Blood levels of glucose and total carbohydrate following intravenous infusions of dextran and hydroxyethylated starches. Fed. Proc. **19**, 103 (1960).
1432. — — — Persistance of starch derivates and dextran when infused after hemorrhage. J. Pharmacol. exp. Ther. **136**, 125 (1962).
1433. —, and R. P. WALTON: Parenteral administration of hydroxyethyl starches. In: Conference on Artificial Colloidal Agents, p. 168. Washington, D. C.: Nat. Acad. Sci. 1962.
1434. — —, and L. LEE-BENNER: Intravascular persistance and urinary excretion of hydroxyethyl starch solutions in normovolemic dogs. Fed. Proc. **23**, 539 (1964).
1435. —, D. H. WAYT, and R. P. WALTON: Bleeding volume of hydroxyethyl starch, dextran, blood and glucose. Proc. Soc. exp. Biol. **115**, 474 (1964).
1436. — Interaction of hydroxyethyl starch and dextran with plasma proteins and erythrocyte envelopes. Biorheology **3**, 49 (1966).
1437. THORÉN, L.: Hypovolemic shock. Viewpoints on treatment. Opuscula med. **7**, 72 (1962).
1438. THORSÉN, G.: Dextran as a plasma substitute. Lancet **I**, 132 (1949).
1439. — Resuscitative effect of dextran Ph after large hemorrhages. An experimental study. Acta chir. scand. **100**, 221 (1950).
1440. —, and H. HINT: Aggregation, sedimentation and intravascular sludging of erythrocytes. Acta chir. scand. suppl. **154** (1950).
1441. — Dextran—position in therapy in Sweden 1953 and problems. Ann. Chir. Gynaec. Fenn. **43**, suppl. 5, 445 (1954).
1442. — The use of dextrans as infusion fluids. Surg. Gynec. Obstet. **109**, 43 (1959).
1443. TINCKLER, L. F., and W. KULKE: Postoperative absorption of water from the small intestine. Gut **4**, 8 (1963).
1444. TOPLEY, E.: Studies on the degree and timing of blood transfusion following trauma. Bibl. haemat. **10**, 453 (1959).

1445. TORII, A., S. NAKANO, and Y. MIYAZATO: The use of gammaglobulin in th( prevention of serum hepatitis. Bibl. haemat. **23**, 1055 (1965).

1446. TOURTELOTTE, D.: Modified fluid gelatin as a new plasma expander. V' Congr. int. Transf. sangu., Paris 1954.

1447. —, and H. E. WILLIAMS: Chemical modifications of gelatin for use as plasm; expander. In: G. STAINSBY: Recent advances in gelatin and glue research p. 246. London: Pergamon Press 1957.

1448. — — Acylated gelatins and their preparations. US Patent 2, 827, 419, 1958. II, 761 (1954).

1449. TOVEY, G. H.: Techniques of blood transfusion. Practitioner **195**, 167 (1965)

1450. TRAENCKNER, K.: Das Schicksal des Periston im menschlichen Körper nach histologischen Untersuchungen. Frankf. Z. Path. **65**, 62 (1954).

1451. — Morphologische Nierenveränderungen nach Periston beim Menschen Frankf. Z. Path. **65**, 80 (1954).

1452. — Zur Frage des Schicksals des Dextrans im menschlichen Körper nach histologischen Untersuchungen. Frankf. Z. Path. **65**, 390 (1954).

1453. — Experimentelle Untersuchungen zur Frage der Periston-Speicherung in den Mitochondrien der Nierentubuli. Z. ges. exp. Med. **123**, 101 (1954).

1454. TREDE, M., E. ROTH, A. ENCKE, O. HALLWACHS, M. WANKE u. F. STÖHRER: Vergleichende Untersuchungen über das Verhalten der Nierenfunktion bei Hochverdünnungsperfusionen mit Glucose, Haemaccel und Rheomacrodex. Arch. klin. Chir. **316**, 642 (1966).

1455. TREGEAR, R. T.: The permeability of skin to albumin, dextrans and polyvinylpyrrolidone. J. invest. Derm. **46**, 24 (1966).

1456. TRINER, L., and M. MRÁZ: Some biochemical changes in the blood after dextrane administration. Physiol. bohemoslov. **12**, 128 (1963).

1457. — —, and M. CHMELAŘOVÁ: The favourable effect of glucose and glucose with insulin administered in a dextrane solution on the course of haemorrhagic shock in rabbits. Physiol. bohemoslov. **13**, 87 (1964).

1458. TROBAUGH, F. E., JR., and F. DE CATALDO: Management of transfusion reactions. Med. Clin. N. Amer. **43**, 1537 (1959).

1459. TRUNIGER, B., S. M. ROSEN u. D. E. OKEN: Renale Hämodynamik und hämorrhagische Hypotension. Klin. Wschr. **44**, 857 (1966).

1460. TSCHIRREN, B.: Künstliche Blutersatzsstoffe. Schweiz. med. Wschr. **93**, 596 (1963).

1461. —, u. P. PFISTNER: Praktische Erfahrungen mit Physiogel als Blutersatzstoff. Helv. chir. Acta **33**, 404 (1966).

1462. TURNER, F. P., B. C. BUTTLER, M. E. SMITH, and J. SCUDDER: Dextran. An experimental plasma substitute. Surg. Gynec. Obstet. **88**, 661 (1949).

1463. UEBERMUTH, H.: Neuere Gesichtspunkte zu Schock und Kollaps. Chir. Praxis **8**, 165 (1964).

1464. UPHAM, H. C., F. W. LOVELL, L. E. DETRICK, D. H. HIGHBY, V. DEBLEY, and T. J. HALEY: Tissue deposition of polyvinylpyrrolidone in normal and irradiated rabbits. Arch. int. Pharmacodyn. **106**, 151 (1956).

1465. URSO, L., e F. BRESCHI: I sostituti del plasma in chirurgia. Sperimentazioni e rilievi clinici a proposito di un nuovo plasmaexpander. Minerva anest. **29**, 352 (1963).

1466. VARS, H. M., W. M. PARKINS, and J. H. PERLMUTT: Various plasma expanders in animals. Ann. N.Y. Acad. Sci. **55**, 496 (1952).

1467. VICKERY, A. L.: The fate of dextran in tissues of the acutely wounded; a study of the histologic localization of dextran in tissues of Korean battle casualties. Amer. J. Path. **32**, 161 (1956).

1468. Viereck, H., u. V. Köhler: Die Bedeutung lokal angewandter Kolloide für die Verhütung von Nachblutungen bei der extrapleuralen Pneumolyse. Klin. Wschr. **31**, 855 (1953).

1469. Villasanta, U.: Therapy in antepartum thrombophlebitis. Obstet. Gynec., N.Y. **26**, 534 (1965).

1470. Vineyard, G. C., B. E. Bradley, A. Defalco, D. Lawson, E. T. A. Wagner, W. K. Pastis, F. A. Nardella, and J. R. Hayes: Effect of hydroxyethyl starch on plasma volume and hematocrit following hemorrhagic shock in dogs. Comparison with dextran, plasma and Ringer's. Ann. Surg. **164**, 891 (1966).

1471. Vorhees, B., H. J. Baker, E. J. Pulaski, and M. Ferguson: Reactions of albino rats to injection of dextran. Proc. Soc. exp. Biol. **76**, 254 (1951).

1472. Vormittag, W.: Vergleichende Untersuchungen der Wirkung von Kochsalz-, Albumin- und Plasmaproteinlösungen als Blutersatzmittel an Ratten. Klin. Med. **21**, 620 (1966).

1473. Walcott, W. W.: Blood volume in experimental hemorrhagic shock. Amer. J. Physiol. **143**, 247 (1945).

1474. — Standardization of experimental hemorrhagic shock. Amer. J. Physiol. **143**, 254 (1945).

1475. Walker, J. B.: Osmolar and electrolyte changes in haemorrhagic shock. Lancet **I**, 662 (1963).

1476. Walker, W. F.: Blood substitutes for transfusion. Practitioner **195**, 187 (1965).

1477. Wallace, J.: Cross-matching of blood in the presence of dextran. Lancet **II**, 761 (1954).

1478. Wallenius, G.: The relief of nephrotic oedema by dextran infusion. Scand. J. clin. lab. Invest. **2**, 228 (1950).

1479. — Renal clearance of dextran as a measure of glomerular permeability. Acta Soc. Med. upsalien. suppl. **4** (1954).

1480. — Det nefrotiska syndromet. Experimentella studier av glomerulusmembranens permeabilitet. Nord. Med. **57**, 283 (1957).

1481. Walters, G., and G. K. McGowan: Significance of oligaemia in hypotensive surgical patients. Lancet **I**, 1236 (1965).

1482. Walton, K. W., and C. R. Ricketts: Anaphylactoid response in Guinea pigs to the parenteral administration of sulphate esters of high molecular weight dextran. Nature (Lond.) **173**, 31 (1954).

1483. Walton, R. P.: Report on further studies on a hydroxyethyl starch solution. In: Second Conference on Artificial Colloidal Agents, p. 118. Washington, D. C.: Nat. Acad. Sci. 1963.

1483a. Wangensteen, S. L., H. B. Hechtmann, L. R. Rose, and C. F. Vor der Bruegge: The army in surgical research. J. surg. Res. **7**, 239 (1967).

1484. Ward, R., S. Krugman, J. Giles, and M. A. Jacobs: Endemic viral hepatitis in an institution: Epidemiology and control. In: F. W. Hartmann, G. A. Lo-Grippo, J. G. Mather, and J. Barron: Hepatitis frontiers, p. 227. Boston: Little, Brown 1957.

1485. Warren, J. V., E. A. Stead jr., A. J. Merrill, and E. S. Brannon: Chemical, clinical and immunological studies on the products of human plasma fractionation. IX. The treatment of shock with concentrated human serum albumin: a preliminary report. J. clin. Invest. **23**, 506 (1944).

1486. Warren, J., J. C. Feder, and J. P. Kent: Serological reactions of human sera and rabbit sera with clinical dextrans and Leuconostoc mesenteroides. Bact. Proc. **52**, 92 (1952).

1487. Wasserman, K., and H. S. Mayerson: Plasma and dextran infusions following hemorrhage in dogs. Fed. Proc. **11**, 168 (1952).

1488. — — Relative importance of dextran molecular size in plasma volume expansion. Amer. J. Physiol. **176**, 104 (1954).

1489. — — Plasma volume changes compared with hematocrit and plasma protein changes after infusion. Amer. J. Physiol. **182**, 419 (1955).

1490. Waters, E. T.: Comparison of isinglass and gelatin as blood substitutes. Canad. med. Ass. J. **45**, 395 (1941).

1491. Waud, R. A.: Blood and hemodynamic changes in dogs following hemorrhagic hypotension and its treatment with dextran. J. Pharmacol. exp. Ther. **119**, 85 (1957).

1492. Weale, F. E.: A simplified theory of shock. Lancet **I**, 973 (1963).

1493. Weatherly-White, R. C. A., B. C. Paton, and B. Sjöström: Experimental studies in cold injury. III. Observations on the treatment of frostbite. Plast. reconstr. Surg. **36**, 10 (1965).

1494. Weese, H.: Blutersatzprobleme. Med. Z. **1**, 19 (1944).

1495. — Blutersatzmittel. Pharmazie **8**, 337 (1948).

1496. Wehner, W., G. Friedrich u. G. Kotz: Klinische Erfahrungen mit niedermolekularem Dextran („Infukoll M 40" des VEB Serumwerk Bernburg). Dtsch. GesundhWes. **21**, 1925 (1966).

1497. Weikel, J. H., jr., and L. Lusky: Pharmacology of the reticulo-endothelial system. I. Blockade by polyvinylpyrrolidone (PVP) as measure with radiochromic phosphate in rabbit. J. Pharmacol. exp. Ther. **118**, 148 (1956).

1498. Weil, M. H.: Current concepts on the management of shock. Circulation **16**, 1097 (1957).

1499. — Circulatory shock, a symposium on advances in the understanding of mechanisms and treatment. Calif. Med. **103**, 310 (1965).

1500. —, H. Shubin, and L. Rosoff: Fluid repletion in circulatory shock. J. Amer. med. Ass. **192**, 668 (1965).

1500a. Weil, M. H., and H. Shubin: Diagnosis and treatment of shock. Baltimore: Williams & Wilkins Co. 1967.

1501. Weil, P. G., and D. R. Webster: Clinical experience with plasma augmenters, dextran and PVP. Surg. Forum **4**, 712 (1954).

1502. —, and R. E. Baldry: Plasma expanders in surgical shock. Canad. Serv. Med. J. **10**, 293 (1954).

1503. Weil, P., and D. Webster: The relationship of abnormal bleeding in surgical patients to administration of dextran, excesses of citrate and to fibrinolysis. Surg. Forum **6**, 88 (1956).

1504. Weiss, H. J.: The effect of clinical dextran on platelet aggregation, adhesion and ADP release in man: in vivo and in vitro studies. J. lab. clin. Med. **69**, 37 (1967).

1505. Wells, R. E.: Rheology of blood in the microvasculature. New Engl. J. Med. **270**, 832, 889 (1964).

1506. — Mechanism of action of dextran. J. clin. Invest. **44**, 1109 (1965).

1507. — Rheology of blood in low flow states. In: L. C. Mills, and J. H. Moyer: Shock and hypotension, p. 80. New York: Grune & Stratton 1965.

1507a. WELLS, R.: Rheology of flow stasis. Thrombosis and the dextrans. Int. Surg. **46,** 71 (1966).
1508. WESTON, R. E., M. JANOTA, S. O. LEVINSON, and H. NECHELES: Studies on hemoconcentration and shock following severe hemorrhage. Amer. J. Physiol. **138,** 450 (1943).
1509. WETTERFORS, J.: Albumin. Investigations into the metabolism, distribution, and transfer of albumin under normal and certain pathological conditions, with special reference to the gastro-intestinal tract. Acta med. scand. suppl. **430** (1965).
1510. WHIPPLE, G. H., and S. C. MADDEN: Hemoglobin, plasma protein and cell protein—their interchange and construction in emergencies. Medicine **23,** 215 (1944).
1511. WIEDERSHEIM, M.: An investigation of oxyethylstarch as a new plasma volume expander in animals. Arch. int. Pharmacodyn. **111,** 353 (1957).
1512. WIEMERS, K.: Schock. Dtsch. med. Wschr. **84,** 1145 (1959).
1513. WIGGERS, C. J.: Physiology of shock. New York: Commonwealth Fund 1950.
1514. WILDEGANS, H.: Kristalloide und kolloidale Blutersatzlösungen. Med. Klin. **47,** 1134 (1952).
1515. WILKINSON, A. W.: Clinical trial of dextran in surgical patients. J. int. Chir. **11,** 186 (1951).
1516. —, and I. D. STOREY: "Reactions" to dextran. Lancet **II,** 956 (1953).
1517. — Dextran without reactions. Lancet **II,** 604 (1956).
1518. WILKINSON, R.: Rheomacrodex nephrosis. In: Symposia on Rheomacrodex, vol. II, p. 21. London: Pharmacia 1964.
1519. WILLENEGGER, H.: Zur Transfusion von konserviertem Plasma. Schweiz. med. Wschr. **74,** 899 (1944).
1520. —, u. H. BRÜTSCH: Klinischer Beitrag zur Wirkung des Plasmaersatzes Periston. Helv. chir. Acta **12,** 296 (1945).
1521. — Der heutige Stand der Blutersatzfrage. Schweiz. med. Wschr. **77,** 614 (1947).
1522. — Das Dextran im Rahmen der Blutersatzfrage. Helv. chir. Acta **17,** 307 (1950).
1523. — La valeur du Macrodex et du Periston comme succédanés du plasma. Vortr. int. Tag. Bluttransfusion Blutersatz, Lissabon 1951.
1524. — Transfusionsprobleme vom Standpunkt des Klinikers. Zbl. Bakt. Paras. Infekt. Hyg. **164,** 356 (1955).
1525. — Zur Therapie des Schocks. Ther. Umsch. **17,** 74, 83 (1960).
1526. WILLIAMS, B. N.: Cerebral injury following cardiac operations. Lancet **I,** 221 (1964).
1527. WILLIAMS, J. A., and J. FINE: Measurement of blood volume with a new apparatus. New Engl. J. Med. **264,** 842 (1961).
1528. —, E. GRABLE, and J. FINE: Semi-automatic instrument for measuring blood volume: further clinical studies and comparison of $I^{131}$ and $I^{125}$ labeled albumin and gamma globulin spaces. J. Amer. med. Ass. **178,** 1097 (1961).
1529. — —, H. A. FRANK, and J. FINE: Blood losses and plasma volume shifts during and following major surgical operations. Ann. Surg. **56,** 648 (1962).
1530. — Blood volume, comments on methodology. Amer Surg. **30,** 375 (1964).
1531. — Peripheral red cell and plasma flows: Observations on the physiologic reality of the whole body to large vessel hematocrit ratio. In: L. C. MILLS, and J. H. MOYER: Shock and hypotension, p. 87. New York: Grune & Stratton 1965.

1532. WILSON, B. J., and K. O. ADWAN: A critical assessment of the use of blooc transfusions during major gastric operations. Arch. Surg. **80,** 760 (1960)
1533. —, and J. A. STIRMAN: Initial treatment of burns. J. Amer. med. Ass. **173** 509 (1960).
1534. WILSON, J. N., J. B. GROW, C. V. DEMONG, A. E. PREVEDEL, and J. C. OWENS Central venous pressure in optimal blood volume maintenance. Arch Surg. **85,** 563 (1962).
1535. — The management of acute circulatory failure. Surg. Clin. N. Amer. **43** 469 (1963).
1536. — Rational approach to management of clinical shock. Arch. Surg. **91,** 9: (1965).
1537. WILSON, J. S., E. H. ESTES, J. T. DOYLE, and W. L. BLOOM: The use of dextran in the treatment of shock. J. clin. Invest. **30,** 682 (1951).
1538. — — — —, and J. V. WARREN: The use of dextran in the treatment oi blood loss and shock. Amer. J. med. Sci. **223,** 364 (1952).
1539. WILSON, R. F., J. S. BASSETT, and J. A. WALT: Five years of experience witl massive blood transfusions. J. Amer. med. Ass. **194,** 851 (1965).
1540. WIN, M. S., and J. LISTER: Role of the kidney and adrenal in homeostatic response to hemorrhage. Surg. Forum **17,** 21 (1966).
1541. WINFREY, E. W., C. B. NABEL, C. G. RHEA, and J. H. FOSTER: Experimental studies of the antithrombogenic properties of low molecular weight dextran. In: Conference on Evaluation of Low Molecular Weight Dextran in Shock, p. 80. Washington, D. C.: Nat. Acad. Sci. 1963.
1542. —, and J. H. FOSTER: Low molecular weight dextran in small artery surgery. Arch. Surg. **88,** 78 (1964).
1543. WINNIE, A. P., and V. J. COLLINS: Pharmacologic adjuncts to the management of shock. In: L. R. ORKIN: Management of the patient in shock. Clin. Anesth. **2,** 59, 1965. Oxford: Blackwell.
1544. WINTROBE, M. M.: Clinical hematology. Philadelphia: Lea & Febiger 1961.
1545. WISE, W., L. R. HEAD, M. MORSE, and J. G. ALLEN: The physiological effects of acute anemia produced by the replacement of serial hemorrhages with dextran, plasma and whole blood. Surg. Forum **8,** 18 (1957).
1546. WITHAM, A. C., J. W. FLEMMING, and W. L. BLOOM: The effect of the intravenous administration of dextran on cardiac output and other circulatory dynamics. J. clin. Invest. **30,** 897 (1951).
1547. WIZNITZER, T., and R. ROZIN: The effect of low molecular weight dextran on endotoxin shock. Exp. Med. Surg. **23,** 340 (1965).
1547a. WOLDOW, A., A. S. GOOCH, and H. GOLDBERG: Dextran effect on lipid metabolism. Circulation **34,** suppl. 3, 34 (1966).
1548. WOLFMAN, E. F., S. A. NEILL, D. K. HEAPS, and G. D. ZUIDEMA: Donor blood and isotonic salt solution. Arch. Surg. **86,** 869 (1963).
1549. WOLFSON, L. J.: Blood loss in trauma. Ann. roy. Coll. Surg. Engl. **33,** 158 (1963).
1550. — The anaesthesist's management of the injured patient. Brit. J. Anaesth. **38,** 274 (1966).
1551. —, and F. TELLER: Intravenous use of gelatin solution in hemorrhage; experimental study. Amer. J. med. Sci. **178,** 562 (1929).
1552. WOLLHEIM, E., K. W. SCHNEIDER, J. ZISSLER u. M. EIFERT: Veränderungen der aktiven Plasma- und Blutmenge nach Plasma- und Bluttransfusionen. Cardiologia **21,** 321 (1952).
1553. — — Untersuchungen zur funktionellen Pathologie und Therapie großer intestinaler Blutungen. Verh. dtsch. Ges. inn. Med. **60,** 333 (1954).

1554. WOLLHEIM, E.: Bluttransfusion und Blutmenge. Bibl. haemat. 6, 73 (1957).
1555. —, G. BECKER u. K. W. SCHNEIDER: Die Bestimmung der aktiven Blutmenge mittels Evans Blue, $P^{32}$ und $Cr^{51}$. Klin. Wschr. 36, 800 (1958).
1556. —, u. K. W. SCHNEIDER: Das Blutvolumen nach Plasma- und Bluttransfusionen. Dtsch. med. Wschr. 83, 1117 (1958).
1557. — — Konservative Behandlung oder Frühoperation bei großen intestinalen Blutungen? Dtsch. med. Wschr. 85, 2169 (1960).
1558. — Use of different dye methods in blood volume determination. In: A. S. CAIN, JR.: World Trends in Cardiology. III: Blood volume and contractile protein in heart muscle, p. 61. New York: Hoeber-Harper 1961.
1559. —, u. K. W. SCHNEIDER: Herz- und Gefäßinsuffizienz. In: P. UHLENBRUCK: Praxis der Herz- und Kreislauferkrankungen, p. 207. München: Lehmann-Verlag 1964.
1560. WRAGE, K. H.: Untersuchungen über die Unterschiede in der Speicherung von Periston und Periston N. Frankf. Z. Path. 66, 246 (1955).
1561. WÜLFING, D.: Intraoperative Blutungen als Folge von Blutgerinnungsstörungen. Actuelle Chir. 1, 141 (1966).
1561a. YANCHICK, V. A.: Urinary excretion of low molecular weight dextran in endotoxin shock. Bull. parent. Drug Ass. 20, 173 (1966).
1562. YAO, S. T., and W. C. SHOEMAKER: Plasma and whole blood viscosity changes in shock and after dextran infusion. Ann. Surg. 164, 973 (1966).
1563. YASARGIL, E. C.: Schockbegriff im Wandel der Zeiten und heute. Schweiz. med. Wschr. 94, 1112, 1143, 1163 (1965).
1564. YEO, R.: A clinical study of surgical shock. Lancet II, 497 (1966).
1565. ZÄBISCH, K.: Beobachtungen über die Verträglichkeit eines Plasmaexpanders auf Gelatinebasis. Schweiz. med. Wschr. 90, 378 (1960).
1566. ZAHLER, P.: Vergleichende Untersuchungen über den Einfluß der Plasmaersatzlösung Physiogel auf die Blutsenkung und die Viskosität von menschlichem Blut. Helv. chir. Acta 33, 348 (1966).
1567. ZEDERFELDT, B.: Studies on wound healing and trauma with special reference to intravascular aggregation of erythrocytes. Acta chir. scand. suppl. 224 (1957).
1568. — The hemodynamic effects of plasma substitutes. Scand. J. clin. lab. Invest. 17, suppl. 86, 93 (1965).
1569. ZIJLSTRA, W. G., and S. G. HEERES: The influence of plasma substitutes on the suspension stability of human blood. Proc. kon. nederl. Akad. Wet. 68, 412 (1965).
1570. ZIMMERMANN, W. E.: Die Beeinflussung der Nieren- und Hirndurchblutung durch Veränderungen des Säure-Basen-Haushaltes im Schock beim schweren Unfall. Hefte Unfallheilk. 87, 125 (1966).
1571. — Die Puffersysteme. In: O. H. JUST u. H. LUTZ: Genese und Therapie des hämorrhagischen Schocks, p. 147. Stuttgart: Thieme 1966.
1572. — Veränderungen des Säure-Basen-Haushaltes beim traumatischen Schock. In: K. LANG, R. FREY u. M. HALMÁGYI: Infusionstherapie, p. 46. Berlin-Heidelberg-New York: Springer 1966.
1573. — Die Hirn- und Nierendurchblutung bei normo- und hypovolämischem Schock. In: K. HUTSCHENREUTER: Anaesthesie und Notfallmedizin, p. 169. Berlin-Heidelberg-New York: Springer 1966.
1574. ZINGG, W.: Surgery 1963—trauma, shock, burns, hyperbaric oxygen. Manitoba med. Rev. 44, 95 (1964).
1575. —, and P. LINDSAY: Rheology of blood-dextran mixtures. Surg. Forum 15, 228 (1964).

1576. Zollinger, H. U.: Anurie bei Chromoproteinurie. Stuttgart: Thieme 1952.
1577. Zolotokrylina, E. S., and S. S. Chistyakov: The feasibility of the thera peutic use of dextran in cases of clinical death caused by rapi exsanguination. Fed. Proc. 25, T645 (1966).
1578. Zozaya, J.: Immunological reactions between dextran polysaccharides an some antibacterial sera. J. exp. Med. 55, 353 (1932).
1579. — Carbohydrates adsorbed on colloids as antigens. J. exp. Med. 55, 32 (1932).
1580. Zuschneid, K.: Vergleichende tierexperimentelle Untersuchungen bei de Behandlung schwerster Schockzustände und der Agonie (Wiederbelebung mit der intraarteriellen und intravenösen Transfusion (IAT und IVT Arch. klin. Chir. 308, 357 (1964).
1581. Zweifach, B. W.: Microcirculatory derangments as a basis for the leth manifestations of experimental shock. Brit. J. Anaesth. 30, 466 (1958).
1582. — Annotated Bibliography on Shock 1950—1962. Washington, D. C.: Na Acad. Sci., Nat. Res. Counc. Publ. 1182 (1963).
1583. — Current concepts of microcirculatory behavior. Bibl. anat. 7, 2 (1965).
1584. — Annotated bibliography on shock 1962—1964, vol. II. Washington, D. C. Nat. Acad. Sci., Nat. Res. Counc. Publ. 1358 (1966).

# Additional Literature

1585. Abel, F. L., J. A. Waldhausen, W. J. Daly, and W. L. Pearce: Pulmonary blood volume in hemorrhagic shock in the dog and primate. Amer. J Physiol. 213, 1072 (1967).
1586. Abildgaard, U., and F. Skjörten: Influence of low molecular weigh dextran and thrombin infusions on blood platelets and fibrinogen. J Atheroscl. Res. 8, 69 (1968).
1587. Abraham, A. S., R. B. Hedworth Whitty, and J. M. Bishop: Effects o acute hypoxia and hypervolaemia singly and together, upon the pulmo nary circulation in patients with chronic bronchitis. Clin. Sci. 33, 371 (1967).
1588. Adamkiewicz, V. W., and P. J. Sacra: Histamine and sugars. Fed. Proc 26, 224 (1967).
1588 a. Adamson, J., and R. S. Hillman: Blood volume and plasma protein replace ment following acute blood loss in normal man. J. Amer. med. Ass. 205 609 (1968).
1589. Adriani, J.: The role of anesthesia and adjunctive drugs. Trans. amer. Acad Ophthal. Otolaryng. 72, 25 (1968).
1589 a. Ahlberg, A.: Trombosprofylax med Macrodex i ett material av kollum frakturer. Nord. Med. 80, 1491 (1968).
1590. Alberts, I.: Die Pufferkapazität kolloidaler und kristalloider Infusions lösungen. Diss. Mainz 1967.
1591. Anderson, R. W., P. M. James, C. E. Bredenberg, J. A. Collins, S. Levitsky, and R. M. Hardaway III: Extracellular fluid and plasma volume studies on casualties in the republic of Vietnam. Surg. Forum 18, 32 (1967).
1592. Ankier, S. I., and M. S. Starr: The importance of plasma kinins in the anaphylactoid reaction in rats. Brit. J. Pharmacol. 31, 331 (1967).
1593. Arfors, K. E., G. Arturson, och O. Tangen: Blodvolymförändringar efter utblödning och substitution med dextran hos vakna och hos sövda hundar. Nord. Med. 79, 90 (1968).

1594. ARTURSON, G., and S. SOEDA: Changes in transcapillary leakage during healing of experimental burns. Acta chir. scand. **133**, 609 (1967).

1595. ASCARI, W. Q., P. C. JOLLY, and P. A. THOMAS: Autologous blood transfusion in pulmonary surgery. Transfusion **8**, 111 (1968).

1596. ATIK, M., P. V. LIU, S. AMINI, and C. ROSENBERG: Pseudomonas exotoxin shock. J. Amer. med. Ass. **200**, 540 (1967).

1596 a. —, P. V. HANSON, B. A. AMINI, and S. ROSENBERG: Pseudomonas exotoxin shock. A preliminary report of studies in dogs. J. Amer. med. Ass. **205**, 134 (1968).

1597. AUKLAND, K., and M. WOLGAST: Effect of hemorrhage and retransfusion on intrarenal distribution of blood flow in dogs. J. clin. Invest. **47**, 488 (1968).

1598. AUSTEN, W. G., and M. J. BUCKLEY: Treatment of various forms of surgical shock. Progr. cardiovasc. Dis. **10**, 97 (1967).

1599. BARNES, A., and T. E. ALLEN: Transfusions subsequent to administration of universal donor blood in Vietnam. J. Amer. med. Ass. **204**, 695 (1968).

1599 a. BARNES, R. W., H. MOHRI, R. J. NELSON, and K. A. MERENDINO: The use of low molecular weight dextran in superior vena caval replacement. Diseases Chest **53**, 390 (1968).

1600. BARNHART, M. I., and C. QUINTANA: Platelet alterations with dextran. Blood **30**, 541 (1967).

1601. BARRAS, J.-P.: Introduction à la rhéologie sanguine. L'écoulement stationnaire du sang dans un tube rigide. Méd. Hyg. **25**, 1394 (1967).

1602. — Viscosité apparente de suspensions d'hématies dans différents substituts du plasma. In: A. HÄSSIG: Plasmaersatzpräparate auf Gelatinebasis. Bibl. haemat. (Karger): in press.

1603. BAUE, A. E., E. T. TRAGUS, and W. M. PARKINS: A comparison of isotonic and hypertonic solutions and blood flow and oxygen consumption in the initial treatment of hemorrhagic shock. J. Trauma **7**, 743 (1967).

1603 a. — Recent developments in the study and treatment of shock. Surg. Gynec. Obstet. **127**, 849 (1968).

1604. BAUER, U. R.: Das Verhalten des zirkulierenden Blutvolumens nach Aderlass sowie anschliessender Substitution durch sogenannte Plasmaexpander. Diss. Düsseldorf 1967.

1604 a. BEHRENS, U., et al.: Microbiological preparation of dextran. EG P. 62647, clg. 6. 7. 64 (EG) as 105352 Pub. 5. 7. 68.

1605. BENNETT, P. N., D. P. DHALL, and N. A. MATHESON: Effect of dextran 70 infusion on platelet adhesiveness after operation. Brit. J. Surg. **55**, 289 (1968).

1606. BERGER, R. L., E. IATRIDES, and T. J. RYAN: The homologous blood reaction of cardiopulmonary bypass; an experimental study on pathogenesis and treatment. Ann. thorac. Surg. **4**, 542 (1967).

1607. BERNSTEIN, E. F., and A. R. CASTANEDA: The importance of low shear rate blood viscometry in extracorporeal circulation. Biorheology **4**, 89 (1967).

1608. BEVAN, G., H. F. TASWELL, and G. J. GLEICH: Serum immunoglobulin levels in blood donors implicated in transmission of hepatitis. J. Amer. med. Ass. **203**, 92 (1968).

1609. BICHER, H. I., and A. M. BEEMER: Induction of ischemic myocardial damage by red blood cell aggregation (sludge) in the rabbit. J. Atheroscl. Res. **7**, 409 (1967).

1610. BLOHMÉ, G., I. KERSTELL, and A. SVANBORG: The effect of dextran on plasma lipids. Acta med. scand. **183**, 481 (1968).

1611. Blood Flow Improvement. Pharmacia, Uppsala 1968.
1611 a. BOBA, A.: Responses to hemorrhage replaced by lactated Ringer solution. Acta anaesth. scand. Suppl. **31** (1968).
1612. BOLLINGER, A.: Bedeutung biophysikalischer Faktoren im venösen Kreislauf. Zbl. Phlebol. **1**, 16 (1968).
1613. —, H. J. SIMON, R. KÖHLER u. E. LÜTHY: Wirkung von niedermolekularem Dextran auf Blutviskosität und Extremitätendurchblutung. Z. Kreisl.-Forsch. **57**, 456 (1968).
1614. BOLOOKI, H., R. I. GOLDBERG, H. I. ANTELL, J. H. STUCKEY, and K. E. KARLSON: Comparison of the effect of low molecular weight dextran on blood flow and peripheral resistance during extracorporeal circulation and hypothermia. J. thorac. cardiovasc. Surg. **54**, 216 (1967).
1615. BOSSART, J.: Bestimmung des Blutzuckers in dextranhaltigem Serum nach einer modifizierten o-Toluidin-Methode. Praxis **56**, 1035 (1967).
1616. BOSWICK, J. A., JR., and N. H. STONE: Methods and materials in managing the severely burned patient. Surg. Clin. N. Amer. **48**, 177 (1968).
1616 a. BOULTON, T. B., and P. V. COLE: Anaesthesia in difficult situations. Anaesthesia **23**, 385 (1968).
1617. BOYAN, C. P.: Hypovolemic shock. Anaesth. Analg. Curr. Res. **46**, 746 (1967).
1618. BRAHMANKAR, D. M., and W. E. CONNOR: Effect of high molecular weight dextran on experimental hypercholesterolemia. Circulat. Res. **21**, 817 (1967).
1619. BRATTEBY, L. E., L. GARBY, F. INTONTI, and S. NORDLUND: Erythrocyte aggregation and sequestration after high-molecular-weight dextran infusion in dogs. Acta chir. scand. **133**, 429 (1967).
1620. BREWER, S. S., JR.: The sthenoplastic effect of dextran on platelets — the mechanism for prevention of thromboembolism. Blood **25**, 601 (1965).
1621. BRISMAN, R., L. C. PARKS, and D. W. BENSON: Pitfalls in the clinical use of central venous pressure. Arch. Surg. **95**, 902 (1967).
1621 a. — —, and J. A. HALLER: Anaphylactoid reactions associated with the clinical use of dextran 70. J. Amer. med. Ass. **204**, 824 (1968).
1622. BROGHAMMER, H.: Therapeutische Wirkung von Gelatine-Plasmaersatzlösungen im experimentellen Schock. In: A. HÄSSIG: Plasmaersatzpräparate auf Gelatinebasis. Bibl. haemat. (Karger): in press.
1623. BROWN, P. B.: The effect of low molecular weight dextran on the microcirculation of skin. Brit J. plast. Surg. **20**, 272 (1967).
1624. BURNS, G. P., and W. G. SCHENK, JR.: The effect of hemorrhage and dextran infusion on blood flow in stenotic arteries. J. thorac. cardiovasc. Surg. **55**, 572 (1968).
1625. BYGDEMAN, S., and R. ELIASSON: Effect of dextrans on platelet adhesiveness and aggregation. Scand. J. clin. Lab. Invest. **20**, 17 (1967).
1626. — Thrombotic diseases with reference to the use of dextrans. Acta chir. scand. Suppl. **387** (1968).
1627. — Prevention and therapy of thromboembolic complications with dextran. Progr. Surg. **7**, 114 (1968).
1627 a. CAILLOUETTE, J. C.: Prevention and early diagnosis of thromboembolic disease in obstetrics and gynecology. Clin. Obstet. Gynecol. **11**, 233 (1968).
1628. CANANI, M. B., V. TRIPODI, D. A. CAPASSO, e M. T. DI TULLIO: Variazioni in vivo dell'adesività piastrinica indotte dal destrano in soggetti normali. Boll. Soc. ital. Biol. sper. **43**, 249 (1967).

1629. CAPASSO, D. A., V. TRIPODI, M. T. DI TULLIO e M. B. CANANI: Azione del destrano, in vitro, sull'adesività piastrinica indotta dall'ADP. Boll. Soc. ital. Biol. sper. **43**, 254 (1967).

1630. CASLEY-SMITH, J. R.: Electron microscopical observations on the dilated lymphatics in oedematous regions and their collapse following hyaluronidase administration. Brit. J. exp. Path. **48**, 680 (1967).

1631. CERNY, L. C., R. C. GRAHAM, and H. JAMES, JR.: Dilute solution properties of hydroxyethyl starch. J. appl. Polymer Sci. **11**, 1941 (1967).

1631 a. —, J. D. GRAUZ, and H. JAMES: The effectiveness of plasma expanders, an osmotic pressure and viscosity study. Biorheology **5**, 103 (1968).

1632. CHIEN, S., S. USAMI, R. J. DELLENBACK, M. I. GREGERSEN, L. B. NANNINGA, and M. M. GUEST: Blood viscosity: Influence of erythrocyte aggregation. Science **157**, 829 (1967).

1633. CHOPRA, P. S., S. SRINIVASAN, T. LUCAS, and P. N. SAWYER: Effects of heparin, protamine and low molecular weight dextran (LMD) on electrokinetic characteristics of canine blood vessel intima in vivo. Bull. N. Y. Acad. Med. **43**, 1206 (1967).

1634. CLAUSS, R. H., and J. F. RAY: Pharmacologic assistance to the failing circulation. Surg. Gynec. Obstet. **126**, 611 (1968).

1635. COHEN, Y., et F. BOISMARE: Action de la pentamidine sur l'oedème au dextran de la patte du rat surrénaloprivé. Thérapie **22**, 829 (1967).

1636. — — Rôles de l'histamine et de la sérotonine dans le développement de l'oedème expérimental chez le rat. Thérapie **22**, 837 (1967).

1637. COLARD, M., et L. DE GEETER: Le problème du shock traumatique. Acta chir. belg. Suppl. **1**, 58 (1967).

1638. Committee on Plasma and Plasma Substitutes: Statement on normal (whole, pooled) human plasma. Transfusion **8**, 57 (1968).

1639. CONN, J., JR., and J. J. BERGAN: Treatment of arterial embolism: The conservative approach. Surg. Clin. N. Amer. **48**, 163 (1968).

1640. COOK, J. R., T. R. SHERROD, and J. C. COOLEY: Myocardial contractile force in hemorrhagic shock. Arch. Surg. **95**, 500 (1967).

1641. COOK, W. A., and W. E. WEBB: Pulmonary changes in hemorrhagic shock. Surgery **64**, 85 (1968).

1641 a. CROCKER, M. C.: Fluids for emergency conditions. A review with special reference to disaster situations. Anaesthesia **23**, 413 (1968).

1642. CUTLER, R. G., and F. X. PALETTA: Effectiveness of dextran in traumatic edema. Amer. J. Surg. **115**, 313 (1968).

1643. DAVIDOV, M., N. KAKAVIATOS, and F. A. FINNERTY, JR.: The lack of importance of plasma volume reduction in the early fall of arterial pressure during drug induced saluresis. Clin. Res. **15**, 200 (1967).

1644. DEDICHEN, H., D. RACE, and W. G. SCHENK, JR.: Hemodilution and concomitant hyperbaric oxygenation. J. thorac. cardiovasc. Surg. **53**, 341 (1967).

1645. DETRICK, L. E., V. DEBLEY, and T. H. HALEY: Tolerance, toxicity and caloric availability of intravenously injected oxypolygelatin solution in rabbits. J. amer. pharm. Ass. **42**, 623 (1953).

1646. DHALL, D. P., P. BENNETT, F. N. MCKENZIE, and N. A. MATHESON: Effects of dextran on human platelets. Bibl. anat. (Karger) **9**, 295 (1967).

1647. —, W. A. J. BRYCE, and N. A. MATHESON: Optical clearing effect of dextran on human platelet suspensions. Nature **216**, 719 (1967).

1648. —, P. N. BENNETT, and N. A. MATHESON: Effect of dextran 70 on platelet behaviour after operation. Brit. J. Surg. **55**, 67 (1968).

1649. Dhall, D. P., and N. A. Matheson: In vitro clumping of human platelets by dextran. Thromb. Diath. haemorrh. **19**, 70 (1968).

1650. Dickinson, P. H., I. F. McNeill, and J. M. Morrison: Aortoiliac occlusion. A review of 100 cases treated by direct arterial surgery. Brit. J. Surg. **54**, 764 (1967).

1650 a. Dickmans, H. A., J. Eisolt, P. Gaehtgens u. H. Hirsch: Über den Einfluß der Erythrocytenaggregation auf das Stromzeitvolumen des isolierten Hundedarmes. Arch. ges. Physiol. **300**, 67 (1968).

1650 b. Dintenfass, L.: Internal viscosity of the red cell and a blood viscosity equation. Nature **219**, 956 (1958).

1651. Dorner, M. M., E. W. Bassett, S. M. Veiser, E. A. Kabat, and S. W. Tannenbaum: Studies on human antibodies. V. Amino acid composition of antidextrans of the same and of differing specificities from several individuals. J. exp. Med. **125**, 823 (1967).

1652. Drucker, W. R., J. Schlatter, and R. P. Drucker: Metabolic factors associated with endotoxin-induced tolerance for hemorrhagic shock. Surgery **64**, 273 (1968).

1653. Ebert, K. H.: Betrachtungen über den Zustand nativer Dextrane in Lösung unter Annahme einer Helix-Konformation. Mh. Chem. **98**, 1128 (1967).

1654. —, and M. Brosche: Origin of branches in native dextrans. Biopolymers **5**, 423 (1967).

1654 a.—, G. Schenk u. R. Scholz: Untersuchungen über das Schicksal von Dextran im Organismus von Meerschweinchen. Z. klin. Chem. **6**, 435 (1968).

1654 b. — — Fermentpolymerisation IX. Kinetik und Mechanismus der enzymatischen Dextransynthese und Wirkung der Akzeptoren auf diese Reaktion. Z. Naturforsch. **23 b**, 788 (1968).

1654 c. — — Mechanisms of biopolymer growth: The formation of dextran and levan. Advan. Enzymol. **30**, 179 (1968).

1654 d. Editorial: World war II: Dextran's origin. J. Amer. med. Ass. **204**, 45 (1968).

1654 e. — Dextran alters hemostasis by 'coating' blood cells, vessels. J. Amer. med. Ass. **204**, 45 (1968).

1654 f. — Dextran prophylaxis. Clinical trial supports role of platelets in embolism. J. Amer. med. Ass. **204**, 38 (1968).

1654 g. — Transmission of disease by blood transfusion. Brit. med. J. **II**, 426 (1966).

1654 h. — Post-transfusion hepatitis. Brit. med. J. **I**, 256 (1967).

1654 i. — Dextran og muligheten for allergiske reaksjoner. T. norske Laegeforen. **88**, 1446 (1968).

1655. Eichholtz, W. u. W. Eger: Über Vorkommen und Häufigkeit der Inokulationshepatitis nach morphologisch-histologischen Untersuchungen. Med. Welt **19**, 119 (1968).

1656. Eisenberg, S,: Failure of low-molecular-weight dextran to alter blood viscosity. Circulation **35/36**, Suppl. 2, 102 (1967).

1657. Engberg, A., and J. L. E. Ericsson: Effects of low molecular weight dextran on renal proximal tubules. Electron microscopic observations. J. Ultrastruct. Res. **20**, 293 (1967).

1658. — — — Osmotisk nefros — en morfologisk studie. Nord. Med. **78**, 1493 1967).

1659. Engeset, J., A. L. Stalker, and N. A. Matheson: Erythrocyte aggregation — studies on the effects of dextran 40 and on the quantitation of aggregation and cohesiveness. Bibl. anat. (Karger) **9**, 282 (1967).

1660. ENGESET, J., A. L. STALKER, and N. A. MATHESON: Effects of dextran 40 on red cell aggregation in rabbits. Cardiovasc. Res. **1**, 379 (1967).

1661. — — — Objective measurement of the dispersing effect of dextran 40 on red cells from man, dog and rabbit. Cardiovasc. Res. **1**, 385 (1967).

1662. —, U. FREYSCHUSS, L. KAIJSER, and P. ÅSÉN: Hemodynamic findings in patients with intravascular red cell aggregation. Acta med. scand. Suppl. **472**, 68 (1967).

1663. ERICSSON, J. L. E., G. ANDRES, A. BERGSTRAND, H. BUCHT, and P.-Å. ÖRSTEN: Further studies on the fine structure of renal tubules in healthy humans. With a note on the effect of the intravenous infusion of low molecular weight dextran. Acta path. microbiol. scand. **69**, 493 (1967).

1664. ESTOUR, E., et P. GAILLARD: Incidence du "sludge" dans les suites opératoires. Intérêt du dextrane de faible poids moléculaire (40.000). Lyon Méd. **218**, 81 (1967).

1665. EVANS, G., and J. F. MUSTARD: Platelet-surface reaction and thrombosis. Surgery **64**, 273 (1968).

1666. EVANS, J. C., and P. V. GABLE: Modifications of tumor microcirculation as an adjunct to hyperbaric oxygen in radiotherapy. Radiology **89**, 140 (1967).

1667. EVANS, W. E., R. T. SHORE, L. C. CAREY, and J. C. DARIN: Effect of intestinal exclusion in escherichia coli endotoxin shock. Arch. Surg. **95**, 511 (1967).

1668. EVARTS, C. M.: Low molecular weight dextran. Med. Clin. N. Amer. **51**, 1285 (1967).

1669. EVONUK, E., and F. J. SULLIVAN: Effects of low molecular weight dextran on cardiovascular and metabolic parameters in dogs. Amer. J. Physiol. **213**, 1512 (1967).

1669 a. FAVRE, H., M. GIROMINI, J. C. GERSTER et X. SAVOY: Anurie associée à l'administration de Dextran de faible poids moléculaire. Schweiz. med. Wschr. **98**, 1982 (1968).

1670. FILLASTRE, J.-P., F. MIGNON, J.-D. SRAER, L. MOREL-MAROGER, et G. RICHET: Insuffisance rénale aiguë réversible après traitement prolongé par le dextran. Presse méd. **75**, 2535 (1967).

1671. FINE, J., C. PALMERIO, and S. RUTENBURG: New developments in therapy of refractory traumatic shock. Arch. Surg. **96**, 163 (1968).

1672. FISCHER, M.: Der Einfluß verschiedener Plasmavolumenersatzmittel (Rheomacrodex und Haemaccel) auf das fibrinolytische System und einige Funktionen der Thrombozyten. In: A. HÄSSIG: Plasmaersatzpräparate auf Gelatinebasis. Bibl. haemat. (Karger): in press.

1672 a. FISHER, B., and E. R. FISHER: Effect of low molecular weight dextran on hepatic metastases in the rabbit. Cancer Res. **28**, 1586 (1968).

1673. FLANNERY, B., and C. W. VENABLES: The effects of low molecular dextran upon ischaemic Roux-en-Y intestinal loops. Brit. J. Surg. **55**, 95 (1968).

1674. FLOTTE, C. T.: Dextran in atherosclerosis. Circulation **35/36**, Suppl. 2, 11 (1967).

1675. FÖRSTER, O., u. E. STOKLASKA: Über die Bedeutung von Proteasen für die Arthus-Reaktion und pharmakologisch induzierte Oedeme in der Rattenpfote. Med. Pharmacol. exp. **17**, 77 (1967).

1676. FOSTER, F. H.: Dextran — manufacture and use. Part 1. Proc. Biochem., 15 (1968).

1677. — Dextran — manufacture and use. Part. 2. Proc. Biochem., 55, 62 (1968).

1677 a. FOURNIER, A., J. M. WATCHI, et R. J. RÉVEILLAUD: Les néphroses dites osmotiques ou vacuolisations hydropiques diffuses des tubes proximaux. Actualités néphrolog., 353 (1968).
1678. FOWLER, N. O., J. C. HOLMES, and T. E. GAFFNEY: Beta sympathetic blockade and the hemodynamic effects of anemia. Clin. Res. **15**, 202 (1967).
1679. GABR, Y., F. SALEEB, and M. OSMAN: Evaluation studies on a 4% gelatin solution containing 1% glycine for intravenous use. Arzneimittelforsch. **17**, 643 (1967).
1680. —, and A. MICHAEL: Evaluation studies on 4% gelatin solutions for intravenous use. Excretion and retention of gelatin in relation to its molecular weight. Arzneimittelforsch. **17**, 1211 (1967).
1681. GARZON, A. A., C. CHENG, B. LERNER, S. LICHTENSTEIN, and K. E. KARLSON: Hydroxyethyl starch (HES) and bleeding. An experimental investigation of its effect on hemostasis. J. Trauma **7**, 757 (1967).
1682. GIEBEL, O., u. K. HORATZ: Therapeutische Ergebnisse bei der Verwendung von Gelatine-Plasmaersatzlösungen in der Anaesthesiologie, Chirurgie, Gynäkologie, Geburtshilfe, Ophthalmologie und Neurochirurgie. In: A. HÄSSIG: Plasmaersatzpräparate auf Gelatinebasis. Bibl. haemat. (Karger): in press.
1683. GIROMINI, M., P. JUNGERS, et H. DUCROT: Anurie provoquée par la perfusion de dextran de faible poids moléculaire. Presse méd. **75**, 2561 (1967).
1684. GÖLTNER, E.: Die Beeinflussung des intravasalen Flüssigkeitsvolumens durch Gelatineinfusionen bei Nichtschwangeren und Schwangeren. In: A. HÄSSIG: Plasmaersatzpräparate auf Gelatinebasis. Bibl. haemat. (Karger): in press.
1684 a. GOLBERT, T. M., G. E. LUCENA, A. E. FALLERONI, B. H. BOOTH, and R. PATTERSON: Treatment of anaphylaxis. To the editor. New Engl. J. Med. **278**, 1180 (1968).
1684 b. GOLLUB, S., and C. SCHAEFER: Structural alteration in canine fibrin produced by colloid plasma expanders. Surg. Gynec. Obstet. **127**, 783 (1968).
1685. GORDON, J. A., and K. P. ROBINSON: The effect of intravenous infusion of Rheomacrodex and normal saline on pulmonary metastases. Brit. J. Surg. **54**, 1016 (1967).
1686. GOWDEY, C. W., and I. E. YOUNG: Cardiorenal effects of large infusions of dextran in dogs. Canad. J. Biochem. Physiol. **32**, 599 (1964).
1686 a. GRABLE, E., and J. A. WILLIAMS: Simplified method for simultaneous determinations of plasma volume and red cell mass with $^{125}$I — labeled albumin and $^{51}$Cr-tagged red cells. J. nucl. Med. **9**, 219 (1968).
1687. GRANATH, K. A., and B. E. KVIST: Molecular weight distribution analysis by gel chromatography on Sephadex. J. Chromat. **28**, 69 (1967).
1688. GREENWOOD, C. T., and D. J. HOURSTON: Physicochemical studies on starches. Part XXXIII: Some physicochemical properties of hydroxyethyl starch used as a volume extender for blood plasma. Stärke **19**, 243 (1967).
1689. GRINDON, A. J., P. V. HOLLAND, and P. J. SCHMIDT: Posttransfusion hepatitis. Amer. Heart J. **74**, 591 (1967).
1690. GRUBER, U. F.: The influence of temperature on the volume effect of dextran 70. Z. ges. exp. Med. **144**, 217 (1967).
1691. — Der Wert der Blutvolumenbestimmung im Schock. 3. int. Fortb.kurs für klin. Anaesth., 77 (Wien. med. Akad., Wien, 1967).
1691 a. GUNNAR, R. M., H. S. LOEB, R. J. PIETRAS, and J. R. TOBIN: Hemodynamic measurements in a coronary care unit. Progr. cardiovasc. Dis. **11**, 29 (1968).

1691 b. Gutelius, J. R., H. M. Shizgal, and G. Lopez: The effect of trauma on extracellular water volume. Arch. Surg. **97**, 206 (1968).
1691 c. Hallwachs, O., u. H. Lutz: Die Nierenfunktion nach Infusion von Dextran- und Gelatine-Präparaten ohne und mit Zusatz von THAM im experimentellen hämorrhagischen Schock. Arch. klin. Chir. **318**, 14 (1968).
1692. Hardaway, R. M.: New concepts of shock and its treatment. Clin. Med. **74**, 33 (1967).
1692 a. — Clinical management of shock. Springfield: Thomas 1968.
1693. Hardcastle, J. D., and H. D. Ritchie: The liver in shock. Brit. J. Surg. **55**, 365 (1968).
1693 a. Hardwicke, J., B. Hulme, J. H. Jones, and C. R. Ricketts: Measurement of glomerular permeability to poly-disperse radioactively-labelled macromolecules in normal rabbits. Clin. Sci. **34**, 505 (1968).
1693 b. Heath, M. L., D. Dunlap, and M. D. Vickers: The effect on the red cell circulation of replacement of operative blood loss with different fluids. Brit. J. Anaesth. **40**, 144 (1968).
1694. Hölscher, B.: Funktionelle und histologische Untersuchungen zur Wirkung eines modifizierten hochmolekularen Gelatinepräparates auf die Niere. Chirurg **39**, 228 (1968).
1694 a. — Über die Wirkung von Volumenersatzmitteln auf die Niere bei akutem Blutvolumenmangel. Chirurg **39**, 178 (1968).
1695. Hopkins, R. W., R. B. Fratianne, J. S. Abrams, and F. A. Simeone: Controlled hypotension for uncontrolled hemorrhage. Arch. Surg. **95**, 517 (1967).
1696. Hopkinson, B. R., J. R. Border, W. C. Heyden, and W. G. Schenk, Jr.: Interstitial fluid pressure changes during hemorrhage and blood replacement with and without hypotension. Surgery **64**, 68 (1968).
1697. Horatz, K.: Plasmaersatzpräparate auf Gelatinebasis. Thieme: Stuttgart 1968.
1697 a. Housset, E., J. Etienne, J. Loeper et J. Cottet: Action du dextran sur l'activité lipoprotéine lipase du plasma humain. Pathol. Biol. Semaine Hôp. **16**, 653 (1968).
1698. Huggins, R. A., E. L. Smith, and S. Deavers: $Cr^{51}$-tagged red cell equilibration in dogs. Amer. J. Physiol. **211**, 283 (1966).
1699. Hunt, P. S., and T. S. Reeve: Experimental arterial thrombus prevention and renal function in sheep after infusion with low molecular weight dextran and dextran 70.000. Ann. Surg. **166**, 51 (1967).
1700. Hunt, T. K., B. H. Zederfeldt, T. K. Goldstick, and W. B. Conolly: Tissue oxygen tensions during controlled hemorrhage. Surg. Forum **18**, 3 (1967).
1700 a. Hutchin, P.: History of blood transfusion: A tercentennial look. Surgery **64**, 685 (1968).
1700 b. Hymes, A. C., M. H. Safavian, A. Arbulu, and P. Baute: A comparison of Pluronic F-68, low molecular weight dextran, mannitol and saline as priming agents in the heart-lung apparatus. Part I. Pluronic F-68: First use as a plasma substitute. J. thorac. cardiovasc. Surg. **56**, 16 (1968).
1700 c. —, and K. Beck: A comparison of Pluronic F-68, low molecular weight dextran, mannitol and saline as priming agents in the heart-lung apparatus. Part II. The in vitro influence on oxygen consumption of certain fluids used as priming agents in a heart-lung bypass apparatus. J. thorac. cadiovasc. Surg. **56**, 23 (1968).

1700 d. Iverius, P. H.: Solubility of low density ($\beta$-) lipoproteins in the presence of dextran. Clin. chim. Acta **20**, 261 (1968).

1701. Jacobson, E. D.: A physiologic approach to shock. New Engl. J. Med. **278**, 834 (1968).

1702. Johansson, B., E. Linder, and T. Seeman: Effects of hematocrit and blood viscosity on myocardial blood flow during temporary coronary occlusions in dogs. Scand. J. thorac. cardiovasc. Surg. **1**, 165 (1967).

1702 a. Johnson, D. C., and T. S. Reeve: The effect and clinical significance of low molecular weight and clinical dextran on an experimental venous thrombus in sheep. Ann. Surg. **168**, 123 (1968).

1703. Johnson, G., Jr., and J. Lambert: Responses to the rapid intravenous administration of an overload of fluid and electrolytes in dogs. Ann. Surg. **167**, 561 (1968).

1704. Johnston, D. G., and W. F. Burgos: Blood volume estimation: development and application to surgical and medical practice. Amer. J. Surg. **113**, 225 (1967).

1705. Jones, C. E., J. W. Crowell, and E. E. Smith: A cause-effect relationship between oxygen deficit and irreversible hemorrhagic shock. Surg. Gynec. Obstet. **127**, 93 (1968).

1706. Juchems, R., u. G. Ammerschläger: Über den Einfluß mäßiger Blutverluste auf das Herzminutenvolumen, Schlagvolumen und den peripheren Gesamtwiderstand. Z. KreislForsch. **56**, 963 (1967).

1707. Kaijser, L., and Å. Rieger: Changes in blood volume and plasma proteins on administration of different substitutes after operations in man. Acta chir. scand. **134**, 15 (1968).

1708. Kalmus, H.: Pharmacogenetics. Scope and limitations of pharmacogenetics. Proc. roy. Soc. Med. **61**, 167 (1968).

1708 a. Kalny, J., and V. Cerny: Case of fatal allergy to Dextran Spofa. Rozhl. Chir. **46**, 699 (1967).

1708 b. Karow, A. M., Jr., O. Carrier Jr., and B. R. Clower: Toxicity of cryoprotective agents at 30°. J. Pharm. Pharmacol. **20**, 297 (1968).

1709. Kavee, D. J., E. Lichtenstein, and H. Laufman: Collateral arterial flow under normotensive and hypotensive conditions. Effects of autotransfusion, normal saline solution infusion and dextran 40 infusion. Arch. Surg. **95**, 395 (1967).

1710. Kho, L. K., and W. C. Shoemaker: Evaluation of therapy in clinical shock by cardiorespiratory measurements. Surg. Gynec. Obstet. **127**, 81 (1968).

1711. Kief, H.: Morphologische Ergebnisse nach ein- und mehrfacher Verabreichung von Plasmaersatzlösungen auf Gelatinebasis. In: A. Hässig: Plasmaersatzpräparate auf Gelatinebasis. Bibl. haemat. (Karger): in press.

1712. —, P. Hajdu u. K. Engelbart: Reabsorptive Vacuolisation (sog. osmotische Nephrose) nach Inulin. Frankf. Z. Path. **77**, 12 (1967).

1712 a. Kief, H., K. Engelhart, G. Arnold u. H. Bähr: Vacuoläre Rückresorbtion von nativer und abgebauter Gelatine (sog. osmotische Nephrose). Virchows Arch. Abt. B. Zellpath. **1**, 240 (1968).

1712 b. Kiselev, A. E.: Test reagents for blood group determination. RU P. 202440, clg. 16. 9. 66 (RU) as 1101632/31-16. Pub. March 1968.

1713. Klütsch, K. u. A. Heidland: Der Einfluß verschiedener Volumenexpander auf die Nierenfunktion bei Hypo- und Normovolämie. In: A. Hässig: Plasmaersatzpräparate auf Gelatinebasis. Bibl. haemat. (Karger): in press.

1714. Knott, H. W., and J. W. Kirklin: Validity of comparison of plasma volumes before and after operation. Surgery **62**, 843 (1967).

1715. KOROLKOV, V. I., and V. B. KOZINER: Myocardial oxygen tension and oxygen supply to the organism in partial blood substitution by dextran. Cor Vasa **9**, 306 (1967).

1716. — — Oxygen supply to the myocardium during acute anemia due to replacement of some part of the blood with polyglucin. Byul. Eksperim. Biol. Med. **62**, 37 (1967).

1717. KRONECKER, H.: Kritisches und Experimentelles über lebensrettende Infusionen von Kochsalzlösungen bei Hunden. Korr. Bl. Schweiz. Ärzte **16**, 447, 486, 500 (1886).

1717 a. KRÜGER, B., W. DISSMANN, R. EISELE, P. LUNKENHEIMER u. W. THIMME: Über den Einfluß des niedermolekularen Dextrans auf die Hämodynamik. Arch. klin. Chir. **322**, 1182 (1968).

1718. KUGNETSOVA, V. M., G. S. SELTSOVSKAIA, and M. E. PREOBRAZHENAKAIA: Effect of variation of the native dextrans on nonspezific resistance to infection. Dokl. Akad. Nauk. S.S.S.R. **175**, 495 (1967).

1719. KUMMER, H., and P. LUNDSGAARD-HANSEN: The influence of clinical dextran and modified gelatin on hemorrhagic diathesis in irradiated, thrombocytopenic dogs. Helv. med. Acta **34**, 244 (1968).

1719 a. KUZNETSOVA, V. M., M. E. PREOBRAZHENSKAYA, and E. L. ROZENFELD: The effect of modified dextran preparations on non-specific resistance to infection. Dokl. Akad. Nauk. SSSR **178**, 492 (1968).

1720. LAAFF, H., H. GIERTZ u. F. HAHN: Zur Frage der Aminbeteiligung beim Dextranoedem. Arch. intern. Pharmacodyn. **168**, 101 (1967).

1720 a. LAMOTTE, M., J. ROUJEAU, J.-M. SEGRESTAA, C. CAULIN et S. MELMAN: Un cas d'anurie par néphropathie osmotique après perfusions de dextrane a faible poids moléculaire. Semaine Hôp. Paris **44**, 187 (1968).

1721. LANGSJOEN, P. H., and T. W. INMON: Rheologic changes in myocardial infarction. Amer. Heart J. **73**, 430 (1967).

1721a. —, S. A. SANCHEZ, D. J. LYNCH, and T. W. INMON: The treatment of myocardial infarction with low molecular weight dextran. Amer. Heart J. **76**, 28 (1968).

1721 b. LANGSJOEN, P. H., and T. W. INMON: Hemorrheologic observations in acute myocardial infarction. Angiology **19**, 247 (1968).

1722. LARCAN, A., F. STREIFF, et B. GENETET: Modifications de quelques caractéristiques hémorhéologiques (viscosité-vitesse de sédimentation-morphologie érythrocytaire) sous l'influence de quelques substituts du plasma. In: A. HÄSSIG: Plasmaersatzpräparate auf Gelatinebasis. Bibl. haemat. (Karger): in press.

1723. LAVER, M. B., A. J. MURPHY, A. SEIFEN, and E. P. REDFORD: Blood oxygen content measurements using the oxygen electrode. J. appl. Physiol. **20**, 1063 (1965).

1724. LEANDOER, L.: Fibrinogen after massive haemorrhage. Acta chir. scand. Suppl. **390** (1968).

1725. LEBRIE, S. J.: Renal peritubular capillary permeability to macromolecules. Amer. J. Physiol. **213**, 1225 (1967).

1726. LECOMTE, J.: Sur les modalités de la tachyphylaxie au dextran chez le rat. C. R. Soc. Biol. **161**, 203 (1967).

1727. —, et J. SALMON: Sur la nature éventuellement anaphylactique de l'hypotension artérielle induite par les dextrans chez le rat. C. R. Soc. Biol. **161**, 481 (1967).

1728. — Comparison des effets pharmacodynamiques généraux de deux dextrans de poids moléculaire différent. C. R. Soc. Biol. **161**, 483 (1967).

1729. Lecomte, J.: Histamine et 5-hydroxytryptamine endogènes dans le déterminisme de l'hypotension artérielle induite par le dextran. Arch. intern. Pharmacodyn. **166**, 200 (1967).
1730. Lee, Y.: Experimental studies of metastases. A review. Part III. Reaction of tumor cells and endothelium in the establishment of metastasis. Missouri Med. **65**, 205 (1968).
1730 a. Lee, W. H., Jr., N. Cooper, M. G. Weidner Jr., and E. S. Murner: Clinical evaluation of a new plasma expander, hydroxyethyl starch. J. Trauma **8**, 381 (1968).
1731. Leikola, J.: Studies of the nature of incomplete anti-Rh antibodies. Int. Arch. Allergy appl. Immunol. **32**, 474 (1967).
1731 a. Lewis, B. A., M. J. St. Cyr, and F. Smith: The structure of Leuconostoc mesenteroides strain C dextran. I. Methylation analysis. II. Fragmentation analysis. J. org. Chem. **33**, 3136 (1968).
1732. Lichardus, B., V. Pliska, V. Uhrin, and T. Barth: The cow as a model for investigating natriuretic activity. Lancet **I**, 127 (1968).
1733. Limet, R., et J. Lecomte: Action inhibitrice de l'indométhacine sur l'oedème généralisé induit par le dextran chez le rat. Arch. intern. Pharmacodyn. **171**, 109 (1968).
1734. Loeb, H. S., A. Cruz, C. Y. Teng, J. Boswell, R. J. Pietras, J. R. Tobin, and R. M. Gunnar: Haemodynamic studies in shock associated with infection. Brit. Heart J. **29**, 883 (1967).
1735. Lösel, H. u. W. Appel: Wirkung von niedermolekularem Dextran (Rheomacrodex) auf den Serumcholesterinspiegel. Fortschr. Med. **85**, 517 (1967).
1736. Long, D. M., Jr., D. B. Todd, R. A. Indeglia, R. L. Varco, and C. W. Lillehei: Clinical use of dextran-40 in extracorporeal circulation — A summary of 5 years' experience. Transfusion **6**, 401 (1966).
1737. Long, D. M., and R. D. Corley: Mechanism of plug flow phenomena in shock and trauma. Surg. Forum **18**, 23 (1967).
1738. Lundsgaard-Hansen, P.: Zum Problem der Plasmaersatzstoffe — Schlußwort. Helv. chir. Acta **34**, 566 (1967).
1738a. —, Grundlagen der Therapie hämorrhagisch-traumatischer Schockzustände mit Plasmaersatzmitteln. Schweiz. med. Wschr. **98**, 1273 (1968).
1739. Lutz, H.: Tierexperimentelle Untersuchungen über die Wirkung von kolloidalen Blutflüssigkeitsersatzmitteln im Entblutungsschock beim Hund. Z. ges. exp. Med. **146**, 383 (1968).
1740. MacCannell, K. L., and N. C. Moran: Pharmacological basis for the use of adrenergic agonists and antagonists in cardiogenic shock and hypotension. Progr. cardiovasc. Dis. **10**, 55 (1967).
1741. Mach, O., and L. Lacko: Density gradient in a dextran medium. Ann. Biochem. **22**, 393 (1968).
1742. MacLean, Ll. D., W. G. Mulligan, A. P. H. McLean, and J. H. Duff: Patterns of septic shock in man — a detailed study of 56 patients. Ann. Surg. **166**, 543 (1967).
1743. Mailloux, L., C. D. Swartz, R. Capizzi, K. E. Kim, G. Onesti, O. Ramirez, and A. N. Brest: Acute renal failure after administration of low-molecular-weight dextran. New. Engl. J. Med. **277**, 1113 (1967).
1743a. Maltby, J. R.: Anaphylactic reaction to dextran. Brit. J. Anaesth. **40**, 552 (1968).
1744. Mandelbaum, I., and H. B. Shumacker: The effect of mannitol and low molecular weight dextran upon renal vascular resistance during controlled renal blood flow. Ann. Surg. **167**, 533 (1968).
1745. Matheson, N. A.: PVP and platelet adhesiveness. Lancet **II**, 1363 (1967).

1745 a. MATHESON, N. A.: Hepatitis-free plasma protein solution. Brit. med. J. II, 615 (1968).

1746. MATSUMOTO, T., R. M. HARDAWAY, and J. E. McCLAIN: Microcirculation in hemorrhagic shock with relationship to blood pressure. Arch. Surg. 95, 911 (1967).

1747. — — —, and P. M. MARGETIS: Microcirculation of dogs in hemorrhagic shock and after treatment. Arch. Surg. 96, 179 (1968).

1748. McDONALD, K. M., R. W. SCHRIER, D. P. LAULER, and R. WELLS: Role of blood viscosity and body fluid distribution in the renal response to extracellular fluid (ECF) volume expansion. Clin. Res. 15, 363 (1967).

1749. McFARLANE, R. M., J. J. LAIRD, R. LAMON, A. J. R. FINLAYSON, and R. JOHNSON: Evaluation of dextran and DMSO to prevent necrosis in experimental pedicule flaps. Plast. reconstr. Surg. 41, 64 (1968).

1750. McLAUGHLIN, J. S., D. SANTOS, H. KHAZEI, S. ATTAR, A. MANSBERGER, and R. A. COWLEY: Clinical shock: A hemodynamic and metabolic assessment of treatment. Amer. Surg. 33, 687 (1967).

1751. MEISELMAN, H. J., and E. W. MERRILL: The effect of the addition of dextran on the rheological properties of blood. Biorheology 4, 89 (1967).

1752. — — Hemorheology: The effect of hemodilution and low molecular weight dextran. Bibl. anat. (Karger) 9, 288 (1967).

1753. MESSMER, K.: Die Wirkung hypertoner Lösungen bei Ratten im irreversiblen Schock. Anaesthesist 17, 295 (1968).

1754. MICHELSON, E.: Anaphylactic reaction to dextrans. New Engl. J. Med. 278, 552 (1968).

1755. MOGENSEN, C. E.: The glomerular permeability determined by dextran clearance using Sephadex gel filtration. Scand. J. clin. Lab. Invest. 21, 77 (1968).

1756. MONSON, D. O., and W. C. SHOEMAKER: Sequence of hemodynamic events after various types of hemorrhage. Surgery 63, 738 (1968).

1757. MORRISON, F. S., P. L. MOLLISON, and D. C. ROBSON: Post-transfusion survival of red cells stored in liquid nitrogen. Brit. J. Haemat. 14, 215 (1968).

1758. MOSS, G. S., C. R. VALERI, and C. E. BRODINE: Clinical experience with the use of frozen blood in combat casualties. New Engl. J. Med. 278, 747 (1968).

1759. MOYER, C. A., and H. R. BUTCHER: Burns, shock, and plasma volume regulation. St. Louis: C. V. Mosby 1967.

1760. MÜLLER, K.-H.: Vergleichende Untersuchungen über die Beeinflussung der Blutgerinnung durch Blutersatzflüssigkeiten in vivo und in vitro. In: A. HÄSSIG: Plasmaersatzpräparate auf Gelatinebasis. Bibl. haemat. (Karger): in press.

1761. NAGER, F.: Therapie des Herzinfarktes. Praxis 57, 332 (1968).

1762. NAHAS, G.: Experimental evaluation of Plasmagel following massive rapid hemorrhage. In: A. HÄSSIG: Plasmaersatzpräparate auf Gelatinebasis. Bibl. haemat. (Karger): in press.

1763. NASHAT, F. S., and R. W. PORTAL: The effects of changes in haematocrit on renal function. J. Physiol. 193, 513 (1967).

1764. NAVARRO, R. U., and C. C. FERGUSON: Treatment of experimental hemorrhagic shock by the combined use of hyperbaric oxygen and low molecular weight dextran. Surgery 63, 775 (1968).

1765. NEUWALD, F.: Haltbarkeit und Lagerfähigkeit von Gelatine-Plasmaersatzlösungen im Hinblick auf ihre militär-medizinische Verwendung. In: A.

HÄSSIG: Plasmaersatzpräparate auf Gelatinebasis. Bibl. haemat. (Karger): in press.

1766. NICHOLLS, J. G., and D. E. WOLFE: Distribution of $^{14}C$-labeled sucrose, inulin, and dextran in extracellular spaces and in cells of the leech central nervous system. J. Neurophysiol. **30**, 1574 (1967).

1767. NICOLL, P. A., and R. FRAYSER: Physiological considerations of the microcirculation as related to shock. Progr. cardiovasc. Dis. **9**, 558 (1967).

1768. NITSCHMANN, H., u. H. R. STOLL: Gelatine als Ausgangsmaterial für die Herstellung von Plasmaersatzmitteln. In: A. HÄSSIG: Plasmaersatzpräparate auf Gelatinebasis. Bibl. haemat. (Karger): in press.

1768 a. NIZET, A.: Influence of serumalbumin and dextran on sodium and water excretion by the isolated dog kidney. Pflügers Arch. ges. Physiol. **301**, 7 (1968).

1769. NUNN, J. F., and J. FREEMAN: Problems of oxygenation and oxygen transport during haemorrhage. Anaesthesia **19**, 206 (1964).

1770. ONEAL, R. M., R. E. KNODE, W. C. GRABB, and R. O. DINGMAN: The effect of low molecular weight dextran on the survival of skin flaps in pigs vascularized either by a single artery and vein or by a subdermal plexus. Plast. reconstr. Surg. **40**, 595 (1967).

1771. PANDELI, A., W. A. NEELY, and J. D. HARDY: Interstitial fluid pressure changes in endotoxin shock. Surgery **63**, 938 (1968).

1772. PARKINSON, T. M.: Metabolism of orally administered dextran and "Sephadex" derivates in the rat. Nature **215**, 415 (1967).

1773. PATEL, J. A., and G. L. PHILLIPS: A guide to physical compatibility of intravenous drug admixtures. Amer. J. Hosp. Pharm. **23**, 409 (1966).

1774. PERÄSALO, O., P. SILTANEN, and E. MERIKALLIO: Use of hemodilution in total body perfusion. J. cardiovasc. Surg. **8**, 442 (1967).

1774 a. PETRIE, J. J. B., P. R. MACLEAN, and J. S. ROBSON: Glomerular permeability to serum proteins and high molecular weight dextrans in glomerulonephritis. Clin. Sci. **34**, 83 (1968).

1775. POWERS, J. C., G. W. SHAFTAN, H. HERBSMAN, K. E. KARLSON, and A. STULBERGER: Red blood cell and plasma distribution during experimental vasodilator hypotension. Surg. Gynec. Obstet. **126**, 1257 (1968).

1776. POYSER, R. H., and G. B. WEST: Structural requirements of sugars as antagonists of the vascular response to dextran in rat skin. Brit. J. Pharmacol. **32**, 219 (1968).

1777. PROUT, W. G., and R. V. JONES: Resuscitation — fluid replacement. Postgrad. med. J. **43**, 592 (1967).

1778. — Relative value of central-venous-pressure monitoring and blood-volume measurement in the mangement of shock. Lancet **I**, 1108 (1968).

1779. PRUITT, B. A., J. A. MONCRIEF, and A. O. MASON: Efficacy of buffered saline as the sole replacement fluid after acute measured hemorrhage in man. J. Trauma **7**, 767 (1967).

1780. QUAADE, F., O. A. LARSEN, N. A. LASSEN, and S. L. NIELSEN: Observations on the influence of glucose upon subcutaneous adipose tissue blood flow. Acta med. scand. **182**, Suppl. 476, 85 (1967).

1781. RACE, D., E. COOPER, and M. ROSENBAUM: Hemorrhagic shock: The effect of prolonged low flow on the regional distribution of blood and its modification by hypothermia. Ann. Surg. **167**, 454 (1968).

1782. REDDING, M., and C. B. MUELLER: Effect of ambient temperature upon responses to hypovolemic insult in the unanesthetized unrestrained albino rat. Surgery **64**, 110 (1968).

1783. Reid, D. J., S. Digerness, and J. W. Kirklin: Intracellular fluid volume in surgical patients measured by the simultaneous determination of total body water and extracellular fluid. Surg. Forum **18**, 29 (1967).

1784. Remmele, W., u. D. Harms: Zur pathologischen Anatomie des Kreislaufschocks beim Menschen. I. Mikrothrombose der peripheren Blutgefäße. Klin. Wschr. **46**, 352 (1968).

1785. Replogle, R. L., and E. W. Merrill: Hemodilution: Rheologic and metabolic consequences in shock. Surg. Forum **18**, 157 (1967).

1786. Reutter, F. W., S. Mazzoni u. T. Wegmann: Die Behandlung des akuten Myokardinfarktes mit niedermolekularem Dextran. Schweiz. med. Wschr. **98**, 1218 (1968).

1786 a. Reynolds, T. B.: Appraisal of the mortality in acute fulminant viral hepatitis. New Engl. J. Med. **278**, 1248 (1968).

1787. Rieger, Å.: Blood volume and plasma protein. Acta chir. scand. Suppl. **379** (1967).

1788. Rigor, B., P. Bosomworth, and B. F. Rush: Replacement of operative blood loss of more than 1 liter with Hartmann's solution. J. Amer. med. Ass. **203**, 399 (1968).

1789. Roesner, J.: "Rheomacrodex 10% mit Sorbit 20%" beim akuten Hirn- und Rückenmarködem. Med. Klin. **62**, 752 (1967).

1790. Roka, L.: Chemie der OPG. In: A. Hässig: Plasmaersatzpräparate auf Gelatinebasis. Bibl. haemat. (Karger): in press.

1791. Rosenblum, W. I.: Effects of dextran 40 on blood viscosity in experimental macroglobulinaemia. Nature **218**, 591 (1968).

1792. Roth, E., L. C. Lax, and J. V. Maloney, Jr.: Changes in extracellular fluid volume during shock and surgical trauma in animals and man. Surg. Forum **18**, 43 (1967).

1793. Rothschild, M. A., M. Oratz, C. D. Evans, and S. S. Schreiber: Role of hepatic interstitial albumin in regulating albumin synthesis. Amer. J. Physiol. 210, 57 (1966).

1794. Rudowski, W., E. Kostrzewska, R. Scharf, L. Konopka, A. Gregor, K. Rechowicz, B. Czartoryska, Z. Klawe, and J. Ostrowski: Haemodynamic properties of low-molecular dextran in experimental clinical conditions. Polsk. Tygod. Lekar. **22**, 1719 (1967).

1795. Ruetz, P. P., S. A. Johnson, R. Callahan, R. C. Meade, and J. J. Smith: Fainting: A review of its mechanisms and a study in blood donors. Medicine **46**, 363 (1967).

1796. Rush, B. F., Jr., and R. Sparks: Extracellular fluid shifts in endotoxin shock. J. Trauma **7**, 884 (1967).

1797. Sachs, V.: Einst und jetzt: Bluttransfusion. Zur Geschichte des Transfusionswesens bis zum zweiten Weltkrieg. Münch. med. Wschr. **110**, 73 (1968).

1798. — Das Bluttransfusionswesen heute und in Zukunft. Münch. med. Wschr. **110**, 218 (1968).

1799. Salsbury, A. J.: Effect of transfusion materials on rouleaux formation and sedimentation rate of erythrocytes. Brit. med. J. **II**, 88 (1967).

1799 a. Salsbury, A. J., and M. Brozovich: Experience with a hepatitis-free plasma protein solution. Brit. med. J. **II**, 352 (1968).

1800. Sanbar, S. S., and G. Smet: Comparison of the hypolipidemic action of dextran and polyvinylpyrrolidone (PVP) in human subjects. J. lab. clin. Med. 70, 890 (1967).

1801. Sanbar, S., A. Zweifler, and G. Smet: In vivo and in vitro effects of polyvinylpyrrolidone on platelet adhesiveness in human blood. Lancet **II**, 917 (1967).

1802. Sandor, S.: The excretion of dextran preparates of different molecular weights with the urine; the molecular weight distribution and excretion of Plasmodex. Acta pharm. hung. **37**, 178 (1967).

1803. Schäfer, H.: Therapie des intravasalen Volumenmangels. Klinischer Erfahrungsbericht über Haemaccel. Med. Klin. **62**, 1992 (1967).

1804. Schaller, F., u. G. Roggen: Haltbarkeit und Lagerfähigkeit von Gelatine-Plasmaersatzlösungen im Hinblick auf ihre militär-medizinische Verwendung. In: A. Hässig: Plasmaersatzpräparate auf Gelatinebasis. Bibl. haemat. (Karger): in press.

1804 a. Schildt, B., and L. Thorén: Combined injuries and shock. Stockholm: Försvarets Forskningsanstalt 1968.

1805. Schloerb, P. R., C. E. Peters, G. K. Cage, J. C. Kearns, and J. K. Lam: Evaluation of the sulfate space as a measure of extracellular fluid. Surg. Forum **18**, 39 (1967).

1805 a. Schmidt, H. D., P. Rentrop u. J. Schmier: Einfluß des Blutersatzmittels auf die Toleranz gegen Anaemieschock. Arch. ges. Physiol. **300**, 75 (1968).

1806. Schmidt, K., u. H. Bökenkamp: Zur Änderung der Sauerstofftransportkapazität nach Osmo- und Onkotherapie. Anaesthesist **16**, 333 (1967).

1807. Schneider, C. H., and A. L. de Weck: The reaction of benzylpenicillin with carbohydrates at neutral pH with a note on the immunogenicity of hapten polysaccharide conjugates. Immunochemistry **4**, 331 (1967).

1807 a. Schrier, R. W., K. M. McDonald, R. A. Marshall, and D. P. Lauler: Absence of natriuretic response to acute hypotonic intravascular volume expansion in dogs. Clin. Sci. **34**, 57 (1968).

1808. Schulze, E., u. H. Löwe: Speicherung von Dextran in Leber und Milz der Ratte bei chronischer Applikation und ihr Einfluß auf Teilfunktionen dieser Organe. Acta Biol. Med. Ger. **18**, 517 (1967).

1809. Schumer, W., and J. C. Kukral: Metabolism of shock. Surgery **63**, 630 (1968).

1810. — Localization of the energy pathway block in shock. Surgery **64**, 55 (1968).

1811. Schwartzkopff, W., M. Seidel, G. Kunkel u. I. Falck: Klinisch-erperimentelle Untersuchungen über einen Gelatine-Plasmaexpander unter Berücksichtigung der Nierenhämodynamik bei Normo- und Hypovolämikern. Z. ges. exp. Med. **147**, 202 (1968).

1812. Schwick, H. G., u. K. Heide: Immunochemie und Immunologie von Kollagenen und Gelatine. In: A. Hässig: Plasmaersatzpräparate auf Gelatinebasis. Bibl. haemat. (Karger): in press.

1812 a. Selye, H., and A. Somogyi: Various connective-tissue reactions as influenced by dextran of different molecular weight. Ann. Allergy **26**, 1 (1968).

1813. Shizgal, H. M., G. A. Lopez, and J. R. Gutelius: Extracellular fluid volume changes following hemorrhagic shock. Surg. Forum **18**, 35 (1967).

1813 a. Shtykhno, Y. M.: The effect of low-molecular dextran on the indices of hemodynamics and water metabolism in conditions of acute lethal blood loss. Pat. Fiziol. éksp. Ter. **12**, 26 (1968).

1813 b. Silvay, J., E. Sujansky, M. Schnorrer, K. Hrubiskova, J. Slezak, I. Gabauer, and J. Styk: The use of gelatinous priming solution for extracorporeal circulation. J. thorac. cardiovasc. Surg. **55**, 350 (1968).

1813 c. Simon, M. A., and W. R. Olsen: The effect of dextran 40 on serum electrolyte concentration in the dog. Arch. Surg. **97**, 478 (1968).

1814. Skillman, J. J., H. K. Awwad, and F. D. Moore: Plasma protein kinetics of the early transcapillary refill after hemorrhage in man. Surg. Gynec. Obstet. **125**, 983 (1967).

1815. —, J. E. Olson, J. H. Lyons, and F. D. Moore: The hemodynamic effect of acute blood loss in normal man, with observations on the effect of the Valsalva maneuver and breath holding. Ann. Surg. **166**, 713 (1967).

1816. —, D. P. Lauler, R. B. Hickler, J. H. Lyons, J. E. Olson, M. R. Ball, and F. D. Moore: Hemorrhage in normal man: Effect on renin, cortisol, aldosterone, and urine composition. Ann. Surg. **166**, 865 (1967).

1817. —, W. K. Eltringham, R. H. Goldensen, and F. D. Moore: Transcapillary refilling after hemorrhage in the splenectomized dog. J. surg. Res. **8**, 57 (1968).

1817 a. Skillman, J. J., W. K. Eltringham, R. M. Zollinger Jr., D. P. Lauler, and F. D. Moore: Phenoxybenzamine-induced vasodilatation: A stimulus to increased plasma volume with reduced central venous pressure and aldosterone hypersecretion in man. Surgery **64**, 368 (1968).

1817 b. Solanke, T. F.: Clinical trial of 6% hydroxyethyl starch (a new plasma expander). Brit. med. J. **II**, 783 (1968).

1818. Somayaji, B. N., W. D. Stone, and P. B. Glover: Risk of anicteric hepatitis following blood transfusion. Gut **8**, 614 (1967).

1819. Sørensen, B., P. Sejrsen, and M. Thomsen: Dextran solutions in the treatment of burn shock. Scand. J. plast. reconstruct. Surg. **1**, 68 (1967).

1819 a. Srinivasan, S., R. Aaron, P. S. Chopra, T. Lucas, and P. N. Sawyer: Effect of thrombotic and antithrombotic drugs on the surface charge characteristics of canine blood vessels: In vivo and in vitro studies. Surgery **64**, 827 (1968).

1820. Stalker, A. L.: The microcirculatory effects of dextran. J. path. Bact. **93**, 191 (1967).

1821. — Histological changes produced by experimental erythrocyte aggregation. J. path. Bact. **93**, 203 (1967).

1822. Stoll, H. R., u. H. Nitschmann: Succinylierte Gelatine als Plasmaexpander. In: A. Hässig: Plasmaersatzpräparate auf Gelatinebasis. Bibl. haemat. (Karger): in press.

1823. — — Vergleichende physiko-chemische Untersuchungen an Plasmaersatzmitteln. In: A. Hässig: Plasmaersatzpräparate auf Gelatinebasis. Bibl. haemat. (Karger): in press.

1824. Strebel, L., and P. E. Siegler: Experience with clinical testing of dextran solutions. Arch. Surg. **96**, 471 (1968).

1825. Streiff, F., B. Genetet, et A. Larcan: Groupes sanguines et substituts du plasma (dextran et Plasmagel). In: A. Hässig: Plasmaersatzpräparate auf Gelatinebasis. Bibl. haemat. (Karger): in press.

1826. Stremple, J. F., M. Muller, J. Lubitz, and A. S. Close: The failure of low molecular weight dextran and Mannitol to preserve renal function after bilateral occlusion of the renal arteries. Surgery **63**, 766 (1968).

1827. Stroër, W. F. H.: On the interaction of dextran molecules with plasma protein and cholesterol. Acta Physiol. Pharmacol. neerl. **14**, 363 (1967).

1828. Swan, K. G., and E. D. Jacobson: Hemodynamics of endotoxin shock in the conscious animal. Surg. Gynec. Obstet. **125**, 1041 (1967).

1829. Swartz, C., K. Kim, L. Mailloux, and A. N. Brest: Acute renal shutdown following low molecular weight dextran infusion. Ann. intern. Med. **66**, 1054 (1967).

1830. Swartz, C., K. Kim, L. Mailloux, A. N. Brest, G. Onesti, O. Ramirez, and A. Brest: Determinants of dextran 40 anuria. Clin. Res. **15**, 373 (1967).

1831. Taborsky, J.: Blockade der Dextran-Anurie bei wasserbelasteten Ratten durch die Serotoninantagonisten Lysergsäurediaethylamid und 1-Methyl-Lysergsäurebutanolamid. Med. Pharmacol. exp. **17**, 6 (1967).

1832. Tarazi, R. C., E. D. Frohlich, and H. P. Dustan: Plasma volume in men with essential hypertension. New Engl. J. Med. **278**, 762 (1968).

1833. Thal, A. P., and J. M. Kinney: On the definition and classification of shock. Progr. cardiovasc. Dis. **9**, 527 (1967).

1834. Theye, R. A., and A. D. Sessler: Effect of halothane anaesthesia on rate of canine oxygen consumption. Anesthesiology **28**, 661 (1967).

1835. Thiercelin, P. C., et R. Monteil: Influence de la température et des ultra-sons sur la conservation d'un soluté de gélatine fluide modifiée (Plasmagel). In: A. Hässig: Plasmaersatzpräparate auf Gelatinebasis. Bibl. haemat. (Karger): in press.

1836. Thompson, J. E., R. W. Vollman, D. J. Austin, and M. M. Kartchner: Prevention of hypotensive and renal complications of aortic surgery using balanced salt solution: Thirteen-year experience with 670 cases. Ann. Surg. **167**, 767 (1968).

1836 a. Tompkins, R. K., A. R. Kraft, and R. M. Zollinger: Alternate routes of surgical fluid administration. J. surg. Res. **8**, 397 (1968).

1837. Torpey, D. J.: Resuscitation and anesthetic management of casualties. J. Amer. med. Ass. **202**, 131 (1967).

1837 a. Tracht, M. E., L. Tallal, and G. D. Tracht: Intrinsic hepatic control of plasma albumin concentration. Life Sci. **6**, 2621 (1967).

1838. Trinkle, J. K., B. F. Rush, and B. Eiseman: Metabolism of lactate following major blood loss. Surgery **63**, 782 (1968).

1839. Tristani, F. E., and J. N. Cohn: Systemic and renal hemodynamics in oliguric hepatic failure: Effect of volume expansion. J. clin. Invest. **46**, 1894 (1967).

1840. — — Renal hemodynamics in clinical shock. Clin. Res. **15**, 52 (1967).

1841. Tschirren, B., u. K. Stampfli: Zur therapeutischen Verwendung des Plasmaersatzpräparates Physiogel in der Anaesthesiologie und Chirurgie. In: A. Hässig: Plasmaersatzpräparate auf Gelatinebasis. Bibl. haemat. (Karger): in press.

1841 a. Turpini, R., e P. L. Cipolli: L'influenza del destrano e di un polimero della gelatina sulla coagulazione del sangue. Soc. ital. Biol. sper. **40**, 736 (1964).

1842. Tzonos, T.: Der Einfluß von niedermolekularem Dextran mit Sorbit und Tris-Puffer auf das experimentelle Hirnödem nach Mikroembolie. Acta neurochir. Wien **16**, 161 (1967).

1843. Veith, F. J., J. W. Hagstrom, A. Panossian, S. L. Nehlsen, and J. W. Wilson: Pulmonary microcirculatory response to shock, transfusion, and pump-oxygenator procedures: A unified mechanism underlying pulmonary damage. Surgery **64**, 95 (1968).

1844. Vineyard, G. C., and D. P. Osborne, Jr.: Simultaneous determination of extracellular water by 35-sulfate and 82-bromide in dogs, with a note on the acute effects of hypotensive shock. Surg. Forum **18**, 37 (1967).

1845. Vogel, A. P., E. L. Frederickson, and T. M. Holder: Massive blood replacement. Arch. Surg. **95**, 38 (1967).

1846. VOGEL, G., u. M. SASS: Ein tierexperimentelles Modell gesteigerter Capillarpermeabilität. Penetration von Polyvinylpyrrolidon durch die Plasma-Lymph-Schranke wacher Ratten im Dextran-Schock. Arch. exp. Pathol. Pharmakol. **258**, 123 (1967).

1846 a. VOIGT, G.: Experimentelle Untersuchungen zur Adhäsionsprophylaxe mit Dextran. Zbl. Chir. **92**, Suppl., 1981 (1967).

1847. WEHINGER, H.: Zur Beeinflussung der Blutgerinnung durch niedermolekulares Dextran (Rheomacrodex). Klin. Wschr. **45**, 1031 (1967).

1847 a. WELLMER, H. K.: Verhalten der Thrombocyten des Hundes im Kreislauf bei Infusionen von kolloidalen Blutersatzmitteln. Arch. klin. Chir. **322**, 1194 (1968).

1848. WELLS, R. E.: Hemorheologic effects of the dextrans on erythrocyte aggregation: hemodilution versus disaggregation. Biorheology **4**, 88 (1967).

1849. WHITMORE, R. L.: The flow behaviour of blood in the circulation. Nature **215**, 123 (1967).

1850. — Plasma expanders. Biorheology **4**, 105 (1967).

1851. WILHELMSEN, L., and E. VARNAUSKAS: Effects of acute plasma expansion on the mechanics of breathing. Clin. Sci. **33**, 29 (1967).

1852. WILKINSON, T. S., W. S. BLACK, T. C. SUTTERFIELD, and H. H. STONE: Experimental prophylaxis and treatment of venous thrombosis with dextran 75. J. surg. Res. **7**, 464 (1967).

1853. WILLIAMS, W. H., C. E. HUGGINS, and W. G. AUSTEN: Correction of heart defects with cardiopulmonary bypass. Report of a case using frozen autologous blood. Arch. Surg. **96**, 317 (1968).

1854. ZEKORN, D.: Verweildauer, Verteilung, Ausscheidung und Abbau von Gelatineplasmaersatzlösungen. In: A. HÄSSIG: Plasmaersatzpräparate auf Gelatinebasis. Bibl. haemat. (Karger): in press.

# Appendix to the Literature

The following references refer to books which give a survey of the present position of research, diagnosis and therapy in the field of shock in general.

## *Books about Shock*

| Author | Year of publication | Reference |
|---|---|---|
| H. K. BEECHER | 1952 | [*115*] |
| A. BOBA | 1968 | [*1611 a*] |
| K. D. BOCK | 1962 | [*182*] |
| J. B. COATES | 1955 | [*284*] |
| M. COLARD | 1967 | [*1637*] |
| A. N. DRURY | 1940 | [*364*] |
| H. DUBOIS-FERRIÈRE | 1945 | [*366*] |
| R. DUESBERG | 1963 | [*371*] |
| B. EISEMAN | 1963 | [*400*] |
| J. FINE | 1954 | [*438*] |
| P. FITZGERALD | 1966 | [*447 a*] |
| E. F. GERSMEYER | 1961 | [*519*] |
| H. D. GREEN | 1952, 1953, 1954, 1955, 1956, 1957 | [*556*] |
| U. F. GRUBER | 1965 | [*597*] |
| R. M. HARDAWAY | 1968 | [*1692 a*] |
| H. HAYASAKA | 1964 | [*680*] |
| S. G. HERSHEY | 1964 | [*704*] |
| J. M. HOWARD | 1955 | [*730*] |
| O. H. JUST | 1964 | [*796*] |
| R. J. MARSHALL | 1966 | [*954*] |
| D. N. MATTHEWS | 1963 | [*968*] |
| Medical Science Publication | 1953 | [*997*] |
| Medical Science Publication | 1954 | [*998*] |
| L. C. MILLS | 1965 | [*1021*] |
| R. W. MINER | 1948 | [*1022*] |
| V. H. MOON | 1942 | [*1037*] |
| F. D. MOORE | 1959 | [*1038*] |
| C. A. MOYER | 1967 | [*1759*] |
| L. R. ORKIN | 1965 | [*1105*] |
| J. H. POLLOCK | 1966 | [*1136*] |
| J. E. RHOADS | 1963 | [*1183*] |
| B. SCHILDT | 1968 | [*1804 a*] |
| J. SCUDDER | 1940 | [*1307*] |
| S. F. SEELEY | 1961 | [*1311*] |
| W. C. SHOEMAKER | 1967 | [*1337 a*] |
| „Sjokk“ | 1966 | [*1349*] |

| Author | Year of publication | Reference |
|---|---|---|
| H. B. Stoner | 1960 | [1391] |
| J. G. Strawitz | 1965 | [1394] |
| M. H. Weil | 1967 | [1500 a] |
| C. J. Wiggers | 1950 | [1513] |
| B. W. Zweifach (provides short summaries of the most important papers in the shock field from 1950—1962 and 1962—1964) | 1963, 1966 | [1582, 1584] |

## *Review Articles on Shock*

| Author | Year of publication | Reference |
|---|---|---|
| F. W. Ahnefeld | 1962 | [12] |
| R. S. Alexander | 1963 | [20] |
| M. Allgöwer | 1967, 1967 | [40, 41] |
| C. P. Artz | 1966 | [81] |
| W. G. Austen | 1967 | [1598] |
| R. J. Baker | 1967 | [96] |
| C. J. Berne | 1962 | [148] |
| J. H. Bloch | 1966 | [172] |
| T. G. Blocker | 1955 | [173] |
| E. Buchborn | 1960, 1962 | [227, 228] |
| E. S. Bücherl | 1964 | [229] |
| J. P. Bull | 1956, 1964 | [233, 235] |
| J. J. Byrne | 1965, 1966 | [252, 253] |
| A. R. Clarke | 1957 | [281] |
| R. H. Clauss | 1968 | [1634] |
| H. E. Cohn | 1964 | [287] |
| H. A. Davis | 1949 | [339] |
| Editorial | 1965 | [387] |
| F. L. Engel | 1952 | [415] |
| H. Eufinger | 1963 | [418] |
| J. Fine | 1963, 1964, 1965, 1968 | [440, 441, 442, 1671] |
| J. Freeman | 1963 | [446] |
| M. I. Gregersen | 1946 | [559] |
| U. F. Gruber | 1964, 1965 | [595, 598] |
| F. N. Gurd | 1955 | [624] |
| H. F. Hamit | 1965 | [637] |
| R. M. Hardaway | 1967 | [1692] |
| H. N. Harkins | 1941 | [653] |
| H. P. Harrfeldt | 1965 | [655] |
| J. M. Howard | 1960 | [704] |
| E. D. Jacobson | 1968 | [1701] |
| E. Kirchner | 1963 | [822] |
| R. C. Lillehei | 1964 | [889] |
| T. O. Lindenschmidt | 1965 | [893] |
| K. L. MacCannell | 1967 | [1740] |

| Author | Year of publication | Reference |
|---|---|---|
| L. D. MacLean | 1966 | [*941*] |
| A. R. Mansberger | 1965 | [*950*] |
| V. C. Marshall | 1965 | [*955*] |
| G. K. McGowan | 1966 | [*991*] |
| R. C. Millican | 1954 | [*1020*] |
| F. D. Moore | 1965, 1965 | [*1042, 1043*] |
| D. P. Morse | 1963 | [*1050*] |
| H. G. Pauli | 1963 | [*1121*] |
| H. A. Ravin | 1963 | [*1162*] |
| J. Rehn | 1962, 1965 | [*1171, 1172*] |
| J. Rhoads | 1966 | [*1184*] |
| D. W. Richards jr. | 1944 | [*1185*] |
| S. M. Rosenthal | 1954 | [*1214*] |
| M. Saegesser | 1965 | [*1237*] |
| K. W. Schneider | 1963, 1966 | [*1273, 1279*] |
| M. Schneider | 1963 | [*1280*] |
| T. Shires | 1966 | [*1322*] |
| W. C. Shoemaker | 1962, 1965 | [*1333, 1336*] |
| F. A. Simeone | 1948, 1959, 1963 | [*1342, 1343, 1344*] |
| L. L. Smith | 1961, 1965 | [*1357, 1361*] |
| W. W. Spink | 1965 | [*1373*] |
| A. P. Thal | 1966, 1967 | [*1425, 1833*] |
| L. Thorén | 1962 | [*1437*] |
| F. E. Weale | 1963 | [*1492*] |
| M. H. Weil | 1957, 1965 | [*1498, 1499*] |
| K. Wiemers | 1959 | [*1512*] |
| J. N. Wilson | 1963, 1965 | [*1535, 1536*] |
| L. J. Wolfson | 1963 | [*1549*] |
| E. C. Yasargil | 1965 | [*1563*] |
| W. Zingg | 1964 | [*1574*] |
| B. W. Zweifach | 1958, 1965 | [*1581, 1583*] |

## *Books, Monographs and Review Articles about Blood Transfusion and Plasma Expanders*

| Author | Year of publication | Reference |
|---|---|---|
| M. Allgöwer | 1964 | [*37*] |
| C. P. Artz | 1962 | [*80*] |
| Bibl. haemat., fasc. 2 | 1955 | |
| Bibl. haemat., fasc. 5 | 1956 | |
| Bibl. haemat., fasc. 6 | 1957 | |
| Bibl. haemat., fasc. 7 | 1958 | |
| Bibl. haemat., fasc. 9 | 1959 | |
| Bibl. haemat., fasc. 10 | 1959 | |
| Bibl. haemat., fasc. 11 | 1960 | |
| Bibl. haemat., fasc. 12 | 1961 | |
| Bibl. haemat., fasc. 13 | 1962 | |
| Bibl. haemat., fasc. 16 | 1963 | |

| Author | Year of publication | Reference |
|---|---|---|
| Bibl. haemat., fasc. 19 | 1964 | |
| Bibl. haemat., fasc. 20 | 1964 | |
| Bibl. haemat., fasc. 23 | 1966 | |
| Bibl. haemat., fasc. 27 | 1967 | |
| Blood flow improvement | 1968 | [*1611*] |
| W. L. Bloom | 1951 | [*285*] |
| J. P. Bull | 1963 | [*176*] |
| J. B. Coates | 1964 | [*234*] |
| Committee on Plasma and Plasma Substitutes | 1965 | [*294*] |
| Division of Med. Sciences | 1962 | [*355*] |
| Division of Med. Sciences | 1963 | [*356*] |
| Division of Med. Sciences | 1965 | [*357*] |
| B. Eiseman | 1963 | [*401*] |
| R. A. Ewald | 1963 | [*427*] |
| A. Grönwall | 1957 | [*575*] |
| A. L. Gropper | 1952 | [*579*] |
| U. F. Gruber | 1964, 1964, 1966, 1966 | [*592, 594, 607, 611*] |
| F. Hahn | 1961 | [*632*] |
| F. W. Hartman | 1952 | [*660*] |
| G. Heberer | 1967 | [*683 a*] |
| K. Horatz | 1964, 1968 | [*783, 1697*] |
| A. Jeanes | 1952 | [*726*] |
| K. Lang | 1943, 1966 | [*851, 852*] |
| Low Molecular Weight Dextran | 1963 | [*922*] |
| P. L. Mollison | 1967 | [*1031*] |
| F. D. Moore | 1963 | [*1039*] |
| S. Mudd | 1942 | [*1055*] |
| E. J. Pulaski | 1952 | [*1148*] |
| H. Reissigl | 1961 | [*1175*] |
| H. R. Robertson | 1954 | [*1201*] |
| S. I. Schwartz | 1964 | [*1297*] |
| A. Segal | 1964 | [*1312*] |
| W. Spielmann | 1967 | [*1372*] |
| J. R. Squire | 1955 | [*1376*] |
| M. M. Strumia | 1963 | [*1396*] |
| Symposia on Rheomacrodex vol. I und II | 1964 | [*1411*] |
| W. L. Thompson | 1960 | [*1430*] |
| H. Willenegger | 1947, 1951 | [*1521, 1523*] |
| M. M. Wintrobe | 1961 | [*1544*] |
| B. Zederfeldt | 1965 | [*1568*] |

*Books and Monographs about Blood Volume Determination*

| Author | Year of publication | Reference |
|---|---|---|
| S. N. Albert | 1963, 1964 | [16, 17] |
| F. J. Dagher | 1965 | [328] |
| H. A. Davis | 1962 | [341] |
| W. Falholt | 1958 | [432] |
| M. I. Gregersen | 1959 | [560] |
| F. D. Moore | 1959, 1963 | [1038, 1041] |
| E. B. Reeve | 1960 | [1166] |
| K. D. Serkes | 1965 | [1319] |
| T. Sjöstrand | 1953, 1962 | [1350, 1351] |
| J. Wetterfors | 1965 | [1509] |

*Publications about Value and Technical Problems of Blood Volume Determination*

| Author | Year of publication | Reference |
|---|---|---|
| F. W. Ahnefeld | 1964 | [13] |
| M. Allgöwer | 1962 | [36] |
| S. B. Andersen | 1964 | [55] |
| D. J. Armstrong | 1967 | [66] |
| C. H. Baker | 1963 | [92] |
| S.-E. Bergentz | 1965 | [133] |
| R. L. Berger | 1964 | [141] |
| S. A. Berson | 1965 | [150] |
| G. Birke | 1966 | [160] |
| S. Birkeland | 1966 | [162] |
| J. A. Buckwalter | 1963 | [231] |
| O. Carrier | 1964 | [263] |
| T. B. Cartmill | 1965 | [264] |
| H. Chaplin jr. | 1952, 1953 | [272, 273] |
| R. Clarke | 1961 | [282] |
| J. A. Crook | 1964 | [317] |
| J. W. L. Davies | 1959, 1966 | [336, 338] |
| S. Deavers | 1963 | [343] |
| J. C. Donovan | 1964 | [360] |
| L. G. Ekelund | 1965 | [403] |
| D. C. Finlayson | 1964 | [444] |
| J. P. Flanagan | 1964 | [448] |
| P. Fuchsig | 1964 | [482] |
| O. Giebel | 1966 | [523] |
| D. J. Gillet | 1966, 1966 | [525, 526] |
| E. Grable | 1963, 1963, 1964 | [544, 545, 546] |
| J. M. Greep | 1963 | [558] |
| U. F. Gruber | 1963, 1964, 1965, 1965, 1967 | [590, 593, 602, 603, 1691] |
| M. Halmágyi | 1966 | [635] |
| G. C. Henegar | 1964 | [702] |
| R. C. Hoye | 1966 | [744] |

| Author | Year of publication | Reference |
|---|---|---|
| D. G. Johnston | 1967 | [*1704*] |
| K. E. Karlson | 1963 | [*810*] |
| E. Kirchner | 1963 | [*823*] |
| H. Knott | 1967 | [*1714*] |
| O. A. Larsen | 1965 | [*866*] |
| A. C. K. Lawrence | 1959 | [*871*] |
| V. C. Marshall | 1965 | [*956*] |
| J. D. McMurrey | 1962 | [*992*] |
| R. S. Moens | 1962 | [*1036*] |
| R. C. Moore | 1965 | [*1045*] |
| F. P. Muldowney | 1964 | [*1058*] |
| E. Myhre | 1963 | [*1070*] |
| M. D. Pareira | 1959 | [*1112*] |
| B. A. Planque | 1965 | [*1135*] |
| J. C. Powers | 1968 | [*1775*] |
| E. B. Reeve | 1957 | [*1165*] |
| H. Rustad | 1966, 1966 | [*1234, 1235*] |
| H. Scholer | 1963, 1963, 1964 | [*1284, 1285, 1286*] |
| L. Y. Senn | 1958 | [*1316*] |
| E. Sneddon | 1964 | [*1365*] |
| W. E. Spoerel | 1962 | [*1375*] |
| J. L. Steinfeld | 1958 | [*1383*] |
| H. Swan | 1960 | [*1402*] |
| R. C. Tarazi | 1968 | [*1832*] |
| J. P. Thomas | 1961 | [*1428*] |
| E. Topley | 1959 | [*1444*] |
| G. Walters | 1965 | [*1481*] |
| K. Wassermann | 1955 | [*1489*] |
| J. A. Williams | 1961, 1961, 1962, 1964, 1965 | [*1527, 1528, 1529, 1530, 1531*] |
| L. J. Wolfson | 1963 | [*1549*] |
| E. Wollheim | 1958, 1961 | [*1555, 1558*] |

# Subject Index

GPSR Compliance

*The European Union's (EU) General Product Safety Regulation (GPSR) is a set of rules that requires consumer products to be safe and our obligations to ensure this.*

*If you have any concerns about our products, you can contact us on ProductSafety@springernature.com*

In case Publisher is established outside the EU, the EU authorized representative is:

Springer Nature Customer Service Center GmbH
Europaplatz 3
69115 Heidelberg, Germany

**Batch number: 10704713**

Printed by Printforce, the Netherlands